Study Guide and Procedure Checklist Manual for

Kinn's The Administrative Medical Assistant

An Applied Learning Approach

Fifteenth Edition

Brigitte Niedzwiecki, MSN, RN, RMA
Medical Assistant Program Director & Instructor
Chippewa Valley Technical College
Eau Claire, Wisconsin

Julie Pepper, BS, CMA (AAMA)
Medical Assistant Instructor
Chippewa Valley Technical College
Eau Claire, Wisconsin

ELSEVIER

ELSEVIER

3251 Riverport Lane
St. Louis, Missouri 63043

Study Guide and Procedure Checklist Manual for Kinn's The Administrative Medical Assistant, Fifteenth Edition ISBN: 978-0-323-87413-7

Notices

ISBN: 978-0-323-87413-7

Publishing Director: Kristin Wilhelm
Content Development Manager: Luke Held/Danielle Frazier
Senior Content Development Specialist: Sarah Vora
Publishing Services Manager: Julie Eddy
Senior Project Manager: Abigail Bradberry
Design Direction: Ryan Cook

Printed in India

Last digit is the print number: 9 8 7 6 5 4 3 2 1

To the Student

This study guide was created to help you to achieve the objectives of each chapter in your text and establish a solid base of knowledge in medical assisting. Completing the exercises in each chapter in this guide will help reinforce the material studied in the textbook and learned in class.

STUDY HINTS FOR ALL STUDENTS

Ask Questions!

There are no stupid questions. If you do not know something or are not sure about it, you need to find out. Other people may be wondering the same thing but are too shy to ask. The answer could be a matter of life or death for your patient. That is certainly more important than feeling embarrassed about asking a question.

Chapter Objectives

At the beginning of each chapter in the textbook are learning objectives that you should have mastered by the time you have finished studying that chapter. Write these objectives in your notebook, leaving a blank space after each. Fill in the answers as you find them while reading the chapter. Review to make sure your answers are correct and complete. Use these answers when you study for tests. You should also do this for separate course objectives that your instructor has listed in your class syllabus.

Vocabulary

At the beginning of each chapter in the textbook are vocabulary terms that you will encounter as you read the chapter. These terms are in bold type the first time they appear in the chapter.

Summary of Learning Objectives

Use the Summary of Learning Objectives at the end of each chapter in the textbook to help you review for exams.

Reading Hints

As you read each chapter in the textbook, look at the subject headings to learn what each section is about. Read first for the general meaning and then reread parts you did not understand. It may help to read those parts aloud. Carefully read the information given in each table and study each figure and its legend.

Concepts

While studying, put difficult concepts into your own words to determine whether you understand them. Check this understanding with another student or the instructor. Write these concepts in your notebook.

Class Notes

When taking lecture notes in class, leave a large margin on the left side of each notebook page and write only on right-hand pages, leaving all left-hand pages blank. Look over your lecture notes soon after each class while your memory is fresh. Fill in missing words, complete sentences and ideas, and underline key phrases, definitions, and concepts. At the top of each page, write the topic of that page. In the left margin, write the key word for that part of your notes. On the opposite left-hand page, write a summary or outline that combines material from the textbook and the lecture. These can be your study notes for review.

Study Groups

Form a study group with other students so that you can help one another. Practice speaking and reading aloud. Ask questions about material you find unclear. Work together to find answers.

ADDITIONAL STUDY HINTS FOR ENGLISH AS A SECOND LANGUAGE (ESL) STUDENTS

Vocabulary

If you find a nontechnical word you do not know (e.g., drowsy), try to guess its meaning from the sentence (e.g., with electrolyte imbalance, the patient may feel fatigued and drowsy). If you are not sure of the meaning or if it seems particularly important, look it up in the dictionary.

Vocabulary Notebook

Keep a small alphabetized notebook or address book in your pocket or purse. Write down new nontechnical words you read or hear along with their meanings and pronunciations. Write each word under its initial letter so you can find it easily, as with a dictionary. For words you do not know or words that have a different meaning in medical assisting, write down how each word is used and how it is pronounced. Look up the meanings of these words in a dictionary or ask your instructor or first-language buddy (see the following section). Then write the different meanings or uses that you have found in your book, including the medical assisting meaning. Continue to add new words as you discover them.

First-Language Buddy

English as a second language (ESL) students should find a first-language buddy—another student who is a native speaker of English and who is willing to answer questions about word meanings, pronunciations, and culture. Maybe, in turn, your buddy would like to learn about your language and culture; this could be useful for their medical assisting career.

Contents

Competency Checklist

Student Name: ______________________________

Admission Cohort: ______________________________

Graduation Date: ______________________________

CAAHEP Competency (2022)	Procedure	Date	Grade / Pass	Initial
I. Anatomy, Physiology, & Pharmacology				
I.P.1.a. Accurately measure and record: blood pressure				
I.P.1.b. Accurately measure and record: temperature				
I.P.1.c. Accurately measure and record: pulse				
I.P.1.d. Accurately measure and record: respirations				
I.P.1.e. Accurately measure and record: height				
I.P.1.f. Accurately measure and record: weight (adult and infant)				
I.P.1.g. Accurately measure and record: length (infant)				
I.P.1.h. Accurately measure and record: head circumference (infant)				
I.P.1.i. Accurately measure and record: oxygen saturation				
I.P.2.a. Perform the following procedure: electrocardiography				
I.P.2.b. Perform the following procedure: venipuncture				
I.P.2.c. Perform the following procedure: capillary puncture				
I.P.2.d. Perform the following procedure: pulmonary function testing				
I.P.3. Perform patient screening following established protocols				
I.P.4.a. Verify the rules of medication administration: right patient				
I.P.4.b. Verify the rules of medication administration: right medication				

CAAHEP Competency (2022)	Procedure	Date	Grade / Pass	Initial
I.P.4.c. Verify the rules of medication administration: right dose				
I.P.4.d. Verify the rules of medication administration: right route				
I.P.4.e. Verify the rules of medication administration: right time				
I.P.4.f. Verify the rules of medication administration: right documentation				
I.P.5. Select proper sites for administering parenteral medication				
I.P.6. Administer oral medications				
I.P.7. Administer parenteral (excluding IV) medications				
I.P.8. Instruct and prepare a patient for a procedure or a treatment				
I.P.9. Assist provider with a patient exam				
I.P.10. Perform a quality control measure				
I.P.11.a. Collect specimens and perform: CLIA-waived hematology test				
I.P.11.b. Collect specimens and perform: CLIA-waived chemistry test				
I.P.11.c. Collect specimens and perform: CLIA-waived urinalysis				
I.P.11.d. Collect specimens and perform: CLIA-waived immunology test				
I.P.11.e. Collect specimens and perform: CLIA-waived microbiology test				
I.P.12. Provide up-to-date documentation of provider/ professional level CPR				
I.P.13.a. Perform first aid procedure for: bleeding	Procedure 21.5			
I.P.13.b. Perform first aid procedure for: diabetic coma or insulin shock	Procedure 21.1			
I.P.13.c. Perform first aid procedure for: stroke	Procedure 21.3			
I.P.13.d. Perform first aid procedure for: seizures	Procedure 21.3			

CAAHEP Competency (2022)	Procedure	Date	Grade / Pass	Initial
I.P.13.e. Perform first aid procedure for: environmental emergency	Procedure 21.1			
I.P.13.f. Perform first aid procedure for: syncope	Procedure 21.5			
II. Applied Mathematics				
II.P.1. Calculate proper dosages of medication for administration				
II.P.2. Record laboratory test results into the patient's record				
II.P.3. Document on a growth chart				
II.P.4. Apply mathematical computations to solve equations				
II.P.5. Convert among measurement systems				
III. Infection Control				
III.P.1. Participate in bloodborne pathogen training				
III.P.2. Select appropriate barrier/ personal protective equipment (PPE)				
III.P.3. Perform handwashing				
III.P.4. Prepare items for autoclaving				
III.P.5. Perform sterilization Procedure				
III.P.6. Prepare a sterile field				
III.P.7. Perform within a sterile field				
III.P.8. Perform wound care				
III.P.9. Perform dressing change				
III.P.10.a. Demonstrate proper disposal of biohazardous material: sharps				
III.P.10.b. Demonstrate proper disposal of biohazardous material: regulated wastes				
IV.P.1. Instruct a patient regarding a dietary change related to patient's special dietary needs				
V. Concepts of Effective Communication				
V.P.1. Respond to nonverbal communication	Procedure 2.1-2.4			
V.P.2. Correctly use and pronounce medical terminology in healthcare interactions				
V.P.3.a. Coach patients regarding: office policies	Procedure 11.3			

CAAHEP Competency (2022)	Procedure	Date	Grade / Pass	Initial
V.P.3.b. Coach patients regarding: medical encounters	Procedure 7.1			
V.P.4. Demonstrate professional telephone techniques	Procedure 10.1			
V.P.5. Document telephone messages accurately	Procedure 10.2			
V.P.6. Using technology, compose clear and correct correspondence	Procedure 9.1-9.5			
V.P.7. Use a list of community resources to facilitate referrals	Procedure 7.2			
V.P.8. Participate in a telehealth interaction with a patient				
VI. Administrative Functions				
VI.P.1. Manage appointment schedule using established priorities	Procedure 11.1, 11.2, 11.4			
VI.P.2. Schedule a patient procedure	Procedure 11.5			
VI.P.3. Input patient data using an electronic system	Procedure 12.1, 12.2			
VI.P.4. Perform an inventory of supplies	Procedure 13.3			
VII. Basic Practice Finances				
VII.P.1.a. Perform accounts receivable Procedure to patient accounts including posting: charges	Procedure 19.1			
VII.P.1.b. Perform accounts receivable Procedure to patient accounts including posting: payments	Procedure 19.1, 19.3			
VII.P.1.c. Perform accounts receivable Procedure to patient accounts including posting: adjustments	Procedure 19.3			
VII.P.2. Input accurate billing information in an electronic system	Procedure 11.2 Procedure 19.1, 19.3			
VII.P.3. Inform a patient of financial obligations for services rendered	Procedure 18.6 Procedure 19.2			
VIII. Third-Party Reimbursement				
VIII.P.1. Interpret information on an insurance card	Procedure 15.1			
VIII.P.2. Verify eligibility for services	Procedure 18.1, 18.6			
VIII.P.3. Obtain precertification or preauthorization including documentation	Procedure 18.1			
VIII.P.4. Complete an insurance claim form	Procedure 18.2, 18.3			

CAAHEP Competency (2022)	Procedure	Date	Grade / Pass	Initial
VIII.P.5. Assist a patient in understanding an Explanation of Benefits (EOB)	Procedure 18.5			
IX. Procedural and Diagnostic Coding				
IX.P.1. Perform procedural coding	Procedure 17.1, 17.2			
IX.P.2. Perform diagnostic coding	Procedure 16.1			
IX.P.3. Utilize medical necessity guidelines	Procedure 18.4			
X. Legal Implications				
X.P.1. Locate a state's legal scope of practice for medical assistants	Procedure 3.2			
X.P.2.a. Apply HIPAA rules in regard to: privacy	Procedure 4.1 Procedure 10.1			
X.P.2.b. Apply HIPAA rules in regard to: release of information	Procedure 4.2			
X.P.3. Document patient care accurately in the medical record	Procedure 10.1, 10.2 Procedure 7.1, 7.2 Procedure 21.1-21.6			
X.P.4. Complete compliance reporting based on public health statutes	Procedure 4.3			
X.P.5. Report an illegal activity following the protocol established by the healthcare setting	Procedure 4.4			
X.P.6. Complete an incident report related to an error in patient care	Procedure 4.5			
XI. Ethical Considerations				
XI.P.1. Demonstrate professional response(s) to ethical issues	Procedure 5.1, 5.2			
XII. Protective Practices				
XII.P.1. Comply with safety practices				
XII.P.2.a. Demonstrate proper use of: eyewash equipment				
XII.P.2.b. Demonstrate proper use of: fire extinguishers	Procedure 13.6			
XII.P.3. Use proper body mechanics	Procedure 13.3			
XII.P.4. Evaluate an environment to identify unsafe conditions	Procedure 13.4			
Affective Competencies				
A.1. Demonstrate critical thinking skills	Procedure 10.1 Procedure 11.2, 11.5 Procedure 18.5, 18.7 Procedure 21.2			

CAAHEP Competency (2022)	Procedure	Date	Grade / Pass	Initial
A.2. Reassure patients				
A.3. Demonstrate empathy for patients' concerns	Procedure 2.1-2.4 Procedure 4.1 Procedure 11.2 Procedure 18.5, 18.6, 18.7 Procedure 19.2			
A.4. Demonstrate active listening	Procedure 2.1-2.4 Procedure 4.1 Procedure 7.1			
A.5. Respect diversity	Procedure 2.1-2.4			
A.6. Recognize personal boundaries	Procedure 2.1-2.4			
A.7. Demonstrate tactfulness	Procedure 17.3 Procedure 18.5, 18.6, 18.7 Procedure 19.2			
A.8. Demonstrate self-awareness	Procedure 13.5			

Student Name________________________________ Date______________

chapter 1 The Professional Medical Assistant and the Healthcare Team

CAAHEP Competencies	Assessments
XI.C.4 Identify professional behaviors of a medical assistant	Skills and Concepts – B. 1
V.C.10 Identify the role of the medical assistant as a patient navigator	Workplace Application – 2
X.C.1. Identify scope of practice and standards of care for medical assistants	Skills and Concepts – C. 1, 2
X.C.2. Understand the provider role in terms of standard of care	Skills and Concepts – C. 1, 2
V.C.9. Identify the principles of self-boundaries	Skills and Concepts – K. 2
ABHES Competencies	**Assessments**
1. General Orientation	Skills and Concepts – A. 1, 2
a. Describe the current employment outlook for the medical assistant	
b. Compare and contrast the allied health professions and understand their relation to medical assisting	Skills and Concepts – H. 1-19
c. Describe and comprehend medical assistant credentialing requirements, the process to obtain the credential and the importance of credentialing	Skills and Concepts – D. 1
d. List the general responsibilities and skills of the medical assistant	Skills and Concepts – A. 3
5. Human Relations	Skills and Concepts – J. 2
f. Demonstrate an understanding of the core competencies for Interprofessional Collaborative Practice; i.e., values/ethics, roles/responsibilities, interprofessional communication, teamwork	
g. Partner with health care teams to attain optimal patient health outcomes	Skills and Concepts – K. 1
h. Display effective interpersonal skills with patients and health care team members	Skills and Concepts – K. 1
i. Demonstrate cultural awareness	Skills and Concepts – B. 1

ABHES Competencies	Assessments
8. Clinical Procedures	Skills and Concepts – G. 3
i. Identify community resources and Complementary and Alternative Medicine practices (CAM)	

VOCABULARY REVIEW

Using the word pool on the right, find the correct word to match the definition. Write the word on the line after the definition.

Group A

1. Adhering to ethical standards or right conduct standards ______________________
2. The way an individual perceives and processes information to learn new material ______________________
3. To learn or memorize beyond the point of proficiency or immediate recall ______________________
4. The process of sorting patients to determine medical need and the priority of care ______________________
5. A person who identifies patients' needs and barriers, then assists by coordinating care and identifying community and healthcare resources to meet the needs ______________________
6. How an individual internalizes new information and makes it their own ______________________
7. A learning device (e.g., an image, a rhyme, or a figure of speech) that a person uses to help them remember information ______________________
8. Meticulous, careful ______________________
9. How an individual looks at information and sees it as real ______________________
10. The process of thinking about new information to create new ways of learning ______________________
11. Harmful ______________________
12. Conduct expected of a reasonably prudent person acting under similar circumstances; it falls below the standards of behavior established by law for the protection of others against unreasonable risk of harm ______________________

Word Pool

- patient navigator
- detrimental
- integrity
- conscientious
- triage
- negligence
- perceiving
- processing
- learning style
- reflection
- overlearn
- mnemonic

Group B

Word Pool
- critical thinking
- contamination
- allopathic
- holistic
- complementary and alternative medicine (CAM)
- hospice
- indicators
- demeanor
- initiative
- reliable
- morale

1. A group of diverse medical and healthcare systems, practices, and products that are not generally considered part of conventional medicine; some are used in combination with conventional medicine and others are used instead of conventional medicine

   ____

2. Emotional or mental condition with respect to cheerfulness or confidence ______________________
3. A system of medical practice that treats disease by the use of remedies such as medications and surgery to produce effects different from those caused by the disease under treatment

   ____

4. Dependable; able to be trusted ______________________
5. The process by which something becomes harmful or unusable through contact with something unclean

   ____

6. The ability to determine what needs to be done and take action on your own ______________________
7. A form of healing that considers the whole person (i.e., body, mind, spirit, and emotions) in individual treatment plans

   ____

8. A concept of care that involves health professionals and volunteers who provide medical, psychological, and spiritual support to terminally ill patients and their loved ones

   ____

9. Behavior toward others; outward manner

   ____

10. The constant practice of considering all aspects of a situation when deciding what to believe or what to do

    ____

11. An important point or group of statistical values that, when evaluated, indicates the quality of care provided in a healthcare facility ______________________

ABBREVIATIONS

Write out what each of the following abbreviations stands for.

1. CAAHEP ______________________
2. CAM ______________________
3. EHR ______________________
4. ECG ______________________
5. CLIA ______________________
6. OSHA ______________________
7. IV ______________________

8. AAMA ________________________________
9. CEU ________________________________
10. AMT ________________________________
11. NHA ________________________________
12. MD ________________________________
13. DO ________________________________
14. OMT ________________________________
15. DC ________________________________
16. NP ________________________________
17. RN ________________________________
18. PA ________________________________
19. IDS ________________________________
20. ED ________________________________
21. PCMH ________________________________
22. AHRQ ________________________________
23. HHS ________________________________
24. IT ________________________________

SKILLS AND CONCEPTS

Answer the following questions. Write your answer on the line or in the space provided.

A. Responsibilities of the Medical Assistant

1. According the U.S. Bureau of Labor Statistics, employment opportunities for medical assistants is expected to grow ____________________ through ____________________.
2. List factors for the expected growth in job opportunities for medical assistants. ____________________

____

____

____

____

____

____

3. List five clinical and five administrative skills that are part of the job description for an entry-level medical assistant.

Clinical skills include: ______________________________

____

____

____

____

____

Administrative skills include: ______________________________

____

____

____

____

____

B. Characteristics of Professional Medical Assistants

1. What methods can the medical assistant use to treat others with courtesy and respect? ______________

____

____

____

____

____

C. Scope of Practice and Standards of Care for Medical Assistants

1. What is the difference between scope of practice and standards of care? ______________

____

____

____

____

____

____

2. Describe the difference between standard of care for a provider and a medical assistant.

3. Identify five practices that are beyond the scope of practice of medical assistants.

D. Professional Medical Assisting Organizations, Credentials, and Continuing Education

1. What are some of the differences between the AAMA and AMT? What credentials can be granted by each?

2. Is the NHA involved in medical assistant program curriculum development or accreditation? What service does this company provide?

E. How to Succeed as a Medical Assistant Student

1. Choose three study skills from your reading and describe how you think they will help you learn.

____

____

____

____

____

2. What test-taking strategies might help you improve your scores? ________________

____

____

____

3. Describe what it means to be a critical thinker. ________________

____

____

____

____

____

F. The History of Medicine

1. Describe how the profession of medical assisting began. Why are medical assistants defined as *multi-skilled* healthcare workers?

____

____

____

____

____

G. Medical Professionals

1. ________________ physicians, or DOs, complete requirements similar to those for MDs to graduate and practice medicine.

2. ________________ provide direct patient care services under the supervision of licensed physicians and are trained to diagnose and treat patients as directed by the physician.

3. Identify five complementary and alternative medicine therapies. ______________________________

____

____

____

____

____

4. Explain the role of the hospitalist. ______________________________

____

____

____

____

____

H. Allied Health Professionals

Match the following descriptions with the appropriate healthcare occupation.

1. _____ Provides services such as injury prevention, assessment, and rehabilitation
2. _____ Is qualified to implement exercise programs designed to reverse or minimize debilitation and enhance the functional capacity of medically stable patients
3. _____ Practices medicine under the direction and responsible supervision of a medical doctor or doctor of osteopathy
4. _____ Performs diagnostic examinations and therapeutic interventions of the heart or blood vessels, both invasive and noninvasive
5. _____ Assists licensed pharmacists by performing duties that do not require the expertise of a pharmacist
6. _____ Assists in developing and implementing the anesthesia care plan
7. _____ Helps improve patient mobility, relieve pain, and prevent or limit permanent physical disabilities
8. _____ Helps patients use their leisure in ways that enhance health, functional abilities, independence, and quality of life
9. _____ Identifies patients who have hearing, balance, and related ear problems
10. _____ Integrates and applies the principles from the science of food, nutrition, biochemistry, food management, and behavior to achieve and maintain health
11. _____ Evaluates, treats, and manages patients of all ages with respiratory illnesses and other cardiopulmonary disorders

a. audiologist
b. diagnostic cardiovascular technologist
c. therapeutic recreation specialist
d. physical therapist
e. pharmacy technician
f. dietetic technician
g. anesthesiology assistant
h. blood bank technology specialist
i. diagnostic medical sonographer
j. kinesiotherapist
k. occupational therapist
l. orthoptist
m. physician assistant
n. surgical technologist
o. respiratory therapist
p. athletic trainer
q. medical technologist
r. emergency medical technician
s. nuclear medicine technologist

12. _____ Evaluates disorders of vision, eye movement, and eye alignment
13. _____ Performs routine and standardized tests in blood center and transfusion services
14. _____Uses equipment that produces sound waves, resulting in images of internal structures
15. _____ Uses the nuclear properties of radioactive and stable nuclides to make diagnostic evaluations of the anatomic or physiologic conditions of the body
16. _____ Helps prepare patients for surgery and maintain the sterile field in the surgical suite, making sure all members of the surgical team follow sterile technique
17. _____ Assists in helping patients compensate for loss of function
18. _____ Performs diagnostic testing on blood, body fluids, and other types of specimens to assist the provider in arriving at a diagnosis
19. _____ Provides medical care to patients who have suffered an injury or illness outside the hospital setting

I. Types of Healthcare Facilities

1. Hospitals are classified according to the type of care and services they provide to patients. Describe the three different levels of hospitalized care.

   a. ____

   ____

   ____

   ____

   b. ____

   ____

   ____

   ____

   c. ____

   ____

   ____

   ____

J. The Healthcare Team

1. Define a patient-centered medical home (PCMH) and its five core functions and attributes. ____________

2. Define *teamwork* in your own words. ____________

K. Professionalism as a Team Member

1. Summarize three obstructions to professionalism.

   a. ____________

   b. ____________

   c. ____________

2. Identify the principles of self-boundaries. How do they relate to the field of medical assisting? ________

____

____

____

____

____

____

____

____

3. Describe four time-management techniques medical assistants can use in the healthcare environment to meet the demands of a busy practice.

   a. ____

   b. ____

   c. ____

   d. ____

CERTIFICATION PREPARATION

Circle the correct answer.

1. The first national organization formed for medical assistants was
   a. CAAHEP.
   b. ABHES.
   c. AMT.
   d. AAMA.

2. Which healthcare professional is trained to practice medicine under the supervision of a physician?
   a. Medical technologist
   b. Paramedic
   c. Medical assistant
   d. Physician assistant

3. The allied health specialist who performs ultrasound diagnostic procedures under the supervision of a physician is called a(n)
   a. cytotechnologist.
   b. diagnostic medical sonographer.
   c. electroneurodiagnostic technologist.
   d. perfusionist.

4. A method of prioritizing patients so that the most urgent cases receive care first is called
   a. case management.
   b. accreditation.
   c. triage.
   d. quality control.

5. The health professional who provides basic patient care services, including diagnosing illnesses and prescribing medications, is a
   a. nurse practitioner.
   b. nurse anesthetist.
   c. licensed practical nurse.
   d. vocational nurse.

6. One factor is absolutely true about all practicing medical assistants—they are not independent practitioners. Whether certified or not, regardless of length of training or experience, every medical assistant must practice under the direct supervision of a physician or other licensed practitioner (e.g., nurse practitioner or physician assistant).
   a. Both statements are true.
   b. Both statements are false.
   c. The first statement is true; the second is false.
   d. The first statement is false; the second is true.

7. Which mind maps would display the cause and effect of events?
   a. Spider map
   b. Fishbone map
   c. Chain-of-events map
   d. Cycle map

8. Which is *not* part of critical thinking?
   a. Sorting out conflicting information
   b. Weighing your knowledge about the information
   c. Deciding on a reasonable belief or action
   d. Incorporating personal beliefs

9. Deciding which tasks are most important is called
   a. modification.
   b. teaching.
   c. prioritizing.
   d. procrastinating.

10. Which statement about professionalism is true?
    a. It must be practiced at all times in the workplace.
    b. It can lead to wage increases and promotions.
    c. Unacceptable behavior is detrimental to the medical assistant's career.
    d. All of the above are true.

WORKPLACE APPLICATIONS

1. You are employed by a primary care physician who is investigating the possibility of forming a PCMH with other practitioners and allied health professionals in the community. Refer to the Department of Health and Human Services PCMH Resource Center at http://pcmh.ahrq.gov/. Research the meaning of PCMH and review the research that supports the PCMH model of care. What did you learn? Share this information with your class.

2. What does it mean to operate as a patient navigator? Why are medical assistants who are skilled in both administrative and clinical areas ideally suited to help patients navigate complex healthcare systems? How could you help the patient described below?

   Mrs. Kate Glasgow is an 82-year-old patient in the family practice where you work. Mrs. Glasgow recently suffered a mild cerebrovascular accident (CVA) and her son is trying to help coordinate her care. Mrs. Glasgow does not understand when or how to take her new medications, she is concerned about whether her health insurance will cover the cost of frequent clinic appointments and assistive devices, she doesn't understand how to prepare for magnetic resonance imaging (MRI) the provider ordered, and she dislikes having to comply with getting blood drawn every week.

3. Martin Smith is a patient who always disrupts the clinic. He constantly complains about everything from the moment he enters until the moment he leaves. Karen is at the desk when he arrives to check out and pay his bill. When she tells him that he has a previous balance from a claim that his insurance did not pay, he argues that Karen filed the claim incorrectly. Karen is not in charge of filing insurance claims and did not handle any part of the claim in question. How can she be courteous to this patient?

INTERNET ACTIVITIES

1. Choose one of the early medical pioneers discussed in this chapter and research the person using the internet. After conducting the research, create a poster presentation, a PowerPoint presentation, or write a paper and present the results of your research to the class.

2. Research professionalism requirements for other health professions. Talk about the ways that those requirements are similar to or different from those of a medical assistant. Compare professionalism in the healthcare industry to that in other professions such as law enforcement or education. Talk about why medical professionalism is so critical.

Student Name____ Date________________

chapter 2 Therapeutic Communication

CAAHEP Competencies	Assessment
V.C.1. Identify types of verbal and nonverbal communication	Skills and Concepts – C. 1, 3-11; D. 1, 4; Certification Preparation – 1, 2
V.C.2. Identify communication barriers	Skills and Concepts – F. 1 a-h; Certification Preparation – 3
V.C.3. Identify techniques for overcoming communication barriers	Skills and Concepts – F. 2-9; Certification Preparation – 4
V.C.4. Identify the steps in the sender-receiver process	Skills and Concepts – D. 2-3
V.C.5. Identify challenges in communication with different age groups	Skills and Concepts – F. 10-12, 21-28
V.C.9. Identify the principles of self-boundaries	Skills and Concepts – H. 1
V.C.11. Identify coping mechanisms	Skills and Concepts – I. 12-20; Certification Preparation – 5; Internet Activities – 4
V.C.13.a. Understand the basic concepts of the following theories: Maslow	Skills and Concepts – I. 1-9 a-h; Certification Preparation – 8-9; Internet Activities – 3
V.C.13.b. Understand the basic concepts of the following theories: Erikson	Skills and Concepts – F. 13-29; Certification Preparation – 6
V.C.13.c. Understand the basic concepts of the following theories: Kübler-Ross	Skills and Concepts – F. 30-35; Certification Preparation – 7
V.C.14. Identify issues associated with diversity as it relates to patient care	Skills and Concepts – B. 1-9
X.C.10.c. Identify: Americans with Disabilities Act Amendments Act (ADAAA)	Skills and Concepts – J. 1
V.P.1. Respond to nonverbal communication	Procedures 2.1, 2.2, 2.3, 2.4
A.3. Demonstrate empathy for patients' concerns	Procedures 2.1, 2.2, 2.3, 2.4
A.4. Demonstrate active listening	Procedures 2.1, 2.2, 2.3, 2.4
A.5. Respect diversity	Procedures 2.1, 2.2, 2.3, 2.4
A.6 Recognize personal boundaries	Procedure 2.5

ABHES Competencies	Assessment
5. Human Relations a. Respond appropriately to patients with abnormal behavior patterns	Skills and Concepts – F. 3, H. 4-5
b. Provide support for terminally ill patients 1) Use empathy when communicating with terminally ill patients	Skills and Concepts – F. 9
2) Identify common stages that terminally ill patients experience	Skills and Concepts – F. 10 a-e
d. Adapt care to address the developmental stages of life	Skills and Concepts – F. 6, 7, 8 a-i; Certification Preparation – 6
e. Analyze the effect of hereditary and environmental influences on behavior	Skills and Concepts – I. 1-3
h. Display effective interpersonal skills with patients and healthcare team members	Procedures 2.1, 2.2, 2.3, 2.4, 2.5
i . Demonstrate cultural awareness	Internet Activities – 1-2; Procedures 2.2, 2.3
7. Administrative Procedures g. Display professionalism through written and verbal communications	Procedures 2.1, 2.2, 2.4
8. Clinical Procedures j. Make adaptations for patients with special needs (psychological or physical limitations)	Review of Concepts – F. 2b-c, e, g, 6
k. Make adaptations to care for patients across their lifespan	Review of Concepts – F. 7, 8a-h

VOCABULARY REVIEW

Using the word pool on the right, find the correct word to match the definition. Write the word on the line after the definition.

1. The ability to understand another's perspective, experiences, or motivations ______________________
2. The act of sticking to something ______________________
3. A type of communication that occurs through body language and expressive behaviors rather than with verbal or written words ______________________
4. The inherent worth or state of being worthy of respect ______________________
5. Having a deep awareness of the suffering of another and the wish to ease it ______________________
6. The differences and similarities in identity, perspective, and points of view among people ______________________
7. Having a composed and self-assured manner ______________________

Word Pool

- adherence
- communication
- compassion
- coping mechanisms
- defense mechanisms
- dignity
- diversity
- empathy
- nonverbal communication
- hierarchy
- poised
- rapport
- respect
- stress
- therapeutic communication

8. A relationship of harmony and accord between the patient and the healthcare professional ______________________
9. To show consideration or appreciation for another person ______________________
10. A condition that causes physical and / or emotional tension ______________________
11. Exchange of information, feelings, and thoughts between two or more people using spoken words or other methods ______________________
12. A process of communicating with patients and family members in healthcare ______________________
13. Things arranged in order or rank ______________________
14. Unconscious mental processes that protect people from anxiety, loss, conflict, or shame ______________________
15. Behavioral and psychological strategies used to deal with or minimize stressful events ______________________

ABBREVIATIONS

Write out what each of the following abbreviations stands for.

1. ADA ______________________
2. ADAAA ______________________

SKILLS AND CONCEPTS

Answer the following questions.

A. Introduction and First Impressions and High-Quality Patient Care

1. ______________________ is a process of communicating with patients and family members in healthcare.
2. What factors are involved in creating a first impression?
   a. Physical appearance or dress
   b. Attitude and compassion
   c. Therapeutic communication skills
   d. All of the above

B. Respecting Diverse Populations

Match the description with the correct type of diversity. Answers can be used more than once.

1. _____ Includes the general customs, norms, values, and beliefs held by a group of people.
2. _____ Can make it more difficult for people to access healthcare and receive quality healthcare.
3. _____ Relates to a common ancestry, culture, religion, traditions, nationality, and language shared by a group of people.
4. _____ Pertains to the country where the person was born and holds citizenship.
5. _____ Can impact patient care if healthcare professionals assume patients will conform to the mainstream values and the patient's health beliefs are not considered.
6. _____ A person's lifestyle choice may influence the care they receive.
7. _____ Pertains to immigrants to the United States who lack insurance for healthcare.
8. _____ Relates to a group of people who have the same physical characteristics.
9. _____ All the ways a person is different from others (e.g., lifestyle, religion, tastes, and preferences).

a. nationality
b. race
c. culture
d. ethnicity
e. social factors
f. culture and ethnicity

Select the correct answer.

10. To show respect, a healthcare professional should
    a. smile and make eye contact if appropriate when first meeting a person.
    b. be courteous, sincere, polite, and welcoming.
    c. use a calm tone of voice and proper grammar without slang.
    d. all of the above

C. Nonverbal Communication

1. We communicate ________________________ through nonverbal behaviors (our body language and expressive behaviors) than through our words.

2. What is involved with nonverbal communication?
    a. Nonverbal behaviors
    b. Nonverbal communication delivery factors
    c. Cultural differences and spatial distance
    d. All of the above

3. Which is considered a negative, closed nonverbal behavior?
    a. Being at the level of the other person and angled toward them
    b. Arms crossed in front of the body or hands behind the person's back
    c. Poised and shoulders relaxed
    d. Light touch on the person's hand

4. Which is considered a positive, open nonverbal behavior?
   a. Professional appearance
   b. Fidgeting and looking at the clock
   c. Lowered eyebrows or one raised eyebrow
   d. Avoiding eye contact

Match the nonverbal delivery factor with the definition.

5. _____ Describes the emotion in the voice.
6. _____ Refers to the speed at which the speaker talks.
7. _____ Pertains to how the word is said.
8. _____ Refers to the loudness of the speaker's voice.
9. _____ Includes the highness and lowness of the voice.
10. _____ Describes the melodic pattern or the pitch variation.
11. _____ Relates to the quality of the voice.

a. rate
b. clarity
c. volume
d. pitch
e. tone
f. intonation
g. pronunciation

Select the correct answer or fill the answer in on the line.

12. Which of the following is *not* a professional expectation when speaking with patients?
    a. Use a moderate rate and volume.
    b. Speak in a clear voice.
    c. Vary your pitch.
    d. Use medical terminology and generational terms.

13. How can a medical assistant respect a person from another cultural group that is unfamiliar?
    a. Follow the other person's lead in terms of nonverbal behaviors and personal space.
    b. Use gestures cautiously.
    c. Refrain from touching a child's head.
    d. All of the above

14. When medical assistants talk with patients, they should be ______________________ away from the patients, which is considered the ______________________ space.

15. When medical assistants perform procedures on patients, they are ______________________ away from patients, which is considered the ______________________ space.

16. A person will move ______________________ if they want to increase the space between themselves and other people.

D. Verbal Communication

1. Two types of verbal communication include ______________________ and ______________________.

2. Describe the steps in the communication cycle (or sender-receiver process).______________________

____

____

3. We decode messages based on ______________________ and ______________________.

4. Which of the following is a type of written communication?
   a. Texts and written phone messages
   b. Letters and emails
   c. Informational flyers
   d. All of the above

Match style of oral communication with the correct description. Answers can be used more than once.

5. _____ When working with this type of communicator, a person should avoid being controlled and respectfully maintain their position.
6. _____ This type of communicator tries to dominate others and may glare, frown, and purposefully invade others' personal space.
7. _____ This type of communicator clearly states their needs and wants.
8. _____ This type of communicator avoid expressing feelings or opinions, fails to assert themselves, and allows others to infringe on their rights.
9. _____ This type of communicator uses a medium pitch, speed, and volume of voice and positive, open nonverbal behaviors.
10. _____ When working with this type of communicator, a person may need to use humor and try to have a positive discussion.
11. _____ This type of communicator is cunning, tries to control others, and maybe demeaning or condescending.
12. _____ This type of communicator denies problems and may speak in a sugary-sweet voice, look innocent, and pretend to be warm and friendly.
13. _____ When working with this type of communicator, a person should remain calm and attempt to see the other person's point of view.
14. _____ This type of communicator speaks in a soft voice, fidgets, and belittles their contribution.
15. _____ A healthcare professional needs to be this type of communicator.
16. _____ When working with this type of communicator, a person should use a firm approach and be assertive.

a. passive communicator
b. aggressive communicator
c. passive-aggressive communicator
d. manipulative communicator
e. assertive communicator

E. Therapeutic Communication

1. What is the advantage of using therapeutic communication in a healthcare setting?
   a. It is an interactive relationship that conveys acceptance and respect without judgment or blame.
   b. It encourages healthcare professionals to build rapport with patients, which is helpful in building the relationship.
   c. When that bond develops and grows, patients are more comfortable expressing their feelings, ideas, and concerns.
   d. All of the above

2. Which is correct regarding active listening and passively hearing what a speaker is saying?
   a. With active listening, we fully concentrate on what is being said and how it is being said.
   b. The speaker can easily see the person is actively listening.
   c. With passive hearing, we hear what the patient is saying, but we are distracted by our own thoughts.
   d. All of the above

3. What is a nonverbal behavior that *cannot* be used during active listening?
   a. Eye contact and nodding your head
   b. Body position and facial expression
   c. Looking at the clock and yawning
   d. All of the above

4. Which is *not* correct regarding closed questions or statements?
   a. Asks for general information or states the topic to be discussed
   b. Closed questions limit the patient's answer to one or two words
   c. Used to confirm specific facts
   d. Answers to closed questions may include yes and no

5. Which is *not* correct regarding open questions or statements?
   a. Used as a communication tool to begin a conversation with a patient
   b. Used to introduce a new section of questions
   c. A poor method to use when wanting additional details from the patient about their problem
   d. Used when a person introduces a new topic

6. ______________________ allows the listener to get additional information.

7. ______________________ or ______________________ means to reword or rephrase a statement to check the meaning and interpretation.

8. ______________________ allows the listener to recap and review what was said.

9. ______________________ allows time to gather thoughts and answer questions.

10. ______________________ means to put words to the person's emotional reaction, which acknowledges the person's feelings.

F. Barriers to Effective Communication

1. For each description below, identify the type of barrier to communication.
   a. Noise, lack of privacy, temperature ______________________
   b. Fear and anxiety related to being judged by the healthcare professional or the inability to explain personal feelings ______________________
   c. Unable to read or write ______________________
   d. Hunger, pain, anger, tiredness ______________________
   e. Unable to see written communication ______________________
   f. Unable to hear verbal communication ______________________
   g. Functioning at a lower age level ______________________
   h. English is not the patient's primary language ______________________

Match the communication barrier with the correct way the medical assistant can help overcome the barrier.

2. _____ Help make the patient comfortable. Provide food and drink if available. Administer pain medications as ordered.
3. _____ Use audio recordings, screen magnifiers, large-print materials, and screen reader software.
4. _____ Provide privacy for patients. Talk with patients in a quiet room with the door closed. Make sure the room temperature is comfortable.
5. _____ Use print materials and written instructions. Use videos with captions. Have text telephones (TTYs) available. Use a sign language interpreter.
6. _____ Use "functioning age" -appropriate language and materials. Provide information also to the guardian/caregiver.
7. _____ Use interpreters and translated materials. Limit medical terminology and define medical terms that must be used. Use culturally appropriate materials and visuals (pictures, graphs, and models).
8. _____ Use pictures and models. Draw pictures and use simple language.
9. _____ Provide a warm, caring environment. Make sure your body language reflects an open and caring manner. Gain the person's trust. Keep voice at normal level.

a. hearing impairment
b. non-English–speaking
c. illiteracy
d. internal distractions
e. environmental distractions
f. visual impairment
g. emotional distraction
h. intellectual disability

Match the challenges in communication with the correct development stage.

10. _____ Does not comprehend cause and effect or the impact in the future
11. _____ Unable to process medical information
12. _____ Understands concrete examples versus hypothetical situations

a. sensory motor
b. preoperational
c. concrete operations

Match the goal of the stage with the correct psychosocial developmental stages.

13. _____ Encouraged to try new activities. Must assume responsibilities and learn new skills. Will make child feel purposeful and increase self-esteem.
14. _____ To know who you are as a person and how you fit into the world around you. Creates a meaningful self-image.
15. _____ Must develop trust, with the ability to mistrust should the need arise.
16. _____ Must seek to finish tasks. Recognition for accomplishments is important.

a. trust versus mistrust
b. autonomy versus shame and doubt
c. initiative versus guilt
d. industry versus inferiority
e. identity versus role confusion
f. intimacy versus isolation
g. generativity versus stagnation
h. ego integrity versus despair

17. _____ Must explore and manipulate things in their "world" to develop autonomy and self-esteem.
18. _____ Develops friendships; takes on commitments.
19. _____ Reflects on one's life and comes to terms with it, instead of regretting the past.
20. _____ Achieves a balance between the concern for the next generation (having a family) and being self-absorbed.

Match the communication tip with the correct psychosocial developmental stages.

21. _____ Use short simple sentences. Encourage questions. Use imitation, play, and role playing.
22. _____ Communicate with dignity and respect. Limit slang and "generational" terms. Use simpler language. Speak clearly. Allow time to respond.
23. _____ Identify motivating factors and use them as needed during communication. Realize person may be juggling a lot of obligations.
24. _____ Use calm and soothing voice, hold child securely. Loud voices and noises can startle a child.
25. _____ Use engaging simple tools to communicate information (videos, gaming software, pamphlets). Encourage discussion and questions.
26. _____ Provide privacy and independence. Encourage responsible decision making. Encourage discussion and questions.
27. _____ Identify motivating factors and use them as needed during communication. Realize person may be juggling a lot of obligations.
28. _____ Use simple language. Allow child to touch and explore objects. Allow child to play and make choices.

a. trust versus mistrust
b. autonomy versus shame and doubt
c. initiative versus guilt
d. industry versus inferiority
e. identity versus role confusion
f. intimacy versus isolation
g. generativity versus stagnation
h. ego integrity versus despair

Answer the following questions.

29. Discuss how Erikson's theory of psychosocial developmental relates to communicating with patients.

____

____

____

30. Discuss how Kübler-Ross's theory relates to communicating with patients. _______________

____

____

____

Match the description with the correct stage of Kübler-Ross's theory.

31. _____ Person feels sad, fearful, and uncertain. May not participate in normal activities. Distances self from others.
32. _____ Refuses to accept the fact (e.g., diagnosis or prognosis). Defense mechanism that allows the person to ignore what is happening.
33. _____ Has come to terms with situation.
34. _____ Can be directed at self or others.
35. _____ Attempts to bargain with the higher power the person believes in (e.g., God).

a. denial
b. anger
c. bargaining
d. depression
e. acceptance

G. Communicating in the Workplace

1. When speaking with providers, what guideline should the medical assistant follow?
   a. Speak confidently, clearly, and concisely.
   b. Start with the patient's name and age if appropriate.
   c. Discuss the situation in an organized manner.
   d. All of the above

2. When speaking with providers, what guideline should the medical assistant follow?
   a. If the situation relates to a series of events, start with what occurred first, then second, and so on.
   b. Write down any information the provider gives.
   c. Read information written down back to the provider to ensure accuracy.
   d. All of the above

H. Personal and Professional Boundaries with Communication

1. What is a principle of self-boundaries (personal boundaries)?
   a. They are also called personal boundaries.
   b. They are the limits people use to protect themselves.
   c. Include mental, emotional, physical, and social factors.
   d. All of the above

2. The relationship between the patient and the medical assistant must be professional. What should the medical assistant do to keep this relationship professional?
   a. Share personal issues, struggles, life stories, or other personal intimate information.
   b. Befriend the patient on social media.
   c. Refrain from contacting the patient outside of the work environment.
   d. All of the above

I. Understanding Behavior

1. What is correct regarding Maslow's Hierarchy of Needs theory?
   a. This is a motivational theory that depicts eight levels of needs.
   b. Each level must be satisfied before we can move up to the next level.
   c. The needs include "Deficiency" needs and "Growth" needs.
   d. All of the above

Match the description with the correct needs from Maslow's Hierarchy of Needs theory. Answers can be used more than once.

2. _____ These needs are considered coping behaviors.
3. _____ Needs must be fulfilled to cope with life and survival.
4. _____ Top four levels of needs.
5. _____ We are all motivated to meet these unmet needs.
6. _____ These needs relate to making ourselves a better person.
7. _____ Fulfillment of these needs leads to long-lasting happiness.
8. _____ Fulfillment of these needs leads to instant short-term gratification.

a. "growth" needs
b. "deficiency" needs

9. For the following descriptions, identify the level of need according to Maslow's theory.
   a. Includes air, food, drink, shelter, and warmth ______________________
   b. Includes friendship and intimacy ______________________
   c. Includes protection form the elements and security ______________________
   d. Includes knowledge, curiosity, and understanding ______________________
   e. The appreciation of and search for beauty and balance ______________________
   f. Includes self-esteem and achievement ______________________
   g. The need to realize one's potential ______________________
   h. Which needs are met by helping others achieve their very best? ______________________
10. ______________________ are unconscious mental processes that protect people from anxiety, loss, conflict, or shame.
11. Identify the defense mechanism based on the following descriptions.
   a. Completely rejects the information. ______________________
   b. The person comes up with various explanations to justify their response. ______________________
   c. Transfers the emotion toward one person to another person or thing. ______________________
   d. Simply forgets something that is bad or hurtful. ______________________

Match the description or coping mechanism with the correct type of coping mechanism. Answers can be used more than once.

12. _____ Reduce the feelings associated with stress for a short time.
13. _____ Improve our functioning level and reduce stress level
14. _____ Hostility and aggression
15. _____ Eat healthy, well-balanced meals
16. _____ Drug and alcohol use
17. _____ Gambling
18. _____ Social withdrawal and isolation
19. _____ Talk and share with others
20. _____ Exercise, drink water, and get plenty of sleep

a. adaptive (healthy) coping mechanisms
b. maladaptive (unhealthy) coping mechanisms

J. Closing Comments

1. Discuss the impact of the Americans with Disabilities Act Amendments Act (ADAAA) in relationship to communication barriers in healthcare.

____

____

____

____

____

2. Discuss three ways that healthcare providers can meet their federal obligation for accommodating patients with communication disabilities.

____

____

____

CERTIFICATION PREPARATION

Circle the correct answer.

1. What is a type of nonverbal communication?
   a. Body language
   b. Oral communication
   c. Email
   d. Letter

2. What is a type of verbal communication?
   a. Written message
   b. Oral communication
   c. Email
   d. All of the above

3. Hunger, pain, anger, and tiredness are considered which type of barrier to communication?
   a. Environmental distractions
   b. Internal distractions
   c. External distractions
   d. Hearing impairment

4. What is a way to overcome environmental distractions?
   a. Help make the patient comfortable.
   b. Use audio recordings and large-print materials.
   c. Provide privacy for patients.
   d. Use pictures and models.

5. What is a maladaptive coping mechanism?
   a. Passive-aggressive behavior
   b. Drug and alcohol use
   c. Denial
   d. All of the above

6. Erikson's theory places a 4-year-old child in which developmental stage?
   a. Trust versus mistrust
   b. Autonomy versus shame and doubt
   c. Initiative versus guilt
   d. Industry versus inferiority

7. According to Kübler-Ross, when a person feels sadness, fear, and uncertainty, they are in which stage of grief?
   a. Denial
   b. Anger
   c. Bargaining
   d. Depression

8. Which level of Maslow's Hierarchy of Needs includes protection from the elements, security, and stability?
   a. Physiologic needs
   b. Safety needs
   c. Love and belongingness needs
   d. Esteem needs

9. Which level of Maslow's Hierarchy of Needs includes knowledge, curiosity, understanding, and exploration?
   a. Cognitive needs
   b. Aesthetic needs
   c. Self-actualization needs
   d. Transcendence needs

10. A person is using which defense mechanism when they revert to an old, immature behavior to express their feelings?
    a. Denial
    b. Repression
    c. Regression
    d. Displacement

WORKPLACE APPLICATIONS

1. When Christi was doing her orientation, she observed Sally rooming patients. With the patient seated in the room, Sally stood near the patient collecting the patient's information. She smiled occasionally as she talked with the patient. Christi noticed Sally had poor posture and yawned several times during the patient interview. At times, Sally used appropriate light touch with the patient and used small hand gestures. Describe the positive nonverbal behaviors that Christi observed.

   ____

   ____

   ____

   ____

2. Using #1 above, list the negative and closed nonverbal behaviors that Christi observed. For each type of negative behavior, indicate the correct positive and open behavior that should have been used.

____

____

____

3. Christi is following Samantha during orientation as they work with a Hmong provider. Most of the patients are Hmong. Describe specific cultural differences with nonverbal behaviors that would apply to the Hmong community.

____

____

____

INTERNET ACTIVITIES

1. Using online resources, research a specific culture different than your own. Create a poster presentation, a PowerPoint presentation, or write a paper summarizing your research. Include the following points in your project:
   a. Description of the culture (e.g., origin, typical family structure)
   b. Culture, beliefs, religion, and ethnic customs that influence healthcare discussions, treatments, and care
   c. Beliefs that impact verbal and nonverbal communication
2. Using online resources, research four cultures different than your own. Focus your research on cultural beliefs that impact communication in the healthcare environment. Create a poster presentation, a PowerPoint presentation, or write a paper summarizing your research. Include tips for a medical assistant to remember when working with a patient from each of the cultures.
3. Research Maslow's Hierarchy of Needs. Create a poster presentation, a PowerPoint presentation, or write a paper summarizing the theory and describe its importance to medical assistants. Cite two appropriate references used.
4. Research adaptive (healthy) and maladaptive (nonadaptive, unhealthy) coping mechanisms. Create a list of eight adaptive and eight maladaptive coping mechanisms. Discuss the importance of using adaptive coping mechanisms. Cite two appropriate references used.

Procedure 2.1 Use Feedback Techniques and Demonstrate Respect for Individual Diversity: Gender and Appearance

Name ______________________________ **Date** ____________ **Score** __________

Tasks: Use feedback techniques (e.g., reflection, restatement, and clarification) to obtain patient information. Respond to nonverbal communication. Communicate respectfully with patients with individual diversity related to gender and appearance. Demonstrate empathy, active listening, and nonverbal communication.

Background: When working with a transgender patient, ask the patient privately which pronouns the person prefers. Make sure to add this information into the patient's health record for future reference.

Scenario: You are rooming Crystal Green. You can see that she has expertly applied her makeup, has long red fingernails, long blonde hair, and is wearing three-inch heels. You are surprised to see that her birth sex is male. This is the first time you have roomed a transgender patient. You are uncomfortable in this situation because you have strong personal beliefs that birth sex should be maintained throughout a person's life.

Directions: Using the scenario, role-play with a peer the rooming process (obtain the patient's chief complaint [main reason for the visit], allergies, pregnancy history, and current medications). The partner (patient) should make up any information required.

Equipment and Supplies:
- Patient health record
- History form (optional) (Work Product 2.1)
- Pen

Standard: Complete the procedure and all critical steps in _______ minutes with a minimum score of 85% within two attempts (*or as indicated by the instructor*).

Scoring: Divide the points earned by the total possible points. Failure to perform a critical step, indicated by an asterisk (*), results in grade no higher than an 84% (*or as indicated by the instructor*).

Time: Began________ Ended________ Total minutes: ________

Steps	Possible Points	Attempt 1	Attempt 2
1. Greet the patient. Identify yourself. Verify the patient's identity with full name and date of birth. Explain the procedure in a manner that is understood by the patient. Answer any questions the patient may have on the procedure.	10		
2. Demonstrate respect for the patient. Be sincere, courteous, polite, and welcoming. Maintain the patient's dignity. Demonstrate professional, nonjudgmental verbal and nonverbal communication. Ask appropriate questions as information is obtained. (*Refer to the Affective Behaviors Checklist –* ***Respect*** *and the Grading Rubric*)	15*		
3. Using appropriate closed and open-ended questions and statements, obtain the patient's chief complaint (main reason for the visit) and history of present illness, allergies, pregnancy history, medical history, and current medications. Document the information in the health record or on the history form.	10		

4. Use feedback techniques, including reflection, restatement, and clarification as information is obtained.	**10***		
5. Respond to the patient's nonverbal communication by using feedback techniques (e.g., reflection). If the patient's nonverbal communication is interpreted differently than the patient's oral statements, clarify the information with the patient.	**10***		
6. Use active listening skills. Remain neutral and refrain from interrupting. Allow for periods of silence. Smile and nod your head to show interest. Use appropriate eye contact. Focus on the patient and avoid distractions (e.g., looking at the clock, fidgeting). (*Refer to the Affective Behaviors Checklist – **Active Listening** and the Grading Rubric*)	**15***		
7. Use professional, positive nonverbal communication behaviors. Use a clear voice, with a moderate rate and volume. Use a varying pitch and an accepting or a neutral tone. Use words the patient can understand. Correctly pronounce the words. Be at the same eye level as the patient's. Smile and have a poised posture. Use light touch on the hand if appropriate. Maintain proper eye contact if culturally appropriate. (*Refer to the Affective Behaviors Checklist – **Nonverbal Communication** and the Grading Rubric*)	**15***		
8. Demonstrate empathy by listening to the patient and learning about their experiences and concerns. Use therapeutic communication techniques and positive nonverbal behaviors. Show your support and respect. (*Refer to the Affective Behaviors Checklist – **Empathy** and the Grading Rubric*)	**15***		
Total Score	**100**		

Affective Behavior	**Affective Behaviors Checklist** **Directions:** *Check behaviors observed during the role-play.*					
Respect	**Negative, Unprofessional Behaviors**	**Attempt**		**Positive, Professional Behaviors**	**Attempt**	
		1	**2**		**1**	**2**
	Rude, unkind, fake/false attitude, disrespectful, impolite, unwelcoming			Courteous, sincere, polite, welcoming		
	Unconcerned with person's dignity; brief, abrupt			Maintained person's dignity; took time with person		
	Unprofessional verbal communication; inappropriate questions			Professional verbal communication		
	Negative nonverbal behaviors, poor eye contact			Positive nonverbal behaviors, proper eye contact		
	Other:			Other:		

Active Listening	Biased, offensive			Remained neutral		
	Interrupted			Refrained from interrupting		
	Did not allow for silence or pauses			Allowed for periods of silence		
	Negative nonverbal behaviors (rolled eyes, yawned, frowned, avoided eye contact)			Positive nonverbal behaviors (smiled, nodded head, appropriate eye contact)		
	Distracted (looked at watch, phone)			Focused on patient, avoided distractions		
	Other:			Other:		
Nonverbal Communication	Muffled voice; rate too fast or slow; too loud or too soft; unaccepting tone			Clear voice with moderate rate and volume; varying pitch; accepting or neutral tone		
	Incorrectly pronounced words; used words the person did not understand (e.g., medical terminology, generational phrases)			Correctly pronounced words; used words person can understand		
	Stood while patient was sitting; slouching, lack of poised posture			Was at the same position of the patient; had a poised posture		
	Frowned, lack of proper eye contact, inappropriate touch			Smiled, maintained proper eye contact, used light touch on hand when appropriate		
	Other:			Other:		
Empathy	Did not listen to patient's responses			Listened to patient; learned about patient		
	Lack of respect and support demonstrated			Showed respect and support		
	Lack of therapeutic communication techniques used			Used therapeutic communication techniques		
	Negative nonverbal behaviors (e.g., positioning, frowning, poor eye contact)			Positive nonverbal behaviors (e.g., at the same level as patient, smiled, good eye contact)		
	Other:			Other:		

Grading Rubric for the Affective Behaviors Checklist **Directions:** *Based on checklist results, identify the points received for the procedure checklist. Indicate how the behaviors demonstrated met the expectations.*		**Points for Procedure Checklist**	**Attempt 1**	**Attempt 2**
Does not meet Expectation	• Response lacked respect, active listening, professional nonverbal communication, and/or empathy. • Student demonstrated more than 2 negative, unprofessional behaviors during the interaction.	0		
Needs Improvement	• Response lacked respect, active listening, professional nonverbal communication, and/or empathy. • Student demonstrated 1 or 2 negative, unprofessional behaviors during the interaction.	0		
Meets Expectation	• Response was respectful and empathetic. Demonstrated active listening, professional nonverbal communication. No negative, unprofessional behaviors observed. • More practice is needed for behavior to appear natural and for student to appear comfortable and at ease.	15		
Occasionally Exceeds Expectation	• Response was respectful and empathetic. Demonstrated active listening, professional nonverbal communication. No negative, unprofessional behaviors observed. • At times student appeared comfortable and at ease; but more practice is needed for behavior to become natural and consistent with a professional medical assistant.	15		
Always Exceeds Expectation	• Response was respectful and empathetic. Demonstrated active listening, professional nonverbal communication. No negative, unprofessional behaviors observed. • Student's behaviors appeared natural and comfortable. Behaviors are consistent with a professional medical assistant.	15		

Comments

CAAHEP Competencies	**Step(s)**
V.P.1. Respond to nonverbal communication	5
A.3. Demonstrate empathy for patients' concerns	8
A.4. Demonstrate active listening	6
A.5. Respect diversity	2
ABHES Competencies	**Step(s)**
5. Human Relations h. Display effective interpersonal skills with patients and healthcare team members	Entire role-play
7. Administrative Procedures g. Display professionalism through written and verbal communications	Entire role-play

Work Product 2.1 History Form for Established Patient

Name ______________________________ **Date** ____________ **Score** __________

(To be used with Procedure 2.1)

<table>
<tr><td>MEDICAL HISTORY FORM</td><td colspan="2">DATE</td><td>MRN:</td></tr>
<tr><td>NAME</td><td>DOB</td><td colspan="2">AGE</td></tr>
<tr><td colspan="4"></td></tr>
<tr><td colspan="4">CHIEF
COMPLAINT</td></tr>
<tr><td colspan="4">HX OF
PRESENT
ILLNESS</td></tr>
<tr><td></td><td colspan="3"></td></tr>
<tr><td>ALLERGIES</td><td colspan="3">CURRENT MEDICATIONS</td></tr>
<tr><td>FEMALES:
PREGNANT YES NO
LMP: __________</td><td colspan="3">UPDATED TO MEDICAL HISTORY SINCE LAST VISIT</td></tr>
<tr><td>Do you feel safe in your home?
YES NO</td><td colspan="3">NICOTINE / TOBACCO
USE: YES NO
PRODUCT:
AMOUNT DAILY:
NUMBER OF YEARS OF USE: :_______</td></tr>
</table>

Procedure 2.2 Use Feedback Techniques and Demonstrate Respect for Individual Diversity: Race

Name ______________________________ **Date** ____________ **Score** __________

Tasks: Use feedback techniques (e.g., reflection, restatement, and clarification) to obtain patient information. Respond to nonverbal communication. Communicate respectfully with patients with individual diversity related to race. Demonstrate empathy, active listening, and nonverbal communication.

Background: When working with an interpreter, allow time for the person to translate the information to the patient. Also, focus on the patient and do not look at the interpreter when speaking to the patient.

Scenario: You are rooming Maria Hernandez. She is always late for her appointments, and today she was 20 minutes late. She also does not speak English and you need to use a Spanish interpreter for the visit. You are uncomfortable in this situation because you have not worked with an interpreter before. You are also feeling rushed because she was late for her appointment.

Directions: Role-play the scenario with two peers. One peer is the patient, and the other peer is the translator. While acting as the translator, the information can be repeated in English. You need to obtain a brief medical history on this patient (e.g., chief complaint, allergies, and current medications). The peer (patient) should make up any information required.

Equipment and Supplies:
- Patient health record
- History form (optional) (Work Product 2.2)
- Pen

Standard: Complete the procedure and all critical steps in _______ minutes with a minimum score of 85% within two attempts (*or as indicated by the instructor*).

Scoring: Divide the points earned by the total possible points. Failure to perform a critical step, indicated by an asterisk (*), results in grade no higher than an 84% (*or as indicated by the instructor*).

Time: Began_________ Ended_________ Total minutes: _________

Steps	Possible Points	Attempt 1	Attempt 2
1. Greet the patient. Identify yourself. Verify the patient's identity with full name and date of birth. Explain the procedure in a manner that is understood by the patient. Answer any questions the patient may have on the procedure.	10		
2. Demonstrate respect for the patient. Focus on the patient, not on the interpreter. Pause to give the interpreter and patient time to answer. Be sincere, courteous, polite, and welcoming. Maintain the patient's dignity. Demonstrate professional, nonjudgmental verbal and nonverbal communication. Ask appropriate questions as information is obtained. *(Refer to the Affective Behaviors Checklist –* ***Respect*** *and the Grading Rubric)*	15*		
3. Using appropriate closed and open-ended questions and statements, obtain the patient's chief complaint (main reason for the visit) and history of present illness, allergies, pregnancy history, medical history, and current medications. Document the information in the health record or on the history form.	10		

4. Use feedback techniques including reflection, restatements, and clarification as information is obtained.	**10***		
5. Respond to the patient's nonverbal communication by using feedback techniques (e.g., reflection). If the patient's nonverbal communication is interpreted differently than the patient's oral statements, clarify the information with the patient.	**10***		
6. Use active listening skills. Remain neutral and refrain from interrupting. Allow for periods of silence. Smile and nod your head to show interest. Use appropriate eye contact. Focus on the patient and avoid distractions (e.g., looking at the clock, fidgeting). *(Refer to the Affective Behaviors Checklist –* ***Active Listening*** *and the Grading Rubric)*	**15***		
7. Use professional, positive nonverbal communication behaviors. Use a clear voice, with a moderate rate and volume. Use a varying pitch and an accepting or a neutral tone. Use words the patient can understand. Correctly pronounce the words. Be at the same position as the patient. Smile and have a poised posture. Use light touch on the hand if appropriate. Maintain proper eye contact if culturally appropriate. *(Refer to the Affective Behaviors Checklist –* ***Nonverbal Communication*** *and the Grading Rubric)*	**15***		
8. Demonstrate empathy by listening to the patient and learning about their experiences and concerns. Use therapeutic communication techniques and positive nonverbal behaviors. Show your support and respect. *(Refer to the Affective Behaviors Checklist –* ***Empathy*** *and the Grading Rubric)*	**15***		
Total Score	**100**		

Affective Behavior	**Affective Behaviors Checklist** **Directions:** *Check behaviors observed during the role-play.*					
Respect	**Negative, Unprofessional Behaviors**	**Attempt**		**Positive, Professional Behaviors**	**Attempt**	
		1	**2**		**1**	**2**
	Rude, unkind, fake/false attitude, disrespectful, impolite, unwelcoming			Courteous, sincere, polite, welcoming		
	Unconcerned with person's dignity; brief, abrupt			Maintained person's dignity; took time with person		
	Focused on the interpreter; rushed the conversation; did not give the patient and interpreter time to talk			Focused on the patient; gave adequate time for the patient and interpreter to respond		
	Unprofessional verbal communication; inappropriate questions			Professional verbal communication		
	Negative nonverbal behaviors, poor eye contact			Positive nonverbal behaviors, proper eye contact		
	Other:			Other:		

Active Listening	Biased, offensive			Remained neutral		
	Interrupted			Refrained from interrupting		
	Did not allow for silence or pauses			Allowed for periods of silence		
	Negative nonverbal behaviors (rolled eyes, yawned, frowned, avoided eye contact)			Positive nonverbal behaviors, smiled, nodded head, appropriate eye contact		
	Distracted (looked at watch, phone)			Focused on patient, avoided distractions		
	Other:			Other:		
Nonverbal Communication	Muffled voice; too fast or slow of rate; too loud or too soft; unaccepting tone			Clear voice with moderate rate and volume; varying pitch; accepting or neutral tone		
	Incorrectly pronounced words; used words the person did not understand (e.g., medical terminology, generational phrases)			Correctly pronounced words; used words person can understand		
	Stood while patient was sitting; slouching, lack of poised posture			Was at the same position as the patient; had a poised posture		
	Frowned, lack of proper eye contact, inappropriate touch			Smiled, maintained proper eye contact, used light touch on hand when appropriate		
	Other:			Other:		
Empathy	Did not listen to patient's responses			Listened to patient; learned about patient		
	Lack of respect and support demonstrated			Showed respect and support		
	Lack of therapeutic communication techniques used			Used therapeutic communication techniques		
	Negative nonverbal behaviors (e.g., positioning, frowning, poor eye contact)			Positive nonverbal behaviors (e.g., at the same level as patient, smiled, good eye contact)		
	Other:			Other:		

Grading Rubric for the Affective Behaviors Checklist **Directions:** *Based on checklist results, identify the points received for the procedure checklist. Indicate how the behaviors demonstrated met the expectations.*		**Points for Procedure Checklist**	**Attempt 1**	**Attempt 2**
Does not meet Expectation	• Response lacked respect, active listening, professional nonverbal communication, and/or empathy. • Student demonstrated more than 2 negative, unprofessional behaviors during the interaction.	0		
Needs Improvement	• Response lacked respect, active listening, professional nonverbal communication, and/or empathy. • Student demonstrated 1 or 2 negative, unprofessional behaviors during the interaction.	0		
Meets Expectation	• Response was respectful and empathetic. Demonstrated active listening, professional nonverbal communication. No negative, unprofessional behaviors observed. • More practice is needed for behavior to appear natural and for student to appear comfortable and at ease.	15		
Occasionally Exceeds Expectation	• Response was respectful and empathetic. Demonstrated active listening, professional nonverbal communication. No negative, unprofessional behaviors observed. • At times student appeared comfortable and at ease; but more practice is needed for behavior to become natural and consistent with a professional medical assistant.	15		
Always Exceeds Expectation	• Response was respectful and empathetic. Demonstrated active listening, professional nonverbal communication. No negative, unprofessional behaviors observed. • Student's behaviors appeared natural and comfortable. Behaviors are consistent with a professional medical assistant.	15		

Comments

CAAHEP Competencies	**Step(s)**
V.P.1. Respond to nonverbal communication	5
A.3. Demonstrate empathy for patients' concerns	8
A.4. Demonstrate active listening	6
A.5. Respect diversity	2
ABHES Competencies	**Step(s)**
5. Human Relations h. Display effective interpersonal skills with patients and healthcare team members	Entire role-play
i. Demonstrate cultural awareness.	Entire role-play
7. Administrative Procedures g. Display professionalism through written and verbal communications	Entire role-play

Work Product 2.2 History Form for Established Patient

Name ______________________________ **Date** ____________ **Score** __________

(To be used with Procedure 2.2)

<table>
<tr><td>MEDICAL HISTORY FORM</td><td colspan="2">DATE</td><td>MRN:</td></tr>
<tr><td>NAME</td><td>DOB</td><td colspan="2">AGE</td></tr>
<tr><td colspan="4"></td></tr>
<tr><td colspan="4">CHIEF
COMPLAINT</td></tr>
<tr><td colspan="4">HX OF
PRESENT
ILLNESS</td></tr>
<tr><td></td><td colspan="3"></td></tr>
<tr><td>ALLERGIES</td><td colspan="3">CURRENT MEDICATIONS</td></tr>
<tr><td>FEMALES:

PREGNANT YES NO

LMP: __________

Do you feel safe in your home?

YES NO</td><td colspan="3">UPDATED TO MEDICAL HISTORY SINCE LAST VISIT

NICOTINE / TOBACCO
USE: YES NO
PRODUCT:

AMOUNT DAILY:

NUMBER OF YEARS OF USE: :_______</td></tr>
</table>

Procedure 2.3 Demonstrate Respect for Individual Diversity: Religion and Appearance

Name ______________________ **Date** ____________ **Score** __________

Tasks: Respond to nonverbal communication. Communicate respectfully with patients with individual diversity related to religion and appearance. Demonstrate empathy, active listening, and nonverbal communication.

Background: The Sikh religion was founded in northern India. Sikhs believe in one god, the equality of males and females, justice, and community service. Turbans and kachera are worn at all times for religious reasons. Turbans or scarves cover the uncut hair. If the turban or scarf needs to be removed, an alternative head covering should be provided. A turban or scarf should be treated with respect. Placing it on the floor or near shoes would be a sign of disrespect. Kachera are undershorts/undergarments, and at least one leg is to remain in the kachera at all times.

Scenario: You are preparing a patient for an examination. The patient is Sikh. The provider always wants the patient to completely undress, wear a gown, and be seated on the exam table before she comes into the room. You are uncomfortable in this situation because you have never worked with a patient who is Sikh.

Directions: Role-play the scenario with a peer. Instruct the peer (patient) how to prepare for the examination.

Equipment and Supplies:
- Gown and drape sheet (optional)
- Exam table (optional)

Standard: Complete the procedure and all critical steps in _______ minutes with a minimum score of 85% within two attempts (*or as indicated by the instructor*).

Scoring: Divide the points earned by the total possible points. Failure to perform a critical step, indicated by an asterisk (*), results in grade no higher than an 84% (*or as indicated by the instructor*).

Time: Began_________ Ended_________ Total minutes: _________

Steps	Possible Points	Attempt 1	Attempt 2
1. Greet the patient. Identify yourself. Verify the patient's identity with full name and date of birth. Explain the procedure (undressing) in a manner that is understood by the patient. Answer any questions the patient may have on the procedure.	**20**		
2. Demonstrate respect for the patient. Be sincere, courteous, polite, and welcoming. Maintain the patient's dignity. Demonstrate professional, nonjudgmental verbal and nonverbal communication. *(Refer to the Affective Behaviors Checklist –* ***Respect*** *and the Grading Rubric)*	**15***		
3. Respond to the patient's nonverbal communication by using feedback techniques (e.g., reflection). If the patient's nonverbal communication is interpreted differently than the patient's oral statements, clarify the information with the patient.	**20***		

4. Use active listening skills. Remain neutral and refrain from interrupting. Smile and nod your head to show interest. Use appropriate eye contact. Focus on the patient and avoid distractions (e.g., looking at the clock, fidgeting). *(Refer to the Affective Behaviors Checklist – **Active Listening** and the Grading Rubric)*	**15***		
5. Use professional, positive nonverbal communication behaviors. Use a clear voice, with a moderate rate and volume. Use a varying pitch and an accepting or a neutral tone. Use words the patient can understand. Correctly pronounce the words. Be at the same eye level as the patient's. Smile and have a poised posture. Use light touch on the hand if appropriate. Maintain proper eye contact if culturally appropriate. *(Refer to the Affective Behaviors Checklist – **Nonverbal Communication** and the Grading Rubric)*	**15***		
6. Demonstrate empathy by listening to the patient and learning about their experiences and concerns. Use therapeutic communication techniques and positive nonverbal behaviors. Show your support and respect. *(Refer to the Affective Behaviors Checklist – **Empathy** and the Grading Rubric)*	**15***		
Total Score	**100**		

Affective Behavior	**Affective Behaviors Checklist** **Directions**: *Check behaviors observed during the role-play.*					
Respect	**Negative, Unprofessional Behaviors**	**Attempt 1**	**Attempt 2**	**Positive, Professional Behaviors**	**Attempt 1**	**Attempt 2**
	Rude, unkind, fake/false attitude, disrespectful, impolite, unwelcoming			Courteous, sincere, polite, welcoming		
	Unconcerned with person's dignity; brief, abrupt			Maintained person's dignity; took time with person		
	Unprofessional verbal communication; inappropriate questions			Professional verbal communication		
	Negative nonverbal behaviors, poor eye contact			Positive nonverbal behaviors, proper eye contact		
	Other:			Other:		
Active Listening	Biased, offensive			Remained neutral		
	Interrupted			Refrained from interrupting		
	Did not allow for silence or pauses			Allowed for periods of silence		
	Negative nonverbal behaviors (rolled eyes, yawned, frowned, avoided eye contact)			Positive nonverbal behaviors, smiled, nodded head, appropriate eye contact		
	Distracted (looked at watch, phone)			Focused on patient, avoided distractions		
	Other:			Other:		

Nonverbal Communication	Muffled voice; too fast or slow of rate; too loud or too soft; unaccepting tone			Clear voice with moderate rate and volume; varying pitch; accepting or neutral tone		
	Incorrectly pronounced words; used words the person did not understand (e.g., medical terminology, generational phrases)			Correctly pronounced words; used words person can understand		
	Stood while patient was sitting; slouching, lack of poised posture			Was at the same position of the patient; had a poised posture		
	Frowned. Lack of proper eye contact. Inappropriate touch.			Smiled. Maintained proper eye contact. Used light touch on hand when appropriate.		
	Other:			Other:		
Empathy	Did not listen to patient's responses			Listened to patient; learned about patient		
	Lack of respect and support demonstrated			Showed respect and support		
	Lack of therapeutic communication techniques used			Used therapeutic communication techniques		
	Negative nonverbal behaviors (e.g., positioning, frowning, poor eye contact)			Positive nonverbal behaviors (e.g., at the same level as patient, smiled, good eye contact)		
	Other:			Other:		

Grading Rubric for the Affective Behaviors Checklist **Directions**: *Based on checklist results, identify the points received for the procedure checklist. Indicate how the behaviors demonstrated met the expectations.*		**Points for Procedure Checklist**	**Attempt 1**	**Attempt 2**
Does not meet Expectation	• Response lacked respect, active listening, professional nonverbal communication, and/or empathy. • Student demonstrated more than 2 negative, unprofessional behaviors during the interaction.	0		
Needs Improvement	• Response lacked respect, active listening, professional nonverbal communication, and/or empathy. • Student demonstrated 1 or 2 negative, unprofessional behaviors during the interaction.	0		
Meets Expectation	• Response was respectful and empathetic. Demonstrated active listening, professional nonverbal communication. No negative, unprofessional behaviors observed. • More practice is needed for behavior to appear natural and for student to appear comfortable and at ease.	15		

Occasionally Exceeds Expectation	• Response was respectful and empathetic. Demonstrated active listening, professional nonverbal communication. No negative, unprofessional behaviors observed. • At times student appeared comfortable and at ease; but more practice is needed for behavior to become natural and consistent with a professional medical assistant.	15		
Always Exceeds Expectation	• Response was respectful and empathetic. Demonstrated active listening, professional nonverbal communication. No negative, unprofessional behaviors observed. • Student's behaviors appeared natural and comfortable. Behaviors are consistent with a professional medical assistant.	15		

Comments

CAAHEP Competencies	Step(s)
V.P.1. Respond to nonverbal communication	3
A.3. Demonstrate empathy for patients' concerns	6
A.4. Demonstrate active listening	4
A.5. Respect diversity	2
ABHES Competencies	**Step(s)**
5. Human Relations h. Display effective interpersonal skills with patients and healthcare team members	Entire role-play

Procedure 2.4 Use Feedback Techniques and Demonstrate Respect for Individual Diversity: Age, Economic Status, and Appearance

Name ______________________ **Date** __________ **Score** __________

Tasks: Use feedback techniques (e.g., reflection, restatement, and clarification) to obtain patient information. Respond to nonverbal communication. Communicate respectfully with patients with individual diversity related to age, economic status, and appearance. Demonstrate empathy, active listening, and nonverbal communication.

Scenario: You are rooming Mr. Abraham Black (79 years old), who has recently been diagnosed with dementia. He likes to talk about things that happened long before you were born, and you are not interested in those events. He also has a hard time hearing your questions, and you frequently repeat questions. Mr. Black has poor personal hygiene. His clothes are dirty and torn. He has an unpleasant body odor. Mr. Black tells you he cannot afford to eat if he buys his medications. He does not believe in government programs and refuses to take "handouts." You have worked with Mr. Black in the past and have heard this all before, numerous times. You would prefer to work with the younger generation and with patients who have better hygiene.

Directions: Using the scenario, role-play the rooming process with a peer (patient). Obtain the patient's chief complaint, allergies, and current medications. The patient should make up any information required.

Equipment and Supplies:
- Patient health record
- History form (optional) (Work Product 2.3)
- Pen

Standard: Complete the procedure and all critical steps in _______ minutes with a minimum score of 85% within two attempts (*or as indicated by the instructor*).

Scoring: Divide the points earned by the total possible points. Failure to perform a critical step, indicated by an asterisk (*), results in grade no higher than an 84% (*or as indicated by the instructor*).

Time: Began_________ Ended_________ Total minutes: _________

Steps	Possible Points	Attempt 1	Attempt 2
1. Greet the patient. Identify yourself. Verify the patient's identity with full name and date of birth. Explain the procedure in a manner that is understood by the patient. Answer any questions the patient may have on the procedure.	10		
2. Demonstrate respect for the patient. Be sincere, courteous, polite, and welcoming. Maintain the patient's dignity. Demonstrate professional, nonjudgmental verbal and nonverbal communication. Ask appropriate questions as information is obtained. *(Refer to the Affective Behaviors Checklist – **Respect** and the Grading Rubric)*	15*		
3. Using appropriate closed and open-ended questions and statements, obtain the patient's chief complaint (main reason for the visit) and history of present illness, allergies, pregnancy history, medical history, and current medications. Document the information in the health record or on the history form.	10		

4. Use feedback techniques including reflection, restatement, and clarification as information is obtained.	**10***		
5. Respond to the patient's nonverbal communication by using feedback techniques (e.g., reflection). If the patient's nonverbal communication is interpreted differently than the patient's oral statements, clarify the information with the patient.	**10***		
6. Use active listening skills. Remain neutral and refrain from interrupting. Allow for periods of silence. Smile and nod your head to show interest. Use appropriate eye contact. Focus on the patient and avoid distractions (e.g., looking at the clock, fidgeting). *(Refer to the Affective Behaviors Checklist – **Active Listening** and the Grading Rubric)*	**15***		
7. Use professional, positive nonverbal communication behaviors. (Use a clear voice, with a moderate rate and volume. Use a varying pitch and an accepting or neutral tone. Use words the patient can understand. Correctly pronounce the words. Be at the same eye level as the patient's. Smile and have a poised posture. Use light touch on the hand if appropriate. Maintain proper eye contact if culturally appropriate. *(Refer to the Affective Behaviors Checklist – **Nonverbal Communication** and the Grading Rubric)*	**15***		
8. Demonstrate empathy by listening to the patient and learning about their experiences and concerns. Use therapeutic communication techniques and positive nonverbal behaviors. Show your support and respect. *(Refer to the Affective Behaviors Checklist – **Empathy** and the Grading Rubric)*	**15***		
Total Score	**100**		

Affective Behavior	**Affective Behaviors Checklist** **Directions:** *Check behaviors observed during the role-play.*					
Respect	**Negative, Unprofessional Behaviors**	**Attempt**		**Positive, Professional Behaviors**	**Attempt**	
		1	**2**		**1**	**2**
	Rude, unkind, fake/false attitude, disrespectful, impolite, unwelcoming			Courteous, sincere, polite, welcoming		
	Unconcerned with person's dignity; brief, abrupt			Maintained person's dignity; took time with person		
	Unprofessional verbal communication; inappropriate questions			Professional verbal communication		
	Negative nonverbal behaviors, poor eye contact			Positive nonverbal behaviors, proper eye contact		
	Other:			Other:		

Active Listening	Biased, offensive			Remained neutral		
	Interrupted			Refrained from interrupting		
	Did not allow for silence or pauses			Allowed for periods of silence		
	Negative nonverbal behaviors (rolled eyes, yawned, frowned, avoided eye contact)			Positive nonverbal behaviors (smiled, nodded head, appropriate eye contact)		
	Distracted (looked at watch, phone)			Focused on patient, avoided distractions		
	Other:			Other:		
Nonverbal Communication	Muffled voice; too fast or slow of rate; too loud or too soft; unaccepting tone			Clear voice with moderate rate and volume; varying pitch; accepting or neutral tone		
	Incorrectly pronounced words; used words the person did not understand (e.g., medical terminology, generational phrases)			Correctly pronounced words; used words person can understand		
	Stood while patient was sitting; slouching, lack of poised posture			Was at the same position of the patient; had a poised posture		
	Frowned. Lack of proper eye contact. Inappropriate touch.			Smiled. Maintained proper eye contact. Used light touch on hand when appropriate.		
	Other:			Other:		
Empathy	Did not listen to patient's responses			Listened to patient; learned about patient		
	Lack of respect and support demonstrated			Showed respect and support		
	Lack of therapeutic communication techniques used			Used therapeutic communication techniques		
	Negative nonverbal behaviors (e.g., positioning, frowning, poor eye contact)			Positive nonverbal behaviors (e.g., at the same level as patient, smiled, good eye contact)		
	Other:			Other:		

Grading Rubric for the Affective Behaviors Checklist **Directions:** *Based on checklist results, identify the points received for the procedure checklist. Indicate how the behaviors demonstrated met the expectations.*		**Points for Procedure Checklist**	**Attempt 1**	**Attempt 2**
Does not meet Expectation	• Response lacked respect, active listening, professional nonverbal communication, and/or empathy. • Student demonstrated more than 2 negative, unprofessional behaviors during the interaction.	0		
Needs Improvement	• Response lacked respect, active listening, professional nonverbal communication, and/or empathy. • Student demonstrated 1 or 2 negative, unprofessional behaviors during the interaction.	0		
Meets Expectation	• Response was respectful and empathetic. Demonstrated active listening, professional nonverbal communication. No negative, unprofessional behaviors observed. • More practice is needed for behavior to appear natural and for student to appear comfortable and at ease.	15		
Occasionally Exceeds Expectation	• Response was respectful and empathetic. Demonstrated active listening, professional nonverbal communication. No negative, unprofessional behaviors observed. • At times student appeared comfortable and at ease; but more practice is needed for behavior to become natural and consistent with a professional medical assistant.	15		
Always Exceeds Expectation	• Response was respectful and empathetic. Demonstrated active listening, professional nonverbal communication. No negative, unprofessional behaviors observed. • Student's behaviors appeared natural and comfortable. Behaviors are consistent with a professional medical assistant.	15		

Comments

CAAHEP Competencies	**Step(s)**
V.P.1. Respond to nonverbal communication	5
A.3. Demonstrate empathy for patients' concerns	8
A.4. Demonstrate: active listening	6
A.5. Respect diversity	2
ABHES Competencies	**Step(s)**
5. Human Relations h. Display effective interpersonal skills with patients and healthcare team members	Entire role-play
7. Administrative Procedures g. Display professionalism through written and verbal communications	Entire role-play

Work Product 2.3 History Form for Established Patient

Name ______________________ **Date** __________ **Score** __________

(To be used with Procedure 2.4)

<table>
<tr><td>MEDICAL HISTORY FORM</td><td colspan="2">DATE</td><td>MRN:</td></tr>
<tr><td>NAME</td><td>DOB</td><td colspan="2">AGE</td></tr>
<tr><td colspan="4"></td></tr>
<tr><td colspan="4">CHIEF
COMPLAINT</td></tr>
<tr><td colspan="4">HX OF
PRESENT
ILLNESS</td></tr>
<tr><td></td><td colspan="3"></td></tr>
<tr><td>ALLERGIES</td><td colspan="3">CURRENT MEDICATIONS</td></tr>
<tr><td>FEMALES:
PREGNANT YES NO
LMP: __________</td><td colspan="3">UPDATED TO MEDICAL HISTORY SINCE LAST VISIT</td></tr>
<tr><td>Do you feel safe in your home?
YES NO</td><td colspan="3">NICOTINE / TOBACCO
USE: YES NO
PRODUCT:
AMOUNT DAILY:
NUMBER OF YEARS OF USE: :_______</td></tr>
</table>

Procedure 2.5 Demonstrate Appropriate Self-Boundaries

Name ______________________________ **Date** ____________ **Score** __________

Task: Use respectful and tactful communication while demonstrating the principles of self-boundaries.

Background: For the medical assistant to have a professional therapeutic relationship with a patient, the medical assistant must guard against crossing self-boundaries, which are also called *professional boundaries*. The relationship between the medical assistant and the patient needs to be professional. It cannot be a dual relationship, where the medical assistant also becomes a friend to the patient. This means the medical assistant cannot share personal intimate information, contact the patient outside of the work environment, befriend the patient on social media, or engage in a flirty or romantic relationship with the patient.

Scenario #1: You are rooming Morgan, who frequently sees the provider you work for. You have gotten to know Morgan over the time you have worked for the provider. Today, Morgan asks you for your personal phone number and social media information.

Scenario #2: You are rooming Sam, whom you have gotten to know well over the time you have worked for your provider. Sam is outgoing, enjoys talking, and has many of the same interests as you do. You have just split up with your significant other and have been feeling a bit down. Sam asks you if you would be available for coffee sometime.

Directions: Role-play the scenarios with a peer. Your peer will play the patient in the scenario and you are the medical assistant.

Standard: Complete the role-play in _______ minutes with a minimum score of 100% within two attempts (*or as indicated by the instructor*).

Scoring: Divide the points earned by the total possible points. Met competency: 100% (10 points). Not met competency: 0% (0 points).

Time: Began_________ Ended_________ Total minutes: _________

<table>
<tr><th>Affective Behavior</th><th colspan="6">Affective Behaviors Checklist
Directions: Check behaviors observed during the role-play.</th></tr>
<tr><td rowspan="7">Respect</td><td rowspan="2">Negative, Unprofessional Behaviors</td><td colspan="2">Attempt</td><td rowspan="2">Positive, Professional Behaviors</td><td colspan="2">Attempt</td></tr>
<tr><td>1</td><td>2</td><td>1</td><td>2</td></tr>
<tr><td>Rude, unkind, disrespectful, and/or impolite</td><td></td><td></td><td>Courteous and polite</td><td></td><td></td></tr>
<tr><td>Unconcerned with person’s dignity</td><td></td><td></td><td>Maintained person’s dignity</td><td></td><td></td></tr>
<tr><td>Poor eye contact</td><td></td><td></td><td>Proper eye contact</td><td></td><td></td></tr>
<tr><td>Negative nonverbal behaviors</td><td></td><td></td><td>Positive nonverbal behaviors</td><td></td><td></td></tr>
<tr><td>Other:</td><td></td><td></td><td>Other:</td><td></td><td></td></tr>
</table>

Tactful	Improper and/or inappropriate.			Proper and appropriate.		
	Spoke and/or acted in a manner that was offensive to others.			Spoke and acted without offending others.		
	Failed to address the self-boundaries/professional boundary issue or followed through on what the patient wanted.			Addressed the self-boundaries/professional boundary issue in a clear and diplomatic way.		
	Failed to show awareness of the patient's personal space; was too close to the patient during the interaction.			Showed awareness of the patient's personal space and maintained a comfortable distance.		
	Lacked courtesy; demonstrated unprofessional behaviors (verbal or nonverbal) during a difficult situation.			Showed courtesy and professionalism in a difficult situation.		
	Other:			Other:		

Grading Rubric for the Affective Behaviors Checklist **Directions:** *Based on checklist results, identify the points received for the procedure checklist. Indicate how the behaviors demonstrated met the expectations.*		**Point Value**	**Attempt 1**	**Attempt 2**
Does Not Meet Expectation	• Response was disrespectful and/or not tactful. • Student demonstrated more than two negative, unprofessional behaviors during the interaction.	0		
Needs Improvement	• Response was disrespectful and/or not tactful. • Student demonstrated one or two negative, unprofessional behaviors during the interaction.	0		
Meets Expectation	• Response was respectful and tactful; no negative, unprofessional behaviors observed. • More practice is needed for behavior to appear natural and for student to appear comfortable and at ease.	10		
Occasionally Exceeds Expectation	• Response was respectful and tactful; no negative, unprofessional behaviors observed. • At times student appeared comfortable and at ease; but more practice is needed for behavior to become natural and consistent with a professional medical assistant.	10		
Always Exceeds Expectation	• Response was respectful and tactful; no negative, unprofessional behaviors observed. • Student's behaviors appeared natural and comfortable. Behaviors are consistent with a professional medical assistant.	10		

Comments

CAAHEP Competencies	Step(s)
A.6 Recognize personal boundaries	Entire role-play
ABHES Competencies	**Step(s)**
5. Human Relations h. Display effective interpersonal skills with patients and healthcare team members	Entire role-play

Student Name______________________________ Date______________

Legal Principles

chapter **3**

CAAHEP Competencies	Assessment
X.C.1. Identify scope of practice and standards of care for medical assistants.	Skills and Concepts – K. 16-17
X.C.2. Identify the provider role in terms of standard of care.	Skills and Concepts – C. 18
X.C.4. Identify the standards outlined in The Patient Care Partnership	Skills and Concepts – J. 2-4
X.C.5. Identify licensure and certification as they apply to healthcare providers	Skills and Concepts – K. 1-7
X.C.6. Identify criminal and civil law as they apply to the practicing medical assistant	Skills and Concepts – B. 9
X.C.7.a. Define: negligence	Skills and Concepts – C. 8
X.C.7.b. Define: malpractice	Skills and Concepts – C. 11
X.C.7.c. Define: statute of limitations	Skills and Concepts – D. 4; Certification Preparation – 2
X.C.8. Identify the purpose of medical malpractice insurance.	Skills and Concepts – F. 1
X.C.13.a. Define the following medical legal terms: informed consent	Skills and Concepts – I. 1
X.C.13.b. Define the following medical legal terms: implied consent	Skills and Concepts – I. 5; Certification Preparation – 10
X.C.13.c. Define the following medical legal terms: expressed consent	Skills and Concepts – I. 2; Certification Preparation – 10
X.C.13.d. Define the following medical legal terms: patient incompetence	Skills and Concepts – G. 12
X.C.13.e. Define the following medical legal terms: emancipated minor	Skills and Concepts – G. 14
X.C.13.f. Define the following medical legal terms: mature minor	Skills and Concepts – I. 3; Certification Preparation – 8
X.C.13.g. Define the following medical legal terms: subpoena duces tecum	Skills and Concepts – E. 16; Certification Preparation – 6

CAAHEP Competencies	Assessment
X.C.13.h. Define the following medical legal terms: respondeat superior	Skills and Concepts - H. 4; Certification Preparation – 9
X.C.13.i. Define the following medical legal terms: res ipsa loquitur	Skills and Concepts – E. 5
X.C.13.j. Define the following medical legal terms: locum tenens	Skills and Concepts – K. 13; Certification Preparation – 7
X.C.13.k. Define the following medical legal terms: defendant-plaintiff	Skills and Concepts - B. 2, 3
X.C.13.l. Define the following medical legal terms: deposition	Skills and Concepts – E. 13
X.C.13.m. Define the following medical legal terms: arbitration-mediation	Skills and Concepts – E. 6, 8; Certification Preparation – 1
X.P.1. Locate a state's legal scope of practice for medical assistants	Procedure 3.2

ABHES Competencies	Assessment
4. Medical Law and Ethics c. Follow established policies when initiating or terminating medical treatment	Skills and Concepts – H. 1-2e
4.d. Distinguish between employer and personal liability coverage	Skills and Concepts – F. 2-6
4.f. Comply with federal, state, and local health laws and regulations 1) Define the scope of practice for the medical assistant within the state where employed	Procedure 3.2
4.f.2) Describe what procedures can and cannot be delegated to the medical assistant and by whom within various employment settings	Skills and Concepts – K. 18a-f

VOCABULARY REVIEW

Using the word pool on the right, find the correct word to match the definition. Write the word on the line after the definition.

Group A

1. Prone to lawsuits ______________________
2. A bill that has passed becomes this; also found in the name of a specific law ______________________
3. A rule of conduct or action prescribed or formally recognized as enforceable by a controlling authority ______________________
4. Used more to refer to the contents of the actual law ______________________
5. A piece of legislation passed by a municipality or local government ______________________
6. A prior court decision that serves as a model for similar legal cases in the future ______________________

Word Pool

- act
- case law
- common law
- constitutional law
- law
- litigious
- ordinance
- precedent
- statute
- statutory law

7. Derived from legal precedents and common law ______________________
8. Derived from the federal and state constitutions, which give power to federal and state governments ______________________
9. Unwritten laws that come from judicial decisions based on societal traditions and customs ______________________
10. Refers to the laws enacted by state and federal legislatures ______________________

Group B

1. Legally responsible or obligated ______________________
2. A strategy used by the defendant to avoid liability in a lawsuit ______________________
3. Lack of actions ______________________
4. Statutes that define actions or omissions (lack of actions) that threaten and/or harm public safety and welfare ______________________
5. Actions or omissions that are prohibited by criminal laws (and the government) ______________________
6. Protect and define private rights ______________________
7. A civil wrongdoing that causes harm to a person or property, excludes breach of contract ______________________
8. The individual or entity who committed the tort, either intentionally or as a result of negligence ______________________
9. Laws related to procedures, regulations, and rules of governmental administrative agencies ______________________
10. A monetary settlement the defendant pays the plaintiff in a civil case for loss or injury ______________________

Word Pool

- civil laws
- crimes
- criminal law
- damages
- defense
- liable
- omissions
- regulatory and administrative law
- tort
- tortfeasor

Group C

1. A court order by which an individual or institution is required to perform or refrain from performing a certain act ______________________
2. A settlement for a specific dollar amount that directly relates to medical bills ______________________
3. A court judgment that defines the legal rights of the parties involved ______________________
4. The process of settling disputes outside of litigation ______________________
5. A legal obligation ______________________
6. The person or company purchasing the insurance policy ______________________

Word Pool

- alternative dispute resolution
- declaratory judgment
- injunction
- insured
- insurer
- legally binding
- nominal damages
- premium
- special damages
- third party

7. Very small settlement because the plaintiff's injury was slight ______________________
8. The payment the insured pays to the insurance company ______________________
9. Another name for the insurance company ______________________
10. When the insurer pays the plaintiff, the plaintiff is known as the ______________________

Group D

1. One party voluntarily agrees with another party's proposition or plan ______________________
2. An agreement between two parties ______________________
3. Person voluntarily gives up license ______________________
4. License is terminated and the person can no longer practice in that occupation in the state ______________________
5. Person's license is monitored for a specific period of time ______________________
6. Person cannot practice in that occupation for a specific period of time ______________________
7. Person is sent a warning or letter of concern ______________________

Word Pool

- contract
- consent
- license revoked
- license surrendered
- license suspended
- probation
- reprimand

ABBREVIATIONS

Write out what each of the following abbreviations stands for.

1. DOB ______________________
2. VIS ______________________
3. CMA ______________________
4. LPN ______________________
5. NP ______________________
6. CNM ______________________
7. RN ______________________
8. PA ______________________
9. MD ______________________
10. DO ______________________
11. OWI ______________________
12. OUI ______________________

13. ADR ______________________________

14. CDC______________________________

15. CAAHEP ______________________________

SKILLS AND CONCEPTS

Answer the following questions. Write your answer on the line or in the space provided.

A. Sources of Law

1. A(n) ____________________ is a rule of conduct or action prescribed or formally recognized as enforceable by a controlling authority.

2. The ____________________ is the supreme law of the United States.

3. The ____________________ branch includes the Supreme Court and interprets laws according to the U.S. Constitution.

4. The ____________________ branch includes Congress and makes new laws.

5. The president administers the ____________________ branch and issues executive orders, appoints judges, and makes treaties with other nations.

6. Case law was derived from legal ____________________ and ____________________.

B. Criminal and Civil Law

1. ____________________ law determines the rights and obligations of the people and ____________________ laws must be followed when investigating and prosecuting unlawful acts.

2. ____________________ is an individual or party who brings the suit to court.

3. ____________________ is an individual or business against whom a lawsuit is filed

4. In criminal law, the wrongdoing is called a(n) ____________________ and in civil law it can be called a(n) ____________________ or a(n) ____________________.

5. A(n) ____________________, a serious criminal offense, is punishable by a substantial fine and ____________________ time ____________________ 1 year.

6. A(n) ____________________, a lesser criminal offense, is punishable by a substantial fine and possible ____________________ time ____________________ 1 year.

7. Contract issues, divorce, child custody, product liability, and accidents are common types of disputes handled in the ____________________ court system.

8. If the matter is brought to court, in the ____________________ court system, most of the time there is a trial by jury; whereas with the ____________________ court system, cases are decided by the judge and many times there is no jury.

9. Describe criminal and civil law as they apply to the practicing medical assistant. Your answer should also provide an example of a criminal and civil matter that relates to medical assistants. (Provide examples other than those in the textbook.)

____

____

____

____

____

C. Tort Law

1. With ______________________ torts, the plaintiff must prove the defendant had specific intent to perform the action that caused the injury and ______________________ or ______________________ torts result when a person's conduct falls below the standard of behavior expected of a reasonable person in the same situation.

Define the following terms by matching the definition with the term.

2. _____ Disclosing private facts without the consent of the individual or intrusion into a person's personal life
3. _____ The intentional restraint of another individual without consent or reason
4. _____ Deceiving or lying to a person or party for monetary gain
5. _____ Intentionally saying something or writing something false about another person that causes harm
6. _____ Written defamation
7. _____ Spoken defamation
8. _____ Failure to act as a reasonably prudent person would under similar circumstances; such conduct falls below the standards of behavior established by law for the protection of others against unreasonable risk of harm
9. _____ Uses reasonable behavior as an objective test to measure another's actions or lack of actions
10. _____ Refers to the level and type of care an ordinary, prudent healthcare professional, having the same training and experience in a similar practice, would have provided under a similar situation.
11. _____ A type of negligence in which a licensed professional fails to provide the standard of care, causing harm to a person
12. _____ Failure to act when one had a legal duty to act
13. _____ Performance of an unlawful, wrongful act
14. _____ Improper performance of a lawful act that causes damage or injury
15. _____ Range of responsibilities and practice guidelines that determine the boundaries within which a healthcare worker practices

a. fraud
b. defamation
c. false imprisonment
d. slander
e. scope of practice
f. invasion of privacy
g. unintentional torts
h. malfeasance
i. nonfeasance
j. misfeasance
k. reasonable person standard
l. malpractice
m. standard of care
n. libel

Answer the following questions.

16. Explain the "reasonable person" standard and how it can determine negligent acts.__________________

____

____

17. How does medical malpractice differ from negligence?____________________________________

____

____

18. Discuss the provider's role in terms of standard of care. ____________________________________

____

____

____

D. Defenses to Liability

1. Which of the following is a type of defense?
   a. Technical
   b. Denial
   c. Affirmative
   d. All of the above

2. Which is a requirement for Good Samaritan Law protection?
   a. A person must provide treatment in a true emergency.
   b. Care must be provided outside of a place with necessary medical equipment.
   c. The provider cannot bill the patient for the care provided.
   d. All of the above

Define the following terms by matching the definition with the term.

3. _____ Latin for "a thing decided;" once a case has been decided by the court, it cannot be litigated again
4. _____ The length of time legal action can be taken after an event has occurred
5. _____ Used when none of the facts are true
6. _____ The defendant can show evidence that the plaintiff knew about the risks involved and consented to proceed with the activity
7. _____ The defendant admits to wrongdoing, but their attorney introduces facts that support the defendant's conduct
8. _____ The plaintiff's action or lack of action caused the injury to a certain percent

a. assumption of risk
b. affirmative defense
c. comparative negligence
d. denial defense
e. *res judicata*
f. statute of limitations

E. Resolving a Civil Lawsuit

Define the following terms by matching the definition with the term.

1. _____ The healthcare professional has a legal obligation to the patient.
2. _____ The breach of duty of care directly causes the patient's injury.
3. _____ A monetary settlement the defendant pays the plaintiff in a civil case for loss or injury. Also, one of the 4 Ds of negligence, meaning the patient suffers a legally recognized injury.
4. _____ The healthcare professional breaches (violates) the duty of care to the patient.
5. _____ A Latin term meaning "the thing speaks for itself." A legal concept under which the plaintiff's burden to prove malpractice is minimal since the jury can clearly understand the details of the injury.
6. _____ The process in which conflicting parties in a dispute submit their differences to a court-appointed person, who submits a legally binding decision.
7. _____ Monetary payment to the plaintiff for losses suffered.
8. _____ The process of facilitating conflicting parties to make an agreement, settlement, or compromise.
9. _____ A person who observed the situation and testifies in court about the facts of the case.
10. _____ Large payments made to the plaintiff by the defendant as ordered by the court and meant to punish the defendant.
11. _____ Monetary payments to the plaintiff for emotional pain and anguish.
12. _____ A person who is educated and knowledgeable in the area of concern and provides their opinion in court.
13. _____ A sworn testimony made before a court-appointed officer; it is used in the discovery process and may be used in the trial.
14. _____ Written or oral questions that must be answered under oath.
15. _____ A court order requiring a person to appear in court at a specific time to testify in a legal case.
16. _____ A legal document commanding a person to bring a piece of evidence (e.g., the plaintiff's health record) to court.

a. dereliction
b. arbitration
c. expert witness
d. fact witness
e. damages
f. *res ipsa loquitur*
g. direct cause
h. duty of care
i. mediation
j. punitive damages
k. compensatory damages
l. general damages
m. interrogatory
n. *subpoena duces tecum*
o. subpoena
p. deposition

F. Professional Liability Insurance

1. Describe the purpose of medical malpractice insurance. ______________________________

____

____

____

____

____

Match the description with the insurance-related term.

2. _____ A type of liability coverage used by professionals to protect themselves against liability suits incurred because of errors and omissions while performing their professional services
3. _____ A type of liability coverage that protects against claims related to harm other than bodily injury
4. _____ A type of liability coverage purchased by companies. It protects businesses from lawsuits for property loss and bodily injury from nonemployees
5. _____ An insurance policy that covers claims made during the policy year
6. _____ An insurance policy that covers claims for wrongful acts that occurred during the policy year

a. general liability insurance
b. occurrence policy
c. personal injury insurance
d. professional liability insurance
e. claims-made policy

G. Contracts

Match the description with the element required for a legally binding contract.

1. _____ The second party agrees to the offer.
2. _____ A person entering a contract must have legal capacity.
3. _____ The consideration must be legal.
4. _____ Made by one party.
5. _____ Each party exchanges something of value.

a. offer
b. consideration
c. competency and capacity
d. legal subject matter
e. acceptance

Select the correct answer.

6. What is a condition related to competency and capacity that would invalidate a contract?
   a. Underage (minor)
   b. Incompetence
   c. Intoxicated or under the influence of drugs
   d. All of the above

7. Which of the following activities can an emancipated minor *not* do?
   a. Be a party in a contract and sue
   b. Vote and buy alcohol
   c. Keep earned income and apply for public benefits
   d. Make all of their own healthcare decisions

Define the following terms by matching the definition with the term.

8. _____ A common law concept that requires specific types of contracts must be in writing to avoid fraud and to be binding.
9. _____ The parties have agreed to the terms of the contract through their actions and behaviors.
10. _____ One who has not reached adulthood.
11. _____ The parties have specifically stated the terms of the contract in writing, orally, or both.
12. _____ A patient who lacks the ability to manage personal affairs due to mental deficiency; an appointed guardian or conservator manages the patient's affairs.
13. _____ Occurs when the terms of the contract are not fulfilled by one party without a legitimate legal reason.
14. _____ A minor who has been granted emancipation by the court; the minor can assume the rights and responsibilities of adulthood.

a. breach of contract
b. implied contract
c. expressed contract
d. patient incompetence
e. emancipated minor
f. statute of frauds
g. minor

H. Provider-Patient Relationship

1. Which is a reason providers terminate the provider-patient relationship?
   a. Retirement or moving
   b. Patient isn't paying for the services provided
   c. Due to patient's behavior or if the patient isn't following the provider's treatment plan
   d. All of the above

2 Complete the description of the termination process for the provider-patient relationship. Write the word or phrase on the line.

   a. _______________ must notify the patient in writing of the withdrawal of care.

   b. A(n) _______________ must be indicated for the termination and there must be an adequate period of coverage to allow the patient to find another provider.

   c. The termination letter should be sent as a(n) _______________ with return receipt requested.

   d. A(n) _______________ and the return receipt need to be placed or scanned into the patient's health record.

   e. _______________ should be notified of the termination date so no appointments are made after that date.

3. Providers can be charged with ______________________ if they do not follow the proper termination procedure.

4. ______________________ is a common law doctrine that means "let the master answer" and means that the employer/provider is liable for actions that the employee did or did not do within the scope of employment.

5. How can a medical assistant protect the provider from charges of patient abandonment? _______________

____

____

I. Consents

Define the following terms by matching the definition with the term.

1. _____ A legal process that ensures the patient or guardian understands the treatment and gives consent for the treatment
2. _____ Consent that is given either by the spoken or written word
3. _____ A person under the age of adulthood who demonstrates the maturity to make a personal healthcare decision and can give informed consent for treatment
4. _____ One party voluntarily agrees with another party's proposition or plan
5. _____ Consent that is inferred based on signs, actions, or conduct of the patient rather than oral communication

a. informed consent
b. implied consent
c. expressed consent
d. consent
e. mature minor

Select the correct answer.

6. The elements that must be present for informed consent include that the patient or guardian
   a. is competent to understand and decide and voluntarily decides to agree to or refuse the treatment.
   b. understands the diagnosis, reason for treatment, proposed treatment, and the risks of the treatment.
   c. understands the alternative treatments available, the risks of the treatments, and the risks if treatment is delayed or not done.
   d. signs a treatment consent form.
   e. All of the above

7. Who can give informed consent?
   a. Adults with sound mind
   b. Married minors and minor parents
   c. Emancipated minors and mature minors
   d. All of the above

8. Who *cannot* give informed consent?
   a. Patients under the influence of alcohol or drugs
   b. A minor
   c. A patient who is mentally incompetent
   d. A patient who speaks little to no English and no interpreter service was provided
   e. All of the above

9. What is the medical assistant's role with informed consent?
   a. Prepare the informed consent form.
   b. Educate the patient on the procedure.
   c. Educate the patient on alternative procedures.
   d. All of the above

J. Patient's Rights and Responsibilities

1. The Affordable Care Act's Patient's Bill of Rights focuses on rights related to ______________________.
2. The ______________________ document helps patients understand the expectations for patients and the patients' rights and responsibilities.
3. The Patient Care Partnership document replaces the ______________________, though it covers the same topics.

4. Which topic(s) is/are included in the Patient's Bill of Rights and the Patient Care Partnership document?
   a. The patient's rights related to medical care, respectful treatment, privacy and confidentiality, identity, explanation of care, informed consent, research projects, and safe environment
   b. The patient's rights to be informed of the facility's conduct rules and regulations
   c. The patient's responsibilities (e.g., providing information, respect and consideration, compliance with medical care, medical records, responsibilities based on the clinic's rules and regulations, and reporting of patient complaints)
   d. All of the above

5. A patient refuses an injection of medication ordered by the provider. Describe the steps that need to be followed by the medical assistant.

____

____

____

____

K. Practice Requirements

Match the licensure and certification for the following healthcare professionals. Answers may be used more than once.

1. _____ Doctor of medicine (MD)
2. _____ Physician assistant (PA)
3. _____ Doctor of osteopathy (DO)
4. _____ Nurse practitioner (NP)
5. _____ Registered nurse (RN)
6. _____ Medical assistant (MA)
7. _____ Licensed practical nurse (LPN)

a. Must pass a licensure exam to practice.
b. National certification exam is optional.
c. Obtains the certification after passing the national exam. Must obtain a state license to practice.
d. Must pass all three parts of the U.S. Medical Licensing Exam and obtain a state license to practice.

Define the following terms by matching the definition with the term.

8. _____ The state's laws and regulations that govern the practice of medicine
9. _____ A voluntary process indicating that a person has met predetermined criteria
10. _____ A state board grants a license to a person who is currently licensed in another state that has the same or stricter standards
11. _____ A state has a written agreement with another state to recognize licenses issued by that state without additional review of the person's credentials
12. _____ People working in a specific occupation have their name entered into an official registry

a. reciprocity
b. Medical Practice Act
c. endorsement
d. *locum tenens*
e. telemedicine
f. certification
g. registration
h. licensure

13. _____ Latin for "to substitute for;" the term refers to physicians or advanced-practice professionals who temporarily contract to provide healthcare services when a facility has a vacancy, vacation, or a leave of absence.
14. _____ A mandatory process established by state law that ensures a person has met the legal standards for practicing an occupation in that state.
15. _____ The use of telecommunication technology to provide healthcare services to patients at a distance; it is usually used in rural communities.

Answer the following questions.

16. Describe the scope of practice for medical assistants. ____

____

____

____

17. Describe the standard of care for medical assistants. ____

____

____

____

18. For the following activities, identify if the medical assistant could be delegated (assigned) by the provider to do the activity. Write "yes" on the line if the medical assistant could be delegated the activity. Write "no" on the line if the medical assistant could not do the activity.
    a. Prepare the informed consent paperwork. _________
    b. Discuss the procedure with the patient for the informed consent. _________
    c. Prepare waived laboratory testing. _________
    d. Answer phone calls. _________
    e. Prescribe medications for the patient's condition. _________
    f. Diagnose the patient's condition. _________

L. Accreditation

1. ______________________ is a recognition granted by a specific organization to educational, healthcare, or managed care organizations that have demonstrated compliance with standards.

Match the organization with its role.

2. _____ Accredits ambulatory care facilities, hospitals, behavioral healthcare facilities, home healthcare agencies, and laboratory services
3. _____ Accredits medical laboratories
4. _____ Accredits health plans

a. National Committee for Quality Assurance
b. The Joint Commission
c. College of American Pathologists Laboratory Accreditation Program

CERTIFICATION PREPARATION

Circle the correct answer.

1. Which is a type of alternative dispute resolution where the final decision is legally binding?
   a. Dereliction
   b. Mediation
   c. Arbitration
   d. Summary judgment

2. Which varies by state and indicates the length of time legal action can be taken after an event has occurred?
   a. *Res judicata*
   b. *Res ipsa loquitur*
   c. Release of tortfeasor
   d. Statute of limitations

3. Which is a negligent act classification that means the person failed to act when he or she had a legal duty to act?
   a. Misfeasance
   b. Nonfeasance
   c. Malpractice
   d. Malfeasance

4. Which type of defense involves the defendant admitting wrongdoing and the defense attorney introduces facts that support the defendant's conduct?
   a. Denial defense
   b. Comparative defense
   c. Technical defense
   d. Affirmative defense

5. Which is not one of the "Ds" of negligence?
   a. Duty of care
   b. Dereliction
   c. Deposition
   d. Damages

6. Which is a legal document ordering a person to bring the plaintiff's health record to court?
   a. Subpoena
   b. *Subpoena duces tecum*
   c. *Res ipsa loquitur*
   d. Statute of limitations

7. Which is a physician or advanced-practice professional temporarily contracted to provide healthcare services when a facility has a vacancy, vacation, or a leave of absence?
   a. Telemedicine
   b. Injunction
   c. *Respondeat superior*
   d. *Locum tenens*

8. A person younger than the age of adulthood who demonstrates the maturity to make a personal healthcare decision and can give informed consent for treatment is called a(n)
   a. mature minor.
   b. emancipated minor.
   c. incompetence.
   d. *respondeat superior*.

9. Which means "let the master answer;" thus, the employer/provider is legally responsible for the wrongful actions or lack of actions of the employees if done within the scope of employment?
   a. Tortfeasor
   b. *Res ipsa loquitur*
   c. *Respondeat superior*
   d. *Res judicata*

10. ______ consent is inferred based on signs or conduct of the patient, whereas ______ consent is given either by the spoken or written word.
    a. Implied; informed
    b. Informed; expressed
    c. Implied; expressed
    d. Expressed; informed

WORKPLACE APPLICATIONS

1. Cara has just graduated from a medical assistant program and decides to take out a professional liability insurance policy. She wants a policy that she can stop paying at retirement and will still be covered for past situations. Describe what type of policy she should purchase.

2. Dr. Smith and Dr. Brown are family practice providers who trained at the same college. Dr. Smith practices in Los Angeles, CA and Dr. Brown practices in Bayfield, WI (a city of fewer than 600 people). Would the standard of care be the same for these two family practice providers? Explain your answer.

3. Jane is a medical assistant who works with Dr. Walden. She identifies herself as "Dr. Walden's nurse" to patients. Discuss how this might impact the standard of care.

4. Ken Thomas was notified by a medical supplier that the mesh that was used for his hernia surgery was faulty. They paid Ken a monetary compensation after Ken signed a release to give up the right to sue the company in the future. Five years later, Ken had to go through surgery to remove the mesh. Ken wanted to sue the company for his pain and suffering. What technical defense would be used to prevent the lawsuit? Discuss this technical defense.

5. Bella, a new CMA, is working with a patient who is undergoing minor surgery. The provider explained the procedure and stepped out of the room. She needs to get the informed consent form signed. When she asks the patient if she has any questions before signing, the patient states she does. How should Bella handle this situation?

INTERNET ACTIVITIES

1. Using the internet, find a local healthcare facility that has their Patient's Bill of Rights posted online. Create a poster presentation or a PowerPoint presentation summarizing the areas addressed in the facility's Patient's Bill of Rights.

2. Using online resources, research how an MD and / or DO can renew their license in your state. Write a brief summary of what is required to renew a medical doctor's license in your state. Cite the website(s) used.

3. Credentialed medical assistants need to maintain their credentials through continuing education. Using online resources, identify two sites that offer continuing education for medical assistants. Briefly summarize your findings and cite the websites used.

Procedure 3.1 Apply the Patient's Bill of Rights

Name ______________________________ **Date** __________ **Score** __________

Tasks: Apply the Patient's Bill of Rights in scenarios related to choice of treatment, consent for treatment, and refusal of treatment. Demonstrate sensitivity to the patients' rights.

Scenario 1 (Choice of treatment): Julia Berkley (DOB 07/05/19XX) saw Dr. Angela Perez during her entire pregnancy. Julia is experiencing some complications. Dr. Perez explained the choices Julia had for delivery. She stated that with the complications, a cesarean delivery (C-section) may be the best option. Because you are working with Dr. Perez, you prepare the consent form for the C-section. You go into the exam room to have Julia sign the consent form. As you discuss the form, Julia tells you that she is fearful of a C-section and wants a vaginal delivery.

Scenario 2 (Consent for treatment): Ken Thomas (DOB 10/25/19XX) sees Jean Burke, NP, before leaving on a week-long trip out of the country. He is leaving in 3 days and wants a hepatitis A vaccine injection. The area he is traveling to has a high risk for hepatitis A. Jean Burke orders immunoglobulin for Ken, which will provide immediate protection against hepatitis A. You prepare the injection and enter the exam room. As you are telling Ken about the side effects of the medication, he asks, "What is immunoglobulin?" You reply that it is a sterile medication made of antibodies from blood. Ken states that he is a Jehovah's Witness and cannot receive blood products.

Scenario 3 (Refusal of treatment): Aaron Jackson (DOB 10/17/20XX) is brought in by his mother for his well-child checkup. His records indicate that he is due for his first varicella vaccine injection. You bring the Varicella (Chickenpox) Vaccine VIS (vaccine information statement) and the vaccine authorization form to the exam room. As you start to discuss the vaccine, Aaron's mother, Patricia, interrupts you and tells you she is not interested in having Aaron get his chickenpox vaccination.

Equipment and Supplies:
- Patient health records
- Patient's Bill of Rights (Figure 3.3)
- General procedure consent form (Figure 3.4)
- Varicella (Chickenpox) VIS (available at ***https://www.cdc.gov***)
- Vaccine authorization form (Figure 3.5)

Standard: Complete the procedure and all critical steps in _______ minutes with a minimum score of 85% within two attempts (*or as indicated by the instructor*).

Scoring: Divide the points earned by the total possible points. Failure to perform a critical step, indicated by an asterisk (*), results in grade no higher than an 84% (*or as indicated by the instructor*).

Time: Began_________ Ended_________ Total minutes: _________

Steps:	**Point Value**	**Attempt 1**	**Attempt 2**
1. Review the Patient's Bill of Rights. Apply the Patient's Bill of Rights as you role-play each of the three scenarios.	**10***		
2. Using Scenario 1, role-play the situation with a peer. You are the medical assistant. Demonstrate how a medical assistant should handle the situation. Apply the Patient's Bill of Rights to the situation by remembering the rights of the patient. a. Show sensitivity to the patient by being respective and professional. Be open and accepting in your verbal and nonverbal body language. *(Refer to the Checklist for Affective Behaviors.)*	**10***		
b. Ask the patient if she has any questions about the procedures. Let the provider know if the patient has questions.	**10**		
c. Ask the patient what she would like to do. Based on her answer, follow up as necessary.	**10***		
d. Using the health record, document the patient's decision and the name of the provider notified.	**5**		
3. Using Scenario 2, role-play the situation with a peer. You are the medical assistant. Demonstrate how a medical assistant should handle the situation. Apply the Patient's Bill of Rights to the situation by remembering the rights of the patient. a. Show sensitivity to the patient regarding his right to refuse. Be respectful and professional. Be open and accepting in your verbal and nonverbal body language. Be accepting of his beliefs and his refusal. *(Refer to the Checklist for Affective Behaviors.)*	**10***		
b. When the patient refuses the medication, be respectful in your body language and words. Notify the provider.	**10***		
c. Using the health record, document the patient's decision and the name of the provider notified.	**5**		
4. Using Scenario 3, role-play the situation with a peer. You are the medical assistant. Demonstrate how a medical assistant should handle the situation. Apply the Patient's Bill of Rights to the situation by remembering the rights of the patient. a. Show sensitivity to the mother of the patient by being respectful and professional. Be open and accepting in your verbal and nonverbal body language. *(Refer to the Checklist for Affective Behaviors.)*	**10***		
b. Ask the mother if she has any questions about the vaccine. Let the provider know if the mother has questions.	**5**		
c. Ask the mother what she would like to do. Based on her answer, follow up as necessary.	**10***		
d. Using the health record, document the mother's decision and the name of the provider notified.	**5**		
Total Points	**100**		

Checklist for Affective Behaviors

Affective Behavior	**Directions:** *Check behaviors observed during the role-play.*					
Sensitivity	**Negative, Unprofessional Behaviors**	**Attempt 1**	**Attempt 2**	**Positive, Professional Behaviors**	**Attempt 1**	**Attempt 2**
	Poor eye contact			Proper eye contact		
	Distracted; not focused on the other person			Focuses full attention on the other person		
	Judgmental attitude; not accepting attitude			Nonjudgmental, accepting attitude		
	Fails to clarify what the person verbally or nonverbally communicated			Uses summarizing or paraphrasing to clarify what the person verbally or nonverbally communicated		
	Fails to acknowledge what the person communicated			Acknowledges what the person communicated		
	Rude, discourteous			Pleasant and courteous		
	Disregards the person's dignity and rights			Maintains the person's dignity and rights		
	Other:			Other:		

Grading for Affective Behaviors		**Point Value**	**Attempt 1**	**Attempt 2**
Does not meet Expectation	• Response lacked sensitivity. • Student demonstrated more than 2 negative, unprofessional behaviors during the interaction.	0		
Needs Improvement	• Response lacked sensitivity. • Student demonstrated 1 or 2 negative, unprofessional behaviors during the interaction.	0		
Meets Expectation	• Response was sensitive; no negative, unprofessional behaviors observed. • More practice is needed for behavior to appear natural and for student to appear comfortable and at ease.	10		
Occasionally Exceeds Expectation	• Response was sensitive; no negative, unprofessional behaviors observed. • At times student appeared comfortable and at ease; but more practice is needed for behavior to become natural and consistent with a professional medical assistant.	10		
Always Exceeds Expectation	• Response was sensitive; no negative, unprofessional behaviors observed. • Student's behaviors appeared natural and comfortable. Behaviors are consistent with a professional medical assistant.	10		

Documentation – Scenario 1

Documentation – Scenario 2

Documentation – Scenario 3

Comments

Procedure 3.2 Locate the Medical Assistant's Legal Scope of Practice

Name ______________________________ **Date** ____________ **Score** ____________

Tasks: Search online to locate the legal scope of practice for a medical assistant practicing in your state. Summarize the scope of practice.

Equipment and Supplies:
- Computer and printer with word processing software and internet access

Standard: Complete the procedure and all critical steps with a minimum score of 85% within two attempts (*or as indicated by the instructor*).

Scoring: Divide the points earned by the total possible points. Failure to perform a critical step, indicated by an asterisk (*), results in grade no higher than an 84% (*or as indicated by the instructor*).

Steps:	**Point Value**	**Attempt 1**	**Attempt 2**
1. Using the internet, search for the medical assistant's scope of practice in your state. Read the scope of practice for your state.	**20**		
2. Using the word processing software, create a short paper summarizing the medical assistant's scope of practice. Address the following points: a. Can medical assistants give injections? If so, what type of injections? b. Can medical assistants give oral, topical, and/or inhaled medications? c. Can medical assistants calculate drug dosages? d. What is the medical assistant's role with prescriptions? e. Describe additional duties that a medical assistant can legally do in your state. f. Include the website address(es) you used for this paper. *Note:* If your instructor does not provide you with different guidelines for the paper, follow these. Create at least a one-page paper, using double line spacing, a 10- or 12-point font, and 1-inch margins.	**70**		
3. After completing the paper, proofread the paper. Use correct spelling, punctuation, sentence structure, and capitalization. Make any changes required. Based on your instructor's directions, submit the paper to the instructor.	**10**		
Total Points	**100**		

Comments

CAAHEP Competencies	Step(s)
X.P.1. Locate a state's legal scope of practice for medical assistants	Entire procedure
ABHES Competencies	**Step(s)**
4. Medical Law and Ethics f. Comply with federal, state, and local health laws and regulations as they relate to healthcare settings. 1) Define the scope of practice for the medical assistant within the state where employed	Entire procedure

Student Name______________________________ Date______________

chapter 4
Healthcare Laws

CAAHEP Competencies	Assessments
X.C.3. Identify components of the Health Information Portability & Accountability Act (HIPAA)	Skills and Concepts – B. 1-8, C. 1-8, D. 1-5; Certification Preparation – 4-7; Workplace Application – 1a-d, 2-3
X.C.7.d. Define: Good Samaritan Act(s)	Skills and Concepts – H. 4; Certification Preparation – 1
X.C.7.e. Define: Uniform Anatomical Gift Act	Skills and Concepts – H. 8; Certification Preparation – 2
X.C.7.h. Define: Patient Self Determination Act (PSDA)	Skills and Concepts – H. 6; Certification Preparation – 1
X.C.7.i. Define: risk management	Skills and Concepts – M. 4
X.C.9. Identify legal and illegal applicant interview questions	Skills and Concepts – K. 4-5; Certification Preparation – 9
X.C.10.a. Identify: Health Information Technology for Economic and Clinical Health (HITECH) Act	Skills and Concepts – E. 1-2
X.C.10.b. Identify: Genetic Information Nondiscrimination Act of 2008 (GINA)	Skills and Concepts–E. 3, K. 2
X.C.10.c. Identify: Americans with Disabilities Act Amendments Act (ADAAA)	Skills and Concepts – L. 3; Certification Preparation – 10
X.C.11.a. Identify the process in compliance reporting: unsafe activities	Skills and Concepts – K. 6
X.C.11.b. Identify the process in compliance reporting: errors in patient care	Skills and Concepts – M. 5
X.C.11.c. Identify the process in compliance reporting: conflicts of interest	Skills and Concepts – J. 9
X.C.11.d. Identify the process in compliance reporting: incident reports	Skills and Concepts – M. 1-3
X.C.12.a. Identify compliance with public health statutes related to: communicable diseases	Skills and Concepts – I. 1-4
X.C.12.b. Identify compliance with public health statutes related to: abuse, neglect, and exploitation	Skills and Concepts – I. 6-10, 12 ; Workplace Application – 4
X.C.12.c. Identify compliance with public health statutes related to: wounds of violence	Skills and Concepts – I. 5
X.P.2.a. Apply HIPAA rules in regard to: privacy	Procedure 4.1

CAAHEP Competencies	Assessments
X.P.2.b. Apply HIPAA rules in regard to: release of information	Procedure 4.2
X.P.4. Perform compliance reporting based on public health statutes	Procedure 4.3
X.P.5. Report an illegal activity following the protocol established by the healthcare setting	Procedure 4.4
X.P.6. Complete an incident report related to an error in patient care	Procedure 4.5
A.3. Demonstrate empathy for patients' concerns.	Procedure 4.1
A.4. Demonstrate active listening.	Procedure 4.1
ABHES Competencies	**Assessments**
4. Medical Law and Ethics b. Institute federal and state guidelines when: 1) Releasing medical records or information	Procedures 4.1, 4.2
4.b.2) Entering orders in and utilizing electronic health records	Procedure 4.3
4.e. Perform risk management procedures	Procedure 4.5
4.f. Comply with federal, state, and local health laws and regulations as they relate to healthcare settings	Procedures 4.1 through 4.4
4.h. Demonstrate compliance with HIPAA guidelines, the ADA Amendments Act, and the Health Information Technology for Economic and Clinical Health (HITECH) Act	Procedures 4.1, 4.2

VOCABULARY REVIEW

Using the word pool on the right, find the correct word to match the definition. Write the word on the line after the definition.

Group A

1. Step-by-step directions ______________________
2. The electronic exchange of information between two agencies to accomplish financial or administrative healthcare activities ______________________
3. An organization that accepts the claim data from the provider, reformats the data to meet the specifications outlined by the insurance plan, and submits the claim ______________________
4. A system designed to use characters (i.e., numbers and letters) to represent something like a medical procedure or a disease ______________________
5. Written principles that provide goals for the employees and the facility ______________________

Word Pool

- claims clearinghouse
- coding system
- confidentiality
- electronic health record
- electronic transaction
- invasion of privacy
- policies
- precedence
- privacy
- procedures

6. Being free from unwanted intrusion ______________________
7. The top priority ______________________
8. A legally protected right of patients ______________________
9. The disclosing of private facts without the consent of the individual ______________________
10. Conforms to nationally recognized standards and contains health-related information about a specific patient; it can be created, managed, and consulted by authorized clinicians and staff from more than one healthcare organization ______________________

Group B

1. Individually identifiable health information stored or transmitted by covered entities or business associates ______________________
2. Protected health information that has had all of the direct patient identifiers removed ______________________
3. Reasons that the health information can be released ______________________
4. Healthcare providers, health (insurance) plans, and claims clearinghouses that transmit protected health information electronically ______________________
5. A form that must be completed by the patient before information can be shared with another person; also called an *authorization to disclose* form ______________________
6. To remove all direct patient identifiers from the PHI information ______________________
7. A form that must be completed by the patient before the patient records can be transferred ______________________
8. A person or business that provides a service to a covered entity that involves access to PHI ______________________
9. Safeguards that include a security officer who is responsible for creating and carrying out security policies and procedures ______________________
10. Safeguards that include facility, workstation, and device security ______________________

Word Pool

- administrative safeguards
- business associate
- covered entities
- de-identify
- disclosure authorization
- limited data set
- permission
- physical safeguards
- protected health information
- record release form

Group C

1. Disclosure of protected health information, without a reason or permission, which compromises the security or privacy of the information ______________________
2. Leaving a place; exit route ______________________
3. Diseases spread from person to person by either direct contact or indirect contact ______________________
4. An action that purposely harms another person ______________________
5. Written instructions about healthcare decisions in case a person is unable to make them ______________________
6. Failure to provide proper attention or care to another person ______________________
7. The act of using another person for one's own advantage ______________________
8. Communication that cannot be disclosed without authorization of the person involved; includes provider-patient and lawyer-client communications ______________________
9. People between the ages of 18 and 64 who have a mental or physical impairment that prevents them from doing normal activities or protecting themselves ______________________
10. Getting back at others for something they did to you ______________________

Word Pool

- abuse
- advance directives
- breach
- communicable diseases
- dependent adults
- egress
- retaliation
- exploitation
- neglect
- privileged communication

Group D

1. Any financial interest, personal or professional activity, or obligation that impacts a person's objectivity when performing the job ______________________
2. Punishment inflicted on someone as vengeance for a wrong or criminal act; the act of taking revenge ______________________
3. A deceitful action that causes another to give up something of value ______________________
4. The employer can end employment at any time for any reason ______________________
5. Legal reason for firing an employee ______________________
6. Employer did not have just cause for firing the employee ______________________
7. Unfair treatment of another person based on the person's age, gender (sex), ethnicity, sexual orientation, disability, marital status, or other selective factors ______________________
8. Continued, unwanted, and annoying actions done to another person ______________________
9. A person (usually an employee) who reports a violation of the law within the organization; the person reports the information to the public or to a person in authority ______________________

Word Pool

- conflict of interest
- discrimination
- employment-at-will
- fraud
- harassment
- just cause
- retribution
- whistleblower
- wrongful termination

ABBREVIATIONS

Write out what each of the following abbreviations stands for.

1. HIPAA ______________________________
2. EHR______________________________
3. HHS______________________________
4. OCR______________________________
5. CPT ______________________________
6. ICD ______________________________
7. NPI ______________________________
8. HPI ______________________________
9. EIN ______________________________
10. PHI ______________________________
11. ePHI ______________________________
12. FDA______________________________
13. DEA______________________________
14. PPSA ______________________________
15. CMS______________________________
16. CLIA ______________________________
17. OSH Act ______________________________
18. OSHA ______________________________
19. OPIM______________________________
20. PPE ______________________________
21. CAPTA ______________________________
22. VAERS ______________________________
23. CDC______________________________
24. VICP ______________________________
25. UDDA______________________________
26. UAGA______________________________
27. NOTA ______________________________
28. OPTN ______________________________

SKILLS AND CONCEPTS

Answer the following questions.

A. Privacy and Confidentiality

1. If your state's confidentiality laws are stricter than the federal laws, the state laws need to be followed. This is known as ______________________.

2. Healthcare professionals have the duty *not* to disclose what type of information unless authorized by the patient?
   a. medical
   b. financial
   c. insurance
   d. all of the above

B. Health Insurance Portability and Accountability Act

Match the following components to the correct HIPAA standard. Answers can be used more than once.

1. _____ Relates to unique identifiers including the National Provider Identifier, Health Plan Identifier, and the Employer Identification Number.
2. _____ Relates to standard transactions for electronic exchange of administrative healthcare information.
3. _____ Relates to the Security Rule.
4. _____ Relates to code sets including CPT and ICD.
5. _____ Relates to the Privacy Rule.

a. Standard 1
b. Standard 2
c. Standard 3
d. Standard 4

Select the correct answer.

6. Which of the following is *not* a covered entity?
   a. Healthcare provider
   b. Nursing home
   c. Pharmacy
   d. Legal firm representing the healthcare facility

7. Which of the following is *not* a business associate?
   a. Insurance company
   b. Accounting firm used by the healthcare facility
   c. Accreditation agency used by the healthcare facility
   d. Claims processing agency used by the healthcare facility

8. Which of the following is *not* a direct patient identifier?
   a. Patient's name
   b. Social Security number
   c. Contact information
   d. Patient's healthcare provider's name

C. Privacy Rule

1. The main purpose of the ______________ is to define and limit the situations in which a patient's information can be used or disclosed.

2. Patients have the right to
   a. examine their health information.
   b. obtain a copy of their health records.
   c. request corrections to be made if information is incorrect.
   d. All of the above

3. Which of the following statements is correct?
   a. Covered entities must comply with the Privacy Rule.
   b. PHI can be given to business associates only after the written agreement regarding the safekeeping of PHI is signed.
   c. Only PHI required for the business associate's job can be given.
   d. All of the above

4. Which of the following do *not* require written authorization from the patient to release the PHI?
   a. Treatment, payment, and healthcare operations
   b. Uses and disclosures with opportunity to agree or object
   c. Incidental use and disclosure
   d. All of the above

5. When patients are being treated for emotional or mental conditions, the ______________ allows providers to use professional judgment to determine if the records should be released to the patients.

6. The only permission that requires written authorization from patients is disclosing the PHI to a(n) ______________.

7. Which of the following parts of a health record must be held to a higher level of confidentiality?
   a. Psychotherapy notes
   b. Substance abuse information
   c. Human immunodeficiency virus information
   d. All of the above

8. The federal statute called ______________ restricts the release and use of patient records that include substance use diagnoses and services.

D. Security Rule

1. The ______________ covers patient records that are created, used, received, and maintained by the covered entities.

Match the description to the safeguard. Answers can be used more than once.

2. _____ Audits to track activities of users
3. _____ Workstation and device security
4. _____ Potential risks to the ePHI are identified
5. _____ Encryption of data on mobile devices

a. physical safeguard
b. administrative safeguard
c. technical safeguard

E. Other Privacy Laws

1. The ______________________ contains provisions that increased the enforcement of the privacy and security of electronic transmission and health information.

2. How did the HITECH Act modify HIPAA?
   a. Prohibited the sale of PHI without the patient's authorization.
   b. Made business associates directly liable for compliance with HIPAA.
   c. Created a tiered violation category with related violation penalties and breach notification requirements.
   d. All of the above

3. The ______________________ modified HIPAA by clarifying that genetic information is health information and prohibited the use and disclosure of genetic information by covered health plans.

F. Drug Laws

1. The ______________________ enforces the Food, Drug, and Cosmetic Act.

2. The ______________________ is responsible for the safety, effectiveness, security, and quality of drugs, cosmetics, and food.

3. The FDA is responsible for which of the following areas?
   a. Medications
   b. Vaccines and blood components
   c. Medical devices and dietary supplements
   d. All of the above

4. The ______________________ enforces the Controlled Substances Act.

5. The ______________________ oversees the manufacturing, importation, possession, use, and distribution of controlled ______________________.

6. Drugs on Schedule _______ have the highest potential for abuse and those on Schedule _______ have the lowest potential for abuse.

7. Each provider prescribing scheduled medications needs to have a unique ______________________ that needs to be renewed every ______________________.

G. Workplace Safety Laws

1. Occupational Safety and Health Act of 1970 is enforced by the ______________________.

2. ______________________ sets workplace standards and conducts inspections to ensure employee safety.

3. The goal of the ______________________ was to reduce the risk of healthcare workers' exposure to bloodborne diseases and this act required OSHA to update its Bloodborne Pathogens Standard.

4. The impact of the Needle Safety and Prevention Act includes
   a. healthcare workers must use safer medical devices.
   b. the Exposure Control Plan must include a sharps injury log documenting all instances of injuries from sharps.
   c. used sharps must be put in sharps disposal containers and PPE must be worn when there is a risk of blood or body fluid exposure.
   d. all of the above

H. Additional Healthcare Laws and Regulations

1. The ______________________ is commonly known as the Affordable Care Act.

2. Which of the following is *not* a goal of the Affordable Care Act?
   a. Provide Americans with affordable health insurance.
   b. Provide confidentiality standards in the healthcare insurance industry.
   c. Attempt to reform the healthcare system and reduce healthcare spending.
   d. All of the above

3. ______________________ establishes quality standards and regulates laboratory testing.

4. ______________________ are state laws that provide legal protection for those assisting an injured person during an emergency.

5. Which of the following relates to Good Samaritan laws?
   a. The injured person does not pay for the care given.
   b. The injured person needs to agree to the help if possible.
   c. The person assisting the injured person must exercise the same standard of care of their profession within the limits of the emergency.
   d. All of the above

6. ______________________ requires most healthcare institutions to inform patients of their right to make decisions and the facility's policies respecting advance directives.

7. ______________________ served as a guide for state lawmakers to create their own laws that define death.

8. The purpose of the ______________________ was to make organ donation easier for people.

9. ______________________ established the Organ Procurement and Transplant Network (OPTN) and also established a national registry for organ matching.

I. Compliance Reporting

For each of the following, match how a provider complies with the public health statutes when a communicable disease is diagnosed.

1. _____ If the disease is an urgent public health concern, what must be done?
2. _____ If the disease is a less urgent communicable disease, what must be done?
3. _____ How are HIV and AIDS reported by the provider?

a. May be reported electronically by mail or fax within 3 days.
b. The provider may need to mail the paperwork to increase confidentiality.
c. Reporting must be done immediately, usually by phone or fax.

Select the correct answer for the following questions.

4. Which of the following is *incorrect* regarding reporting communicable diseases?
   a. The state's public health department must be notified.
   b. The notification process is called *disease reporting*.
   c. Only the provider can report the new reportable disease case.
   d. The reporting process can vary by each state.

5. Which of the following is correct regarding compliance with wounds of violence reporting?
   a. State statutes vary from state to state regarding wounds of violence reporting.
   b. Reportable cases include wounds caused by gunshots and stabbing.
   c. Reportable cases include specific types of burns and nonaccidental wounds caused by a knife, an axe, or a sharp-pointed instrument.
   d. All of the above

6. Which of the following is *incorrect* regarding compliance reporting child abuse, neglect, and exploitation?
   a. Only some states require child maltreatment to be reported.
   b. In most states, healthcare providers need to report any child maltreatment.
   c. Most state statutes do not consider abuse and neglect information as privileged communication.
   d. The Child Welfare Information Gateway website can be used as a resource for state reporting information.

For each of the following, match the type of child maltreatment.

7. _____ Failure to provide adequate nutrition, clothing, shelter, and hygiene.
8. _____ Failure to provide needed care for injury, impairment, or illness.
9. _____ Fractures or burns that are unexplained or do not match the explanation given.
10. _____ Failure to enroll child in school or to home-school child.

a. physical abuse
b. sexual abuse
c. medical neglect
d. educational neglect
e. physical neglect

Select the correct answer or fill in the blank for the following questions.

11. The purpose of the ______________________ was to maintain the rights and dignity of the older person.

12. Which of the following do all states have?
    a. Adult or elder protective services statutes that provide reporting and investigating procedures for elder abuse in the state.
    b. Statutes that establish a Long-Term Care Ombudsman Program that advocates for the safety and rights of long-term care facility residents.
    c. General criminal statutes on fraud, sexual assault, battery, and other abuses that can relate to elder abuse.
    d. All of the above

13. The ______________________ will dictate who are mandated reporters, when to report, and how to report the situation.

14. ______________________ is a national surveillance program that monitors vaccine safety by collecting information on unusual vaccine side effects.

15. The ______________________ provides compensation for children injured by childhood vaccines.

J. Compliance Programs

1. A(n) ______________________ or corporate compliance is a program within a business that detects and prevents violations of state and federal laws.

2. ______________________ occurs when someone sells or uses another person's personal information for financial gain.

3. ______________________ relates to any financial interest, personal or professional activity, or obligation that affects a person's objectivity when performing the job.

4. The ______________________ prohibits intentionally receiving or giving anything of value to get referrals or generate federal healthcare program business.

5. The ______________________ prohibits a person from submitting false or fraudulent Medicare or Medicaid claims for payment.

6. The ______________________ prohibits a healthcare provider from referring a Medicare patient for services to a facility in which the provider or the provider's immediate family has a financial relationship.

7. The ______________________ prohibits intentionally defrauding any healthcare benefit program.

8. Describe the process in compliance reporting for violations or illegal activities related to fraud.

____

____

____

9. Describe the process in compliance reporting for a conflict of interest. ______________________

____

____

____

K. Employment Concerns

1. The ______________________ prohibits employment discrimination based on color, race, gender, religion, or national origin.

2. The ______________________ prohibits employment discrimination based on the person's genetic information.

3. Describe how a medical assistant should handle violations noticed in the workplace. ______________

____

____

4. Which of the following questions would be considered illegal to ask during an interview?
   a. "Are you eligible to work in this state?"
   b. "Are you pregnant?"
   c. "What medications are you taking?"
   d. b and c

5. Which of the following questions would be considered legal to ask during an interview?
   a. "Can you work on Sundays?"
   b. "How old are you?"
   c. "Have you ever been arrested?"
   d. "What diseases or conditions do you have?"

6. Describe how a medical assistant should handle unsafe activities or practices in the workplace.

____

____

____

L. Laws Protecting Patients Against Discrimination

1. The ______________________ prohibits discrimination against individuals with disabilities in everyday activities, including getting healthcare.

2. The ______________________ prohibits discrimination against individuals with disabilities in services that receive federal financial assistance and requires that healthcare agencies make their services accessible to people with disabilities.

3. The ______________________ expanded the meaning and interpretation of the definition of disability and ensures that individuals with disabilities and certain conditions, such as cancer and diabetes, receive protection under the law.

M. Incident Reports and Risk Management

1. Which of the following is correct regarding incident reports?
   a. An incident report is an internal document that needs to be completed whenever an unexpected event occurs.
   b. The purpose is to gather information about the situation in case of a future lawsuit.
   c. The purpose is to communicate issues for risk-management procedures.
   d. All of the above

2. Which of the following is *incorrect*?
   a. An incident report should be completed for patient complaints, medication errors, and medical device malfunction.
   b. List the facts and your conclusions when completing an incident report.
   c. Do not mention the incident report in the patient's health record.
   d. Complete the incident report by the end of the day when the situation occurred.

3. Usually, the incident report is given to the ______________________ to review before it is sent to the risk-management team.

4. ______________________ involves techniques used to reduce or eliminate accidental loss to the healthcare facility and involves identifying, assessing, and controlling risks.

5. The wrong medication was given to the patient. Describe the process in compliance reporting for errors in patient care.

____

____

____

CERTIFICATION PREPARATION

Circle the correct answer.

1. Which state law provides legal protection for those assisting an injured person during an emergency?
   a. Uniform Anatomical Gift Act
   b. Good Samaritan Act
   c. Patient Self-Determination Act
   d. Genetic Information Nondiscrimination Act

2. Which act makes organ donation easier?
   a. Uniform Determination of Death Act
   b. National Organ Transplant Act
   c. Uniform Anatomical Gift Act
   d. Patient Self-Determination Act

3. Which act requires most healthcare institutions to inform patients of their rights to make decisions and the facility's policies about advance directives?
   a. Uniform Determination of Death Act
   b. National Organ Transplant Act
   c. Uniform Anatomical Gift Act
   d. Patient Self-Determination Act

4. Which HIPAA standard requires healthcare facilities, insurance companies, and others to protect patient information that is electronically stored and transmitted?
   a. Standard 1 related to transactions and code sets
   b. Standard 2 related to the Privacy Rule
   c. Standard 3 related to the Security Rule
   d. Standard 4 related to unique identifiers

5. Individually identifiable health information stored or transmitted by covered entities or business associates is the definition of which term?
   a. Permission
   b. PHI
   c. Covered entities
   d. Limited data set

6. Under HIPAA, healthcare providers, health (insurance) plans, and claims clearinghouses must transmit PHI electronically. What are these entities called under HIPAA?
   a. Covered entities
   b. PHI
   c. Business associates
   d. Permission

7. Under HIPAA, which is a reason for releasing or disclosing patient information?
   a. De-identify
   b. Business associates
   c. PHI
   d. Permission

8. Which psychotherapy notes are held at a higher level of confidentiality?
   a. Prescriptions for medications treating mental health disorders
   b. Results of the clinical tests related to mental health disorders
   c. Types and frequency of treatments ordered for mental health disorders
   d. What the patient said during the session and the provider's analysis of the statements and the situation

9. Which question is illegal during an interview?
   a. "Are you eligible to work in this state?"
   b. "Can you perform the essential job functions of a medical assistant with or without reasonable accommodation?"
   c. "When did you move to the United States?"
   d. "Can you work on weekends?"

10. Which act expanded the meaning and interpretation of the definition of disability and included people with cancer, diabetes, attention-deficit/hyperactivity disorder, learning disabilities, and epilepsy?
    a. ADA
    b. OSHA
    c. ADAAA
    d. Stark Law

WORKPLACE APPLICATIONS

1. The billing department supervisor at Walden-Martin Family Medical Clinic wants to hire ACE Coders to assist with the billing processes. Answer the following questions using this scenario.

   a. Who is the covered entity? ____________________

   b. Who is the business associate? ____________________

   c. What must be in done before the business associate obtains patient information? ____________________

   ____

   d. Can the business associates have unlimited access to all patient information? Explain why or why not.

   ____

   ____

2. Mrs. Smith asked Bella to call and talk with her daughter, Rosie. Mrs. Smith wanted Bella to tell Rosie the results of her blood test. Mrs. Smith stated that Rosie was a nurse and would understand the information. Can Bella give Mrs. Smith's information to Rosie? If not, what could be done so Rosie could get the information?

   ____

   ____

3. Mr. Green had before-and-after pictures taken as he was going through bariatric surgery and weight loss. He requests that these pictures be given to his new provider. What is the typical process to transfer pictures to another agency?

   ____

   ____

4. Mr. Thomas is a 39-year-old dependent adult. During the rooming process, the medical assistant suspects that Mr. Thomas is a victim of neglect. What should the medical assistant do?

   ____

   ____

INTERNET ACTIVITIES

1. Using the internet, research your state's disease reporting public health statutes. Create a poster presentation, PowerPoint presentation, or paper summarizing the reporting process for each category of diseases (e.g., urgent public health concern, less urgent, and HIV and AIDS). List three diseases for the urgent and less urgent categories.

2. Using the internet, review the Child Welfare Information Gateway website (www.childwelfare.gov) for content related to your state. You can also use government websites from your state. Create a poster presentation, PowerPoint presentation, or paper summarizing child protection in your state. Focus on related statutes, the reporting process, and who mandatory reporters are.

3. Using the internet, research prevention of elder abuse, neglect, and exploitation. Focus on resources in your state. Briefly summarize your findings and cite the websites used.

Procedure 4.1 Protecting a Patient's Privacy

Name ______________________________ **Date** ____________ **Score** __________

Tasks: Apply HIPAA rules and protect a patient's privacy. Demonstrate active listening skills and empathy to a patient.

Scenario: Ken Thomas (date of birth [DOB] 10/25/19XX) saw Jean Burke, nurse practitioner (NP), this past week. He was diagnosed with acute leukemia after several tests. You work with Ms. Burke, and you were involved with arranging Ken's tests. Today, Ken's adult child, Alex Thomas, calls you. Alex wants to know what is going on with Ken. You look at Ken's health record and see that Alex is not on the disclosure authorization form. Per the facility's policy, for information to be given to a patient's family, a disclosure authorization form must be completed.

Later Ken calls and asks why you did not update Alex on his condition. He sounds upset while he is talking with you.

Directions: Role-play the scenario with a peer. You are the medical assistant in the scenario. Your peer will play Alex and then Ken.

Equipment and Supplies:
- Patient's health record
- Disclosure authorization form (electronic or paper) (See Figure 4.2)

Standard: Complete the procedure and all critical steps in _______ minutes with a minimum score of 85% within two attempts (*or as indicated by the instructor*).

Scoring: Divide the points earned by the total possible points. Failure to perform a critical step, indicated by an asterisk (*), results in grade no higher than an 84% (*or as indicated by the instructor*).

Time: Began_________ Ended_________ Total minutes: _________

Steps:	**Point Value**	**Attempt 1**	**Attempt 2**
1. You realized that Alex is not on the disclosure authorization form. Inform Alex that his name is not on a disclosure authorization form. Discuss the purpose of the disclosure authorization form. Be professional and respectful as you apply HIPAA rules to the situation. *(Refer to the Affective Behaviors Checklist – **Respect** and the Grading Rubric)*	**20***		
2. Explain to Alex how you would be able to give him information. Encourage Alex to talk with his father about the situation.	**15**		
***Scenario update*:** Your peer will now play the part of Ken, the patient. 3. When Ken calls, be professional and empathetic as you listen to his complaints. Inform Ken that you understand his frustration. Be respectful to his feelings and his rights. Explain why you could not give information to Alex. *(Refer to the Affective Behaviors Checklist – **Empathy** and the Grading Rubric)*	**20***		

4. Demonstrate active listening skills when interacting with Ken. Remain neutral and refrain from interrupting. Keep your voice even and do not raise the volume. Focus on the patient and avoid distractions. *(Refer to the Affective Behaviors Checklist –* ***Active Listening*** *and the Grading Rubric)*	**20***		
5. Discuss with Ken how you could prepare the disclosure authorization form. Make plans for how Ken would sign the form.	**10**		
6. Document the phone call with Alex and Ken. Describe the facts and the plan to complete the disclosure authorization form.	**15**		
Total Points	**100**		

Affective Behavior	**Affective Behaviors Checklist** **Directions:** *Check behaviors observed during the role-play.*					
Respect	**Negative, Unprofessional Behaviors**	**Attempt 1**	**Attempt 2**	**Positive, Professional Behaviors**	**Attempt 1**	**Attempt 2**
	Rude, unkind, fake/false attitude, disrespectful, impolite, unwelcoming			Courteous, sincere, polite, welcoming		
	Unconcerned with person's dignity; brief, abrupt			Maintained person's dignity; took time with person		
	Unprofessional verbal communication; inappropriate questions			Professional verbal communication		
	Negative nonverbal behaviors, poor eye contact			Positive nonverbal behaviors, proper eye contact		
	Other:			Other:		
Active Listening	Biased, offensive; raised volume of voice			Remained neutral, kept voice even and did not raise volume		
	Interrupted			Refrained from interrupting		
	Did not allow for silence or pauses			Allowed for periods of silence		
	Distracted			Focused on patient, avoided distractions		
	Other:			Other:		
Empathy	Did not listen to patient's responses			Listened to patient		
	Lack of respect and support demonstrated			Showed respect and support		
	Lack of therapeutic communication techniques used			Used therapeutic communication techniques		
	Other:			Other:		

Grading Rubric for the Affective Behaviors Checklist **Directions:** *Based on checklist results, identify the points received for the procedure checklist. Indicate how the behaviors demonstrated met the expectations.*		**Points for Procedure Checklist**	**Attempt 1**	**Attempt 2**
Does not meet Expectation	• Response lacked respect, active listening, and/or empathy. • Student demonstrated more than 2 negative, unprofessional behaviors during the interaction.	0		
Needs Improvement	• Response lacked respect, active listening, and/or empathy. • Student demonstrated 1 or 2 negative, unprofessional behaviors during the interaction.	0		
Meets Expectation	• Response was respectful and empathetic. Demonstrated active listening. No negative, unprofessional behaviors observed. • More practice is needed for behavior to appear natural and for student to appear comfortable and at ease.	20		
Occasionally Exceeds Expectation	• Response was respectful and empathetic. Demonstrated active listening. No negative, unprofessional behaviors observed. • At times student appeared comfortable and at ease; but more practice is needed for behavior to become natural and consistent with a professional medical assistant.	20		
Always Exceeds Expectation	• Response was respectful and empathetic. Demonstrated active listening. No negative, unprofessional behaviors observed. • Student's behaviors appeared natural and comfortable. Behaviors are consistent with a professional medical assistant.	20		

Documentation

Comments

CAAHEP Competencies	Step(s)
X.P.2.a. Apply HIPAA rules in regard to: privacy	1-3, 5
A.3. Demonstrate empathy for patients' concerns.	3
A.4. Demonstrate active listening.	4
ABHES Competencies	**Step(s)**
4. Medical Law and Ethics b. Institute federal and state guidelines when: 1) Releasing medical records or information	Entire procedure
4.f. Comply with federal, state, and local health laws and regulations as they relate to healthcare settings	1-3, 6
4.h. Demonstrate compliance with HIPAA guidelines, the ADA Amendments Act, and the Health Information Technology for Economic and Clinical Health (HITECH) Act	1-3, 6

Procedure 4.2 Completing a Release of Record Form for a Release of Information

Name ______________________________ **Date** __________ **Score** __________

Tasks: Apply HIPAA rules and complete a release of record form for a release of information.

Scenario: Aaron Jackson was seen at Walden Hospital for a high fever. You need to help Aaron's mother complete a records release form so his record from the emergency department visit can be sent to the clinic. She needs to request all records from the visit on the first of this month. The clinic information is on the form. The release will expire in 1 month.

AARON'S INFORMATION	WALDEN HOSPITAL'S INFORMATION
Date of birth: 10/17/20XX Social Security number: 164-72-4618 Address: 555 McArthur Avenue Anytown, AL 12345-1234 Phone: (123) 814-7844 Mother: Patricia Jackson	Address: Walden Hospital 123 Healing Way Anywhere, AL 12345-1234 Phone: (123) 814-4563 Fax: (123) 814-6544

Directions: You will complete the medical record release form. You will role-play the scenario with you as the medical assistant and a peer as the mother.

Equipment and Supplies:
- Records release form (electronic or paper) (See Work Product 4.1)
- Patient's health record

Standard: Complete the procedure and all critical steps in _______ minutes with a minimum score of 85% within two attempts (*or as indicated by the instructor*).

Scoring: Divide the points earned by the total possible points. Failure to perform a critical step, indicated by an asterisk (*), results in grade no higher than an 84% (*or as indicated by the instructor*).

Time: Began_________ Ended_________ Total minutes: _________

Steps:	**Point Value**	**Attempt 1**	**Attempt 2**
1. Using the medical record release form, complete the patient information (Work Product 4.1). Add the patient's name, DOB, and social security number (SSN). Include the current address and phone number that is found in the patient's health record. If an electronic form is used, select the correct patient and the fields will auto-populate.	10*		
2. Complete the parts of the form that specify who authorizes the release and who is to release the information.	15*		
3. Check the box(es) of the information that needs to be released. If required, write in what other records need to be released.	15*		
4. Add the date of the visit. Add the name and contact information for the facility where the records need to be sent.	15*		
5. Indicate how the released information will be used.	15		

6. Indicate when the authorization should expire. Proofread the form for accuracy. If using an electronic form, save the form to the patient's record. Print the form so the mother can sign.	**10**		
7. During a role-play with the patient's mother, explain what the provider is requesting. Ensure she can understand and read English. Have the mother read the form.	**10**		
8. Ask the mother if she has any questions. Answer any questions and then explain where she needs to sign if she agrees with the documentation.	**10**		
Total Points	**100**		

Comments

CAAHEP Competencies	**Step(s)**
X.P.2.b. Apply HIPAA rules in regard to: release of information	Entire procedure
ABHES Competencies	**Step(s)**
4. Medical Law and Ethics b. Institute federal and state guidelines when: 1) Releasing medical records or information	Entire procedure
4. f. Comply with federal, state, and local health laws and regulations as they relate to healthcare settings	Entire procedure
4.h. Demonstrate compliance with HIPAA guidelines, the ADA Amendments Act, and the Health Information Technology for Economic and Clinical Health (HITECH) Act	Entire procedure

Work Product 4.1 Records Release Form

Name ______________________ Date __________ Score __________

WALDEN-MARTIN
FAMILY MEDICAL CLINIC
1234 ANYSTREET | ANYTOWN, ANYSTATE 12345
PHONE 123-123-1234 | FAX 123-123-5678

Medical Records Release

Patient Name: ______________ **Date of Birth:** ______________

SSN: ______________ **Phone:** ______________

Address:

I, ______________ **authorize** ______________

to disclose/release the following information (check all applicable):

- ☐ All Records
- ☐ Abstract/Summary
- ☐ Laboratory/pathology records
- ☐ Pharmacy/prescription records
- ☐ X-ray/radiology records
- ☐ Other
- ☐ Billing records

****Note:*** *If these records contain any information from previous providers or information about HIV/AIDS status, cancer diagnosis, drug alcohol abuse, or sexually transmitted disease, you are hereby authorizing disclosure of this information. A copy of this signed authorization must be given to the individual.*

These records are for services provided on the following date(s): ______________

Please send the records listed above to (use additional sheets if necessary):

Name: ______________ **Phone:** ______________

Address: **Fax:** ______________

The information may be used/disclosed for each of the following purposes:

- ☐ At patient's request
- ☐ For employment purposes
- ☐ For patient's health care
- ☐ Other
- ☐ For payment/insurance

This authorization shall expire no later than: _______ **or upon the following event** _______ **, and may not be valid for greater than one year from the date of signature for medical records.**

I understand that after the custodian of records discloses my health information, it may no longer be protected by federal privacy laws. I understand that this authorization is voluntary and I may refuse to sign this authorization which will not affect my ability to obtain treatment; receive payment; or eligibility for benefits unless allowed by law. By signing below I represent and warrant that I have authority to sign this document and authorize the use or disclosure of protected health information and that there are no claims or orders that would prohibit, limit, or otherwise restrict my ability to authorize the use or disclosure of this protected health information.

______________________________	______________________________
Patient signature **(or patient's personal representative)**	**Date**
______________________________	______________________________
Printed name of patient representative	**Representative's authority to sign for patient** *(i.e. parent, guardian, power of attorney, executor)*

Procedure 4.3 Perform Disease Reporting

Name ______________________________ **Date** ____________ **Score** __________

Tasks: Research the state's disease reporting public health statutes and complete the disease reporting paperwork based on public health statutes. Document the activity in the patient's health record.

Scenario: Jean Burke, NP, received the test results for Ken Thomas. He tested positive for gonorrhea. She wants you to file the report with the public health department. Here is the information from his health record and the clinic. For any missing information, follow the instructor's directions (or if no directions are provided for this exercise, make up the information).

Patient Information	Provider and Lab Information	Health Record Information
Ken Thomas 398 Larkin Avenue Anytown, AL 12345-1234 Anycounty Email: k.thomas@anytown.mail Phone: (123) 784-1118 DOB: 10/25/19XX Race: Multiple races Ethnicity: Unknown Marital status: Single, living with Sandy Brown, who was not treated	**Provider:** Jean Burke, N.P. Walden-Martin Family Medical Clinic 1234 Anystreet Anytown, AL 12345-1234 Phone: (123) 123-1234 Fax: (123) 123-5678 **Lab:** Walden-Martin Family Medical Clinic Lab	**Diagnosis:** Gonorrhea **Symptoms:** Started 5 days ago, greenish discharge from penis, burning with urination **Test:** Urine specimen was collected yesterday; gonorrhea nucleic acid amplification test NAAT test done yesterday, results are positive **Treatment:** Patient treated today with ceftriaxone 250 mg intramuscular (IM) single dose and azithromycin 1 g orally single dose

Equipment and Supplies:
- Computer with internet access and printer
- Patient's health record (see table with information)
- Black pen

Standard: Complete the procedure and all critical steps in _______ minutes with a minimum score of 85% within two attempts (*or as indicated by the instructor*).

Scoring: Divide the points earned by the total possible points. Failure to perform a critical step, indicated by an asterisk (*), results in grade no higher than an 84% (*or as indicated by the instructor*).

Time: Began_________ Ended_________ Total minutes: _________

Steps:	**Point Value**	**Attempt 1**	**Attempt 2**
1. Using the internet, search for the disease reporting procedure in your state's public health department or similar facility. Read the procedure.	**10**		
2. Identify which form is required based on the patient's diagnosis. Print the form.	**10**		

3. Use a black pen to complete the form. Neatly complete the patient's demographic information section using the information from the health record.	**25**		
4. Complete the diagnosis, symptoms, testing, and treatment information.	**25**		
5. Complete the rest of the form. Review the form for accuracy. Make any changes required before submitting the form to the instructor.	**20**		
6. Document in the patient's health record that the disease reporting paperwork was completed and submitted.	**10**		
Total Points	**100**		

Documentation

Comments

CAAHEP Competencies	Step(s)
X.P.4. Perform compliance reporting based on public health statutes	Entire procedure
ABHES Competencies	**Step(s)**
4. Medical Law and Ethics f. Comply with federal, state, and local health laws and regulations as they relate to healthcare settings	Entire procedure
4.b.2) Entering orders in and utilizing electronic health records	6

Procedure 4.4 Report Illegal Activity

Name ______________________________ **Date** ____________ **Score** __________

Task: Report an illegal activity in the healthcare setting following proper protocol.

Scenario: You witness a coworker, Sally Brown, taking medical samples from the supply cabinet. You see her sticking them into her purse. She sees you and states, "This was the same medication I had to pay $200 for the last time I was sick. I don't see why we need to pay for medications when we have samples that we give free to patients. We should be able to use them also." You know the facility's professional policy prohibits taking medical samples from the sample cabinet for personal reasons.

Facility's Compliance Reporting Protocol:

Walden-Martin Family Medical Clinic's Compliance Program has a phone number and email address for employees to report suspected violations, suspected illegal activity, fraud, abuse, theft, and workplace safety concerns. Concerns can be left on the voicemail or emailed without fear of retribution or retaliation. Please include as many details as possible, including dates, names, and the situation.

Any employee who seeks retribution or retaliation against another employee for reporting an offense needs to be aware of criminal penalties for such actions.

Equipment and Supplies:
- Computer with email and internet access or phone
- Instructor's email address or voicemail phone number
- Pen and paper
- Facility's compliance reporting protocol (See box)

Standard: Complete the procedure and all critical steps with a minimum score of 85% within two attempts (*or as indicated by the instructor*).

Scoring: Divide the points earned by the total possible points. Failure to perform a critical step, indicated by an asterisk (*), results in grade no higher than an 84% (*or as indicated by the instructor*).

Steps:	Point Value	Attempt 1	Attempt 2
1. Read the facility's corporate compliance reporting protocol.	10		
2. Using the paper and pen, write down the facts of what you witnessed.	10		
3. Using the paper and pen, compose the message you want to email or leave on the voicemail for the compliance office.	30		
4. Proofread the message and make any changes required. Make sure to include the date, names of people involved, and the details of the situation.	20		
5. Using your email or phone, send a message to the corporate compliance office. Use the email address or phone number provided by your instructor.	30		
Total Points	**100**		

Comments

CAAHEP Competencies	Step(s)
X.P.5. Report an illegal activity following the protocol established by the healthcare setting	Entire procedure
ABHES Competencies	**Step(s)**
4. Medical Law and Ethics f. Comply with federal, state, and local health laws and regulations as they relate to healthcare settings	Entire procedure

Procedure 4.5 Complete Incident Report

Name ______________________________ **Date** ____________ **Score** __________

Task: Complete an incident report form for a medication error.

Scenario: Johnny Parker (DOB 06/15/20XX) sees Jean Burke, NP, for a well-child visit. Johnny is off-schedule with his hepatitis B vaccine series, and today he is to get his last hepatitis B booster. You (a medical assistant) prepare the medication and give the injection in his right deltoid muscle. Later in the day, you realize that hepatitis B has been out of stock for 1 week. You must have given a hepatitis A booster to Johnny. You realize that you failed to read the label three times during preparation of the medication. You report the mistake to Jean Burke, NP, and your supervisor. Your supervisor calls Lisa Parker, Johnny's mother. They will come back next week for the hepatitis B vaccine. You need to complete the incident report.

Equipment and Supplies:

- Incident report form (Work Product 4.2) and black pen or computer with internet access and SimChart for the Medical Office (SCMO)

Standard: Complete the procedure and all critical steps in _______ minutes with a minimum score of 85% within two attempts (*or as indicated by the instructor*).

Scoring: Divide the points earned by the total possible points. Failure to perform a critical step, indicated by an asterisk (*), results in grade no higher than an 84% (*or as indicated by the instructor*).

Time: Began_________ Ended_________ Total minutes: _________

Steps:	**Point Value**	**Attempt 1**	**Attempt 2**
1. **SCMO method:** Access SCMO and enter the Simulation Playground. If a popup window appears, select "Return to previous session with saved patient information" and click Start. On the Calendar screen, click on the Form Repository icon. Click on Office Forms on the left Info Panel and select Incident Report. **For both methods:** Accurately complete the information from the date down to the reason for the patient's visit.	20		
2. **For both methods:** Specify the incident description, immediate action and outcome, and contributing factors, and fill in the prevention boxes. Provide as much detail as possible. Be honest and concise with your facts.	20		
3. **For both methods:** Complete the reported by, position, and contact phone number sections. Your information should be in these fields. (For this exercise, make up a contact phone number.)	20		
4. **For both methods:** Complete the other persons involved, position, and contact phone number sections. Jean Burke's information should be in these fields. (Make up her contact phone number.)	20		
5. **For both methods:** Review the form for accuracy. Make any changes required before submitting the form to the instructor. (**For the SCMO method**: Save or print the form based on your instructor's directions.)	20		
Total Points	**100**		

Comments

CAAHEP Competencies	Step(s)
X.P.6. Complete an incident report related to an error in patient care	Entire procedure
ABHES Competencies	**Step(s)**
4. Medical Law and Ethics e. Perform risk management procedures	Entire procedure

Work Product 4.2 Incident Report Form

Name ____________________ Date __________ Score __________

WALDEN-MARTIN
FAMILY MEDICAL CLINIC
1234 ANYSTREET | ANYTOWN, ANYSTATE 12345
PHONE 123-123-1234 | FAX 123-123-5678

Incident Report

Date: ____________ **Time:** ____________

Incident Type: ☐ Staff ☐ Patient ☐ Visitor ☐ Equipment/Property

Witness: ☐ Staff ☐ Patient ☐ Visitor

Department: ____________ **Exact Location:** ____________

Medical Team: ____________

Patient Reason for Visit: ____________ **Medication Incident:** ☐ Yes ☐ No

Incident Description: [ ] **Immediate Actions and Outcome:** [ ]

Contributing Factors: [ ] **Prevention:** [ ]

Next of kin / guardian notified / patient? ☐ Yes ☐ No ☐ N/A **Medical staff notified?** ☐ Yes ☐ No ☐ N/A

Reported By: ____________ **Position:** ____________

Contact Phone Number: ____________

Other Persons Involved: ____________ **Position:** ____________

Contact Phone Number: ____________

Medical Report (Document patient's assessment and list investigations and treatments):

Provider: ____________ **Designation:** ____________

Provider Signature: ____________ **Date/Time:** ____________

Student Name______________________________ Date______________

Healthcare Ethics

chapter 5

CAAHEP Competencies	Assessment
V.C.13.c. Identify the basic concepts of the following theories: Kübler-Ross	Skills and Concepts – I. 1-8; Certification Preparation – 6
X.C.7.e. Define: Uniform Anatomical Gift Act	Skills and Concepts – M. 1; Certification Preparation – 10
X.C.7.f. Define: living will/advanced directives	Vocabulary Review – D. 3, 5; Skills and Concepts – J. 2-3; Certification Preparation – 7
X.C.7.g. Define: medical durable power of attorney	Vocabulary Review – D. 4; Skills and Concepts – J. 5
X.C.7.h. Define: Patient Self Determination Act (PSDA)	Skills and Concepts – J. 1
XI.C.1.a. Define: ethics	Vocabulary Review – D. 1; Certification Preparation – 1
XI.C.1.b. Define: morals	Vocabulary Review – D. 2; Certification Preparation – 2
XI.C.2. Identify personal and professional ethics	Vocabulary Review – A. 1, 5; Skills and Concepts – A. 1-2; B. 1-2, 4; Certification Preparation – 3
XI.C.3. Identify potential effects of personal morals on professional performance	Skills and Concepts – A. 3
XI.P.1. Demonstrate professional response(s) to ethical issues	Procedures 5.1, 5.2

ABHES Competencies	Assessment
4. Medical Law and Ethics g. Display compliance with the Code of Ethics of the profession	Skills and Concepts – B. 4; Procedures 5.1, 5.2

VOCABULARY REVIEW

Using the word pool on the right, find the correct word to match the definition. Write the word on the line after the definition.

Group A

1. Codes of conduct stated by an employer or professional association ____________________
2. Basic units of heredity ____________________
3. Rod-shaped structures found in the cell's nucleus; they contain genetic information ____________________
4. A set of rules about good and bad behavior ____________________
5. An individual's code of conduct ____________________
6. The freedom to determine one's own actions and decisions ____________________
7. People who study the ethical effect of biomedical advances ____________________
8. To treat patients fairly and give them care that is due and appropriate ____________________
9. The moral obligation to act for the good or benefit of others ____________________
10. To do no harm ____________________

Word Pool

- autonomy
- beneficence
- bioethicists
- chromosomes
- code of ethics
- genes
- justice
- nonmaleficence
- personal ethics
- professional ethics

Group B

1. The inability to get pregnant after 1 year of unprotected intercourse ____________________
2. Nonreproductive cells; they do not include sperm and egg cells ____________________
3. Cells can make copies of themselves ____________________
4. Sperm and egg cells ____________________
5. Cells can develop into specialized cells ____________________
6. The process of creating a genetically identical biological entity ____________________
7. The entire genetic makeup of an organism ____________________
8. A branch of medicine involved with using patients' genomic information as part of their clinical care ____________________
9. A branch of pharmacology that studies the genetic factors that influence a person's response to a medication ____________________
10. The manipulation of genetic material in cells to change hereditary traits or produce a specific result ____________________

Word Pool

- cloning
- differentiate
- genetic engineering
- genome
- genomic medicine
- germline cells
- infertility
- pharmacogenomics
- self-renew
- somatic cells

Group C

Word Pool

- cessation
- cryopreservation
- discipline
- ethics committees
- euthanasia
- evidence-based practices
- healthcare proxy
- hospice
- in vitro fertilization
- oocyte
- palliative
- *parens patriae*
- passive euthanasia
- resident
- surrogate
- xenotransplantation

1. A competent adult can appoint a person to make healthcare decisions in the event they are unable to do so ______________________
2. Withholding a life-saving treatment (e.g., feeding tube) and letting the person die ______________________
3. A branch of knowledge, learning, or instruction; for instance, medicine, nursing, social work, and physical therapy ______________________
4. Incorporating the most current and valid research results into the practice of healthcare, thus providing the best patient care ______________________
5. Latin for "father of the country," a doctrine that gives the courts the power to make decisions for people who cannot make their own decisions ______________________
6. Involves removing egg cells from a female's ovaries, fertilizing them with sperm outside of the body, and then implanting the fertilized egg in the uterus ______________________
7. To help relieve the symptoms of a serious illness ______________________
8. A type of palliative care for people who have about 6 months or less to live ______________________
9. Bringing to an end ______________________
10. The act of killing a person who is suffering from an incurable disease ______________________
11. To preserve by freezing at low temperatures ______________________
12. A physician who has graduated from medical school and is finishing specialized clinical training ______________________
13. An immature ovum ______________________
14. A person who acts on behalf of another person or takes the place of another person ______________________
15. A group composed of members from a variety of disciplines that analyzes ethical issues ______________________
16. Any procedure where nonhuman cells, tissues, or organs are implanted or infused into a person ______________________

Group D

Fill in the blank with the word or phrase that is defined.

1. ______________________ are rules of conduct that differentiate between acceptable and unacceptable behavior.
2. ______________________ are internal principles that distinguish between right and wrong.
3. ______________________ are written instructions about healthcare decisions should a person be unable to make them.

4. _______________________ is similar to a living will but includes all healthcare decisions.

5. _______________________ provides instructions about life-sustaining medical treatment to be administered or withheld when the patient has a terminal condition.

ABBREVIATIONS

Write out what each of the following abbreviations stands for.

1. AMA _______________________
2. CEJA _______________________
3. AAMA _______________________
4. GMOs _______________________
5. FDA _______________________
6. ART _______________________
7. IUI _______________________
8. STI _______________________
9. PSDA _______________________
10. DNR _______________________
11. CPR _______________________
12. POLST _______________________
13. UDDA _______________________
14. UAGA _______________________
15. NOTA _______________________
16. OPTN _______________________

SKILLS AND CONCEPTS

Answer the following questions.

A. Personal Ethics

1. _______________________ includes an individual's honesty, fairness, commitment, integrity, and accountability; it also includes doing what one considers to be correct.

2. Our _______________________ affect how we conduct ourselves or, in other words, our personal ethics.

3. Which of the following statements is correct regarding personal morals and professional performance?
   a. Personal morals affect professional performance.
   b. Personal morals that align with professional characteristics will positively affect one's professional performance.
   c. Personal morals can negatively affect professional performance.
   d. All of the above

B. Professional Ethics

1. ______________________ are codes of conduct stated by an employer or a professional association.

2. Which of the following statements is *incorrect* regarding professional ethics?
   a. The employee handbook may indicate how employees need to conduct themselves in the workplace.
   b. Codes of ethics are published by professional associations.
   c. Professional ethics can be violated without consequences.
   d. A code of ethics exists for medical assistants.

3. Which of the following statements is correct?
   a. The care a medical assistant provides must reflect respect for that patient.
   b. The medical assistant is legally and ethically obligated to keep patient information confidential.
   c. The medical assistant must uphold the standards of the profession.
   d. All of the above

4. Which of the following points is *not* included in the Medical Assistant Code of Ethics?
   a. Render service with full respect for the dignity of humanity.
   b. Respect confidential information obtained through employment unless legally authorized or required by responsible performance of duty to divulge such information.
   c. Uphold the honor and high principles of the profession and accept its disciplines.
   d. Endeavor to be more effective and aspire to render greater service.

C. Separation Plan

1. How can a medical assistant approach a situation if it involves their biases? ______________________

   ____

   ____

2. When looking for employment, why is it important to consider one's biases before applying for certain jobs?

   ____

   ____

D. Principles of Healthcare Ethics

Match the ethical principle with the description. Answers may be used more than once.

1. _____ Healthcare professionals promote health in patients and assist patients to recover from illness.
2. _____ Healthcare professionals are obligated not to inflict intentional harm on patients.
3. _____ The medical assistant ensures the environment is both physically and psychologically safe for others and that safety hazards are reported and corrected.
4. _____ The medical assistant promotes health and prevention of diseases.

a. autonomy
b. nonmaleficence
c. beneficence
d. justice

5. _____ The medical assistant must protect patients' privacy.
6. _____ Professional behaviors of the medical assistant include providing equal respect and courtesy to all people.
7. _____ Healthcare professionals must respect and honor the patient's decision.

E. Ethical Issues Related to Genetics

1. Which of the following is an important advance in genomic medicine?
   a. Pharmacogenetics
   b. Stem cell transplants
   c. Genetic testing
   d. All of the above

2. Which of the following is *not* a type of genetic testing?
   a. Newborn screening
   b. Prenatal testing
   c. Bariatric testing
   d. Carrier testing

3. Which of the following is correct regarding stem cells?
   a. Embryonic stem cells are derived from bone marrow, brain, skin, and heart tissue.
   b. Embryonic stem cells are derived from umbilical cord blood.
   c. Adult stem cells are thought to cause fewer rejection issues with transplants if a person's own stem cells are used.
   d. All of the above

4. ______________________ is currently an experimental technique that uses genes to prevent or treat diseases.

5. ______________________, or genome editing, is a specific gene therapy that can remove, add, or alter sections of the gene.

F. Reproductive Ethical Issues

Match the term with the correct description.

1. _____ Specially prepared sperm is placed into a woman's uterus using a long, narrow tube
2. _____ A woman carries and gives birth for another couple
3. _____ Egg freezing or egg banking
4. _____ The deliberate termination of a pregnancy
5. _____ Occurs when the egg is from a surrogate and the sperm is from the father
6. _____ Occurs when the sperm and egg come from the intended parents or are donated, and the surrogate is not related to the baby

a. surrogacy
b. cryopreservation of oocytes
c. gestational surrogacy
d. traditional surrogacy
e. intrauterine insemination
f. elective abortion

G. Childhood Ethical Issues

Match the term with the correct description.

1. _____ No contact between the adoptive parents and the birth parents
2. _____ Used for children or adults who are incompetent and when parents refuse healthcare for a child
3. _____ Allows a person to give up an unwanted infant anonymously
4. _____ Adoptive parents meet and may stay in contact with the birth parents

a. closed adoption
b. open adoption
c. *parens patriae*
d. Safe Haven infant protection laws

H. Research Trials and Ethical Issues

Match the description with the correct answer. Answers may be used more than once.

1. _____ Addressed the importance of human research, the obligations of the physicians involved, the importance of informed consent, and the protection of the participants
2. _____ Human experiments require voluntary consent, the results must be for the good of society, and the experiments must be based on prior knowledge and should avoid all unnecessary physical and mental suffering
3. _____ Researched the natural history of syphilis on African American men
4. _____ Outlined what was legal when conducting human experiments
5. _____ Identified basic ethical principles and guidelines regarding human subject research

a. Nuremberg Code
b. Belmont Report
c. Declaration of Helsinki
d. Tuskegee Study

I. End-of-Life Issues

Match the description and emotions with the correct state of grief and dying. Answers may be used more than once.

1. _____ Tom blames the drug company for his cancer.
2. _____ Tia feels sad, fearful, and uncertain as her mother is dying.
3. _____ Dan experienced disbelief and numbness when he heard the prognosis.
4. _____ Sally makes a deal with God so she can live for another 6 months.
5. _____ John, diagnosed with incurable cancer, distances himself from his friends.
6. _____ Sam's mother is dying of cancer. He has come to terms with the situation.
7. _____ Alice refuses to accept the breast cancer diagnosis.

a. denial
b. anger
c. bargaining
d. depression
e. acceptance

Select the correct answer.

8. Which of the following is correct regarding the stages of grief and dying as defined by Dr. Elisabeth Kübler-Ross?
   a. The grieving stages include denial, anger, bargaining, depression, and acceptance.
   b. Some people may not experience all of the grieving stages.
   c. People may move through the stages differently, and some may switch back and forth among the stages.
   d. All of the above

J. Patient Self-Determination Act

1. The Patient Self-Determination Act requires
   a. healthcare institutions to provide patients with a written document of their rights to make decisions and the facility's policies respecting advance directives.
   b. that patients are asked if they have advance directives at the time of admission.
   c. documentation of the patient's advance directive status in the health record.
   d. all of the above

2. ______________________ are written instructions about healthcare decisions should a person be unable to make them.

3. A(n) ______________________ provides instructions about life-sustaining medical treatment to be administered or withheld when the patient has a terminal condition.

4. With a(n) ______________________, a competent adult can appoint a person to make healthcare decisions in the event they are unable to do so.

5. The ______________________ is similar to a living will but includes all healthcare decisions, names a healthcare proxy, and can include healthcare wishes.

6. ______________________ the person refuses cardiopulmonary resuscitation if they stop breathing or have no pulse.

K. Ethical Issues Related to Dying

1. The Uniform Determination of Death Act
   a. served as a guide for federal lawmakers.
   b. provided a definition of death.
   c. declared death if reversible cessation of circulatory and respiratory functions occurs.
   d. declared death if reversible cessation of all function of the brain occurs.

2. If providers have questions regarding life-sustaining treatments, they should
   a. support the decision of the patient or surrogate.
   b. review the patient's advance directive.
   c. seek advice from an ethics committee.
   d. all of the above

Match the types of euthanasia with the description.

3. _____ The patient consents to the euthanasia action.
4. _____ Another person kills the patient.
5. _____ Killing the person using an injection.
6. _____ The patient does not consent to the action.
7. _____ Withholding a lifesaving treatment and letting the person die.
8. _____ The patient kills him- or herself.
9. _____ The patient kills him- or herself with the assistance of another person.

a. active euthanasia
b. passive euthanasia
c. voluntary euthanasia
d. involuntary euthanasia
e. self-administered euthanasia
f. other-administered euthanasia
g. assisted euthanasia

L. Organ Donation and Ethical Issues

1. Which of the following organs and tissues can be donated?
   a. Intestines, pancreas, and lung
   b. Tendons, bone marrow, and corneas
   c. Kidney, liver, and heart
   d. All of the above

2. With ________________________, the donor specifically names the person to receive the donation.

3. In ________________________, a pair of organs is involved and the transplant candidates do not match the donor they know, but match the other donor; thus, the organs are swapped or traded.

4. With ________________________, the organ donor does not know the person nor is related to the person.

M. Organ Donation Laws

1. The Uniform Anatomical Gift Act
   a. makes it easier for people to donate organs.
   b. was enacted by states and differences exist among states.
   c. provides uniformity in organ and tissue donations across the nation.
   d. all of the above

2. The National Organ Transplant Act
   a. established the Organ Procurement and Transplant Network.
   b. established a national registry for organ matching.
   c. was passed by Congress in 1984.
   d. all of the above

CERTIFICATION PREPARATION

Circle the correct answer.

1. Which term means "rules of conduct that differentiate between acceptable and unacceptable behavior"?
   a. Ethics
   b. Justice
   c. Morals
   d. Code of ethics

2. Which term means "internal principles that distinguish between right and wrong"?
   a. Ethics
   b. Morals
   c. Justice
   d. Nonmaleficence

3. ______ are codes of conduct stated by an employer or professional association.
   a. Personal ethics
   b. Morals
   c. Professional ethics
   d. Code of ethics

4. Which term means "to do no harm"?
   a. Autonomy
   b. Justice
   c. Nonmaleficence
   d. Beneficence

5. What is the process of creating a genetically identical biological entity?
   a. Genetic engineering
   b. Cloning
   c. Genetic testing
   d. Pharmacogenetics

6. Which Kübler-Ross stage of grief and dying involves the person refusing to accept the fact?
   a. Anger
   b. Depression
   c. Bargaining
   d. Denial

7. Which advance directive provides instructions about life-sustaining medical treatment to be administered or withheld when the patient has a terminal condition?
   a. Medical durable power of attorney
   b. Healthcare proxy
   c. Living will
   d. Organ donation

8. Which advance directive allows a competent adult to appoint a person (called a proxy or agent) to make healthcare decisions in the event the patient is unable to do so?
   a. Medical durable power of attorney
   b. Healthcare proxy
   c. Living will
   d. Organ donation

9. Which is the type of euthanasia where the patient consents to the action?
   a. Active
   b. Passive
   c. Voluntary
   d. Involuntary

10. Which act provides uniformity in organ and tissue donations across the nation?
    a. Patient Self-Determination Act
    b. Uniform Anatomical Gift Act
    c. Uniform Determination of Death Act
    d. National Organ Transplant Act

WORKPLACE APPLICATIONS

1. Mrs. Johnson called Walden-Martin Family Medical Clinic and Daniela answered the phone. Mrs. Johnson requested an appointment. She stated that she has experienced sleep changes, difficulty concentrating, sadness, and appetite changes since her husband died. Based on what you have read in this chapter, what might be occurring with Mrs. Johnson?

   ____

   ____

2. Jean is graduating from a medical assistant program. During her practicum, she heard about the dangers of narcotic medications. She does not believe that patients should receive narcotic medications. Jean is an advocate of alternative medications and feels there are reasonable alternatives to narcotic medications. How should Jean approach finding a job, given her bias?

   ____

   ____

3. Jan, a certified medical assistant, was discussing advance directives with a patient. The patient asked Jan to explain the importance of advance directives. How would you explain the importance of advance directives?

   ____

   ____

   ____

INTERNET ACTIVITIES

1. Using the internet, research your state's advance directive forms. Create a poster presentation, PowerPoint presentation, or paper summarizing the topic areas on the advance directive forms. Cite your resource(s).
2. Using the internet, research your state's Safe Haven laws for children. If your state does not have these laws, select a state that does. Create a poster presentation, PowerPoint presentation, or paper summarizing the Safe Haven laws. Focus on related statutes, maximum age of the child, and locations where the child can be brought. Cite your resource(s).
3. Using the internet, research an ethical issue. Create a poster presentation, PowerPoint presentation, or paper summarizing your findings. In your project, summarize the ethical issue and provide the advocates' and opponents' views of the issue.

Procedure 5.1 Developing an Ethics Separation Plan

Name ______________________________ **Date** ____________ **Score** __________

Task: To develop a plan for separation of personal and professional ethics.

Scenario: You are working at WMFM Clinic. Your provider sees many children, including teens. New state laws allow confidential healthcare for minors. The agency has now adopted policies and procedures to allow providers to see teens 16 years or older without parental consent. The teens can be seen for sexually transmitted infections (STIs) and reproductive issues (including birth control). All health records related to these visits are confidential, meaning parents cannot be told about their child's visit.

Your personal belief is that parents should always be allowed to know what is occurring with their children. They are responsible for the child until age 18, and they pay the bills. You also believe that children under 18 are too young to be in an intimate relationship, which should be reserved for adults who are committed to each other. You do not believe in birth control.

Equipment and Supplies:
- Paper and pen
- Medical Assisting Code of Ethics (see box in the textbook)

Standard: Complete the procedure and all critical steps with a minimum score of 85% within two attempts (*or as indicated by the instructor*).

Scoring: Divide the points earned by the total possible points. Failure to perform a critical step, indicated by an asterisk (*), results in grade no higher than an 84% (*or as indicated by the instructor*).

Steps/Criteria:	Point Value	Attempt 1	Attempt 2
1. Read the code of ethics for medical assistants. Write down key themes or phrases.	15		
2. Using the scenario, write down the professional ethics involved in the situation.	15		
3. Using the scenario, write down the personal ethics involved in the situation.	15		
4. Compare the lists. Identify the personal ethics that conflict with the code of ethics and the professional ethics of the agency.	15		
5. For each area of conflict, create a plan for how you will separate your personal and professional ethics. Remember, as a professional, you need to follow the professional ethics of the agency and the profession. Address how you will handle the situation and what your options would be if you were in the situation.	20*		
6. Describe how the personal ethics and morals in this scenario would impact patient care. • Describe how a medical assistant's personal ethics and morals could impact how that person provides care. • Describe how patient care may be altered or not up to the standard of care required. • Describe how a medical assistant could respond in a professional manner and maintain the standard of care and personal integrity.	20*		
Total Points	**100**		

Comments

CAAHEP Competencies	Step(s)
XI.P.1. Demonstrate professional response(s) to ethical issues	5
ABHES Competencies	**Step(s)**
4. Medical Law and Ethics g. Display compliance with the Code of Ethics of the profession	5

Procedure 5.2 Demonstrate Appropriate Response to Ethical Issues

Name ______________________________ **Date** __________ **Score** __________

Tasks: Identify ethical issues and demonstrate professional responses. Recognize the impact of personal ethics and morals on the delivery of healthcare.

Scenario 1: You are working at WMFM Clinic. You are responsible for collecting payments from patients. Mr. Smythe, who is visually impaired, paid for his visit in cash. He gives you $500 for a $402 bill. You make change and give him a receipt. At the end of the day, you notice that you have $60 more than what you should have, and some of the bills were mixed up in the cashbox. You realize you gave Mr. Smythe the incorrect amount of money.

Scenario 2: You are setting up a laceration repair tray for Dr. Martin to use. As you are preparing the sterile equipment, one of the instruments becomes contaminated. You know Dr. Martin urgently needs the tray. You do nothing about the contamination, which you realize can cause an infection. You finish setting up the tray.

Equipment and Supplies:
- Paper and pen

Standard: Complete the procedure and all critical steps in _______ minutes with a minimum score of 85% within two attempts (*or as indicated by the instructor*).

Scoring: Divide the points earned by the total possible points. Failure to perform a critical step, indicated by an asterisk (*), results in grade no higher than an 84% (*or as indicated by the instructor*).

Time: Began_________ Ended_________ Total minutes: _________

Steps:	**Point Value**	**Attempt 1**	**Attempt 2**
1. Read both scenarios. Identify and write down the ethical issues involved.	20		
2. With a peer, role-play scenario 1. Demonstrate a professional and appropriate ethical response to this situation. a. Explain the situation to the supervisor. b. Describe how you felt the error occurred and who received the incorrect change. c. Explain how you would like to handle the situation and correct the error.	30		
3. With a peer, role-play scenario 2. During the role-play, demonstrate a professional and appropriate ethical response to this situation.	30		
4. In a written response, discuss the potential implication for the patient's health related to not reporting or correcting the error in scenario 2.	20		
Total Points	100		

- Ethical issue(s) identified in scenario 1:______________________________

  ____

  ____

  ____

- Ethical issue(s) identified in scenario 2:____

____

____

____

- Discuss the potential implication for the patient's health related to not reporting or correcting the error.

____

____

____

____

____

____

____

____

____

Comments

CAAHEP Competencies	Step(s)
XI.P.1. Demonstrate professional response(s) to ethical issues	1-3
ABHES Competencies	**Step(s)**
4. Medical Law and Ethics g. Display compliance with the Code of Ethics of the profession	Entire procedure

Student Name________________________________ Date________________

Introduction to Medical Terminology and Anatomy

chapter 6

CAAHEP Competencies	Assessment
I.C.1. Identify structural organization of the human body	Skills and Concepts D. 11-14; Certification Preparation – 6; Case Scenario – 4
I.C.2. Identify body systems	Skills and Concepts – B. 14-25
I.C.3.a. Identify: body planes	Skills and Concepts – E. 2-5; Certification Preparation – 7
I.C.3.b. Identify: directional terms	Skills and Concepts – E. 6-15; Certification Preparation – 8
I.C.3.c. Identify: quadrants	Skills and Concepts – E. 25-28; Certification Preparation – 9
I.C.3.d. Identify: body cavities	Skills and Concepts – E. 17-24; Certification Preparation – 10
I.C.4. Identify major organs in each body system	Skills and Concepts – B. 1-13
V.C.8.a. Identify the following related to body systems: medical terms	Skills and Concepts – B. 26-36; C. 1-70

ABHES Competencies	Assessment
3. Medical Terminology a. Define and use the entire basic structure of medical terminology and be able to accurately identify the correct context (i.e., root, prefix, suffix, combinations, spelling and definitions)	Skills and Concepts – A. 1-61; B. 26-36; C. 1-70; Certification Preparation – 1-5; Workplace Applications – 1-2; Internet Activities – 1-2
3b. Build and dissect medical terminology from roots and suffixes to understand the word element combinations	Skills and Concepts – C. 1-48
3c. Apply medical terminology for each specialty	Skills and Concepts – B. 26-36; C. 1-70; Certification Preparation – 3, 5; Workplace Applications – 2; Internet Activities – 2
3d. Define and use medical abbreviations when appropriate and acceptable	Abbreviations – 1-6

VOCABULARY REVIEW

Using the word pool on the right, find the correct word to match the definition. Write the word on the line after the definition.

Group A

1. An abbreviation formed from the first letter of each word of a phrase and pronounced as a word ____________________
2. A word that come from the name of a person, place, or thing associated with the word ____________________
3. A shortened version of a word or phrase ____________________
4. Picture that represents a word or phrase ____________________
5. A word part found at the beginning of the word ____________________
6. A word part found at the end of the word ____________________
7. A word part that is the foundation of the term ____________________
8. A vowel that links the root to the suffix or a root to a root ____________________
9. A root and a combining vowel ____________________
10. A steady state that is created by all the body systems working together to provide a consistent and unvarying internal environment ____________________

Word Pool

- abbreviation
- acronym
- combining form
- combining vowel
- eponym
- homeostasis
- prefix
- root
- suffix
- symbol

Group B

1. Outer covering surrounding the cell that allows certain substances to enter the cell and blocks other substances ____________________
2. Study of disease ____________________
3. Wavelike motion ____________________
4. The microscopic study of body tissues ____________________
5. Rod-shaped structures found in the cell's nucleus; contain genetic information ____________________
6. Tests and procedures used to help diagnose or monitor a condition ____________________
7. A group of similar cells from the same source that together carry out a specific function ____________________
8. Structures inside of the cell ____________________
9. Jelly-like substance the surrounds the nucleus and fills the cells ____________________
10. A cell division process by which two daughter cells are formed from one parent cell ____________________

Word Pool

- chromosomes
- cytoplasm
- diagnostic procedures
- histology
- mitosis
- organelles
- pathology
- peristalsis
- plasma membrane
- tissue

Group C

1. A broad, dome-shaped muscle used for breathing that separates the thoracic and abdominopelvic cavities ______________________
2. Work to prevent changes in the pH ______________________
3. Reflects the number of newly diagnosed people with the disease ______________________
4. The cause of the disorder or disease ______________________
5. How often the disease occurs ______________________
6. A severe, sudden onset of a disease ______________________
7. Something that is only perceived by the patient; called *subjective data* ______________________
8. Substances that stimulate the production of an antibody when introduced into the body ______________________
9. A disease-causing organism ______________________
10. Something that is measured or observed by others; called *objective data* ______________________

Word Pool
- acute
- antigens
- buffers
- diaphragm
- etiology
- incidence
- pathogen
- prevalence
- signs
- symptoms

Group D

1. Substances created by microorganisms, plants, or animals and poisonous to humans ______________________
2. A rapidly dividing cancer cell that has little to no similarity to normal cells ______________________
3. A physician specially trained in the nature and cause of disease ______________________
4. Process of viewing living tissue that has been removed for the purpose of diagnosis or treatment ______________________
5. To spread from one part of the body (the primary tumor) to another part of the body forming a secondary tumor ______________________
6. Protein substances produced in the blood or tissues in response to a specific antigen that destroy or weaken the antigen ______________________
7. Describes how malignant tissue or cells looks like the normal tissue or cells it came from ______________________
8. A specially trained physician who diagnoses and treats cancer ______________________
9. Refers to how abnormal the malignant cells look ______________________
10. Refers to the extent of the cancer, including the size and if it has spread ______________________

Word Pool
- anaplastic
- antibodies
- biopsy
- differentiated
- grade
- metastasize
- oncologist
- pathologist
- toxins
- stage

ABBREVIATIONS

Write out what each of the following abbreviations stands for.

1. BP ____________________
2. CBC ____________________
3. HTN ____________________
4. AIDS ____________________
5. HIPAA ____________________
6. SIDS ____________________

SKILLS AND CONCEPTS

Answer the following questions.

A. Medical Terminology

1. Write the meaning of the following symbols.
   a. $\bar{s}$ ____________________
   b. $\bar{p}$ ____________________
   c. $\bar{a}$ ____________________

For the following word parts, write the definition.

2. ec- ____________________
3. contra- ____________________
4. end- ____________________
5. brady- ____________________
6. endo- ____________________
7. anti- ____________________
8. dia- ____________________
9. epi- ____________________
10. ante- ____________________
11. ana- ____________________
12. dys- ____________________
13. macro- ____________________
14. per- ____________________

15. hypo-__________
16. supra- __________
17. hyper- __________
18. megalo-__________
19. micro- __________
20. tachy- __________
21. mal-__________
22. -ac __________
23. -is__________
24. -stasis __________
25. -ary __________
26. -tension__________
27. -phagia __________
28. -al__________
29. -ism __________
30. -pathy __________
31. -plegia__________
32. -ent __________
33. -osis__________
34. -pnea__________
35. -ic__________
36. -dipsia__________

For the following definitions, write the medical terminology word part.

37. out __________
38. within __________
39. outside of __________
40. between __________
41. near, beside __________
42. four __________
43. together, with __________

44. beyond ____________________
45. one ____________________
46. through, across ____________________
47. instrument to record ____________________
48. instrument to view ____________________
49. tumor, mass ____________________
50. abnormal condition of hardening ____________________
51. process of, condition ____________________
52. process of recording ____________________
53. process of viewing ____________________
54. surgical fixation ____________________
55. to cut ____________________
56. new opening ____________________
57. one who specializes ____________________
58. study of ____________________
59. towards ____________________
60. crushing ____________________
61. suture repair ____________________

B. Combining Forms

Match the body system to the correct major organs and structures it includes.

1. _____ Mouth, tongue, teeth, pharynx, esophagus, stomach, small intestine, large intestine, liver, gallbladder, pancreas, and appendix
2. _____ Ovaries, fallopian tubes, uterus, vagina, vulva, mammary glands, and ovum
3. _____ Brain, spinal cord, neurons, neuroglia cells, peripheral nerves, and autonomic nerves
4. _____ Heart, valves, arteries, arterioles, veins, and venules
5. _____ Lymph, lymph vessels, lymph nodes, thymus, tonsils, spleen, lymphocytes, and antibodies
6. _____ Skin, subcutaneous tissue, sweat and sebaceous glands, hair, nails, and sense receptors
7. _____ Pituitary gland, pineal gland, hypothalamus, thyroid gland, pancreas, adrenal cortex and medulla, parathyroid gland, thymus gland, ovaries, and testes
8. _____ Bones, joints, tendons, ligaments, and cartilage
9. _____ Epididymis vas deferens, prostate gland, testes, scrotum, penis, urethra, and sperm
10. _____ Nephron unit, kidneys, ureters, bladder, and urethra
11. _____ Nose, sinuses, pharynx, larynx, trachea, bronchi, lungs, bronchioles, and alveoli
12. _____ Eyes, ears, taste buds, olfactory receptors, and sensory receptors
13. _____ Muscles

a. cardiovascular system
b. endocrine system
c. gastrointestinal system
d. integumentary system
e. lymphatic and immune system
f. muscular system
g. nervous system
h. reproductive system (female)
i. reproductive system (male)
j. respiratory system
k. sensory system
l. urinary system
m. skeletal system

Match the description of the body system to the correct body system.

14. _____ Produces hormones and is involved with reproduction.
15. _____ Produces hormones that circulate in the blood to target tissues that stimulate a particular action.
16. _____ Protects the body, acts as a sense organ, helps to retain body fluids, protects against infection, and helps regulate the body temperature.
17. _____ Involved with movement, regulation of blood calcium, and the formation of blood cells.
18. _____ Transport materials in the blood through the body. The components in the blood also fight infections and form clots.
19. _____ Breaks down, digests, and absorbs nutrients from food eaten.
20. _____ Controls body structures to maintain homeostasis and receives and processes information from other body structures.
21. _____ Eliminates nitrogenous waste and maintains the electrolyte, water, and acid-base balances.
22. _____ Delivers oxygen to the cells and removes carbon dioxide from the body.
23. _____ Gathers information through the sense of vision, hearing, balance, taste, and smell.
24. _____ Involved with heat production, and muscle contraction, tone, and posture.
25. _____ Maintains fluid balance, provides immunity to some diseases, and protects the internal environment of the body.

a. cardiovascular system
b. endocrine system
c. gastrointestinal system
d. integumentary system
e. lymphatic and immune system
f. skeletal system
g. nervous system
h. reproductive system
i. respiratory system
j. sensory system
k. urinary system
l. muscular system

For the following questions, write your answer on the line.

26. For the following cardiovascular system word parts, write the definition.

    a. aort/o ______________________________

    b. arteri/o ______________________________

    c. coron/o ______________________________

    d. phleb/o ______________________________

    e. plasm/o ______________________________

27. For the following endocrine system word parts, write the definition.

    a. hypophys/o ______________________________

    b. oophor/o ______________________________

    c. pancreat/o ______________________________

    d. parathyroid/o ______________________________

    e. thyroid/o ______________________________

28. For the following gastrointestinal system word parts, write the definition.
    a. col/o ____________________
    b. esophag/o____________________
    c. gastr/o____________________
    d. hepat/o ____________________
    e. pancreat/o ____________________
29. For the following integumentary system word parts, write the definition.
    a. cutane/o ____________________
    b. derm/o ____________________
    c. onych/o____________________
    d. pil/o____________________
    e. seb/o ____________________
30. For the following lymphatic system and immune system word parts, write the definition.
    a. lymph/o ____________________
    b. lymphangi/o ____________________
    c. myel/o____________________
    d. splen/o ____________________
    e. thym/o ____________________
31. For the following musculoskeletal system word parts, write the definition.
    a. arthr/o____________________
    b. crani/o____________________
    c. ligament/o ____________________
    d. lumb/o ____________________
    e. my/o ____________________
    f. oste/o ____________________
    g. stern/o____________________
    h. ten/o ____________________
    i. thorac/o ____________________
    j. vertebr/o____________________

32. For the following nervous system word parts, write the definition.

    a. cerebell/o ____________________

    b. cerebr/o ____________________

    c. encephal/o ____________________

    d. myel/o ____________________

    e. neur/o ____________________

33. For the following reproductive system word parts, write the definition.

    a. cervic/o ____________________

    b. colp/o ____________________

    c. mamm/o ____________________

    d. orch/o ____________________

    e. uter/o ____________________

34. For the following respiratory system word parts, write the definition.

    a. bronch/o ____________________

    b. cyan/o ____________________

    c. nas/o ____________________

    d. pulmon/o ____________________

    e. sin/o ____________________

35. For the following sensory system word parts, write the definition.

    a. audi/o ____________________

    b. blephar/o ____________________

    c. corne/o ____________________

    d. ot/o ____________________

    e. scler/o ____________________

36. For the following urinary system word parts, write the definition.

    a. cyst/o ____________________

    b. vesic/o ____________________

    c. nephr/o ____________________

    d. ren/o ____________________

    e. ureter/o ____________________

C. Building, Defining, and Pronouncing Medical Terms

In the table, combine the word parts and write in the new word and its definition.

Combining Form	Suffix	New Word	Definition
1. arteri/o	-stenosis		
2. cardi/o	-megaly		
3. angi/o	-oma		
4. angi/o	-graphy		
5. phleb/o	-itis		
6. epiglott/o	-itis		
7. valv/o	-itis		
8. arteri/o	-ole		
9. pneumon/o	-ia		
10. blephar/o	-itis		
11. mast/o	-itis		
12. an/o	-plasty		
13. col/o	-stomy		
14. col/o	-scopy		
15. thorac/o	-algia		
16. myel/o	-oma		
17. trache/o	-stenosis		
18. cyst/o	-itis		
19. enter/o	-rrhaphy		
20. glycos/o	-uria		
21. chondr/o	-malacia		
22. ankyl/o	-osis		
23. scler/o	-malacia		
24. appendic/o	-itis		

Combining Form	Suffix	New Word	Definition
25. irid/o	-plegia		
26. abdomen/o	-centesis		
27. col/o	-ectomy		
28. gastr/o	-stomy		
29. gingiv/o	-ectomy		
30. nephr/o	-oma		
31. rhin/o	-rrhagia		

Prefix	Combining Form	Suffix	New Word	Definition
32. endo-	cardi/o	-tis		
33. dys-	men/o	-rrhea		
34. brady-	cardi/o	-ia		
35. tachy-	cardi/o	-ia		
36. a-	men/o	-rrhea		
37. inter-	ventricul/o	-ar		

Combining Form	Combining Form	Suffix	New Word	Definition
38. my/o	cardi/o	-tis		
39. rhin/o	myc/o	-osis		
40. gastr/o	enter/o	-tis		

For the following words, split the word apart into word parts. Label each word part (e.g., prefix, suffix, and combining form). Define each word part.

41. efferent ____________________

42. proximal ____________________

43. unilateral ____________________

44. ventral ____________________

45. popliteal ____________________

46. gluteal ____________________

47. antecubital ____________________

48. ocular ____________________

For each of the following words, write the pluralized word on the line.

49. septum ____________________

50. ruga ____________________

51. fimbria ____________________

52. testis ____________________

53. alveolus ____________________

54. sulcus ____________________

55. canthus ____________________

56. conjunctiva ____________________

57. bacterium ____________________

58. labium ____________________

59. coccus ____________________

60. embolus ____________________

61. prognosis ____________________

62. scapula ____________________

63. acetabulum ____________________

64. diverticulum ____________________

65. axilla ____________________

66. glomerulus ____________________

67. phalanx ____________________

68. meniscus ____________________

69. verruca vulgaris ____________________

70. stratum ____________________

D. Structural Organization of the Body

1. The ____________________ is the basic unit of life.

2. Relate each of the parts of a cell to something found in a city. For instance, the plasma membrane would be the city limits or the walls of the city. In the space provided, draw the "Cell City" and label the structures. Use the cell parts listed in the textbook.

3. ____________________ is the process where one cell splits into two identical daughter cells.

4. At what stage of mitosis is the genetic information replicated?____________________

Match the phases of mitosis with the correct description.

5. _____ Spindle fibers pull the sister chromatids apart.
6. _____ The membrane around the nucleus starts to break down. Centrioles produce spindle fibers and start to move toward opposite sides of the cell.
7. _____ The nucleus reforms around each set of chromosomes. The cell continues to separate into two daughter cells.
8. _____ Each pair of chromatids lines up, and each chromatid is attached to a spindle fiber.

a. prophase
b. metaphase
c. anaphase
d. telophase

Write your answer on the line.

9. ____________________ is the jelly-like substance that surrounds the organelles and fills the cell.

10. ____________________ attach to the endoplasmic reticulum, giving the ER a rough appearance.

11. ____________________ are a group of similar cells from the same source that together carry out a specific function.

12. ____________________ is a structure composed of two or more types of tissue.

13. A(n) ______________________ is composed of several organs and their related structures.

14. Put the following in order from the simplest to the most complex: organism, organs, cells, body systems, tissue

    ____

E. Anatomical Position, Planes, Cavities and Quadrants

1. The ______________________ is a standard frame of reference. This means the body stands erect with the face forward, arms at the sides, palms forward, and toes pointed forward.
2. ______________________ are imaginary cuts or sections through the body.
3. The ______________________ or frontal plane divides the body into front and back portions.
4. The ______________________ or median plane divides the body into equal right and left halves.
5. The ______________________ or horizontal plane divides the body horizontally into an upper part and a lower part.

Match the following terms with the correct definition.

6. _____ Opposite of anterior and refers to the back
7. _____ Pertains to the midline
8. _____ Carrying toward a structure
9. _____ Front of body
10. _____ Far from the origin or farthest from the trunk of the body
11. _____ Towards the surface of the body
12. _____ Near the origin or toward the trunk of the body
13. _____ Away from the surface of the body
14. _____ Downward
15. _____ Opposite side

a. deep
b. anterior or ventral
c. interior
d. posterior or dorsal
e. afferent
f. distal
g. contralateral
h. medial
i. proximal
j. superficial

Write your answers on the line.

16. Using the directional and positional terms listed in this chapter, write four sentences that use a term in reference to the body. Use four different terms. Example: The fingers are distal to the elbows.

    ____

    ____

    ____

    ____

Match the cavity with the correct description.

17. _____ Contains the heart, lungs, esophagus, and trachea
18. _____ Contains the abdominal and pelvic cavities
19. _____ Contains the spinal cord
20. _____ Contains the thoracic and abdominopelvic cavities
21. _____ Contains the brain
22. _____ Contains the cranial and spinal cavities
23. _____ Contains the stomach, liver, gallbladder, and intestines
24. _____ Contains the urinary bladder and the reproductive organs

a. dorsal body cavity
b. ventral body cavity
c. cranial cavity
d. spinal cavity
e. thoracic cavity
f. abdominopelvic cavity
g. pelvic cavity
h. abdominal cavity

Match the quadrant with the organs found within the quadrant.

25. _____ The appendix, cecum, right ovary, right ureter, right spermatic cord, large intestine (ascending colon), right kidney
26. _____ The stomach, spleen, left lobe of liver, pancreas, left kidney, and large intestine (transverse and descending colon)
27. _____ The small intestine, large intestine (descending and sigmoid colon), left ovary, left ureter, left spermatic cord, and left kidney
28. _____ The right lobe of liver, gallbladder, right kidney, small intestine (duodenum), large intestine (ascending and transverse colon), head of pancreas

a. left upper quadrant
b. right upper quadrant
c. left lower quadrant
d. right lower quadrant

F. Acid-Base Balance

1. A solution with a pH under 7 is a(n) ______________________ solution.
2. A solution with a pH over 7 is a(n) ______________________ solution.
3. For the body to maintain homeostasis, a pH between ______________________ and ______________________ must be maintained in the blood.
4. Which of the following helps maintain the acid-base balance in the body?
   a. Urinary system
   b. Respiratory system
   c. Chemical buffers
   d. All of the above

G. Pathology Basics

Match the definition with the correct term.

1. _____ Something that is measured or observed by others; called *objective data*
2. _____ How often the disease occurs
3. _____ A severe, sudden onset of a disease
4. _____ Something that is only perceived by the patient; called *subjective data*
5. _____ A disease, disorder, or syndrome that lasts longer than 6 months
6. _____ Death
7. _____ Reflects the number of newly diagnosed people with the disease
8. _____ Illness

a. prevalence
b. incidence
c. morbidity
d. mortality
e. acute
f. chronic
g. sign
h. symptom

H. Causes of Disease

Match the definition with the correct term.

1. _____ Cellular structure is the same as the surrounding tissue. The tumor is encapsulated and grows slowly.
2. _____ Have anaplastic changes and are poorly differentiated; infiltrates and metastasizes. May grow at a slow, rapid, or very rapid rate.
3. _____ Refers to how abnormal the malignant cells look.
4. _____ A disease that cannot be transmitted from one person to another.
5. _____ Refers to the extent of the cancer, including the size and if it has spread.
6. _____ A disease that can be transmitted from one person to another.

a. grade
b. communicable disease
c. stage
d. benign tumor
e. malignant tumor
f. noncommunicable disease

CERTIFICATION PREPARATION

Circle the correct answer.

1. What does the prefix "sub-" mean?
   a. Forward, before
   b. Before, in front of
   c. Upward, above
   d. Under, less than

2. What does the suffix "-osis" mean?
   a. Tumor, mass
   b. Softening
   c. Abnormal condition
   d. Disease condition

3. What does the combining form "thromb/o" mean?
   a. Blood
   b. Clot
   c. Artery
   d. Blood cell

4. What does the combining form "olig/o" mean?
   a. Night
   b. Water
   c. Pain
   d. Scanty

5. What does the combining form "hemat/o" mean?
   a. Vein
   b. Blood
   c. Plasma
   d. Valve

6. What is the structural organization of the body from the simplest to the most complex?
   a. Organism, body system, tissues, organs, and cells
   b. Cells, organs, tissues, and body systems
   c. Cells, tissues, organs, body systems, and organism
   d. Cells, tissues, body systems, organs, and organism

7. Which plane divides the body horizontally into upper and lower sections?
   a. Frontal plane
   b. Median plane
   c. Midsagittal plane
   d. Transverse plane

8. ______ pertains to closer to the midline and ______ pertains to farther away from the midline.
   a. Anterior, posterior
   b. Superior, inferior
   c. Ipsilateral, contralateral
   d. Medial, lateral

9. Which quadrant contains the stomach, spleen, left lobe of the liver, pancreas, and left kidney?
   a. RUQ
   b. LUQ
   c. RLQ
   d. LLQ

10. Which cavity is part of the ventral body cavity and contains the heart and lungs?
    a. Spinal cavity
    b. Thoracic cavity
    c. Abdominopelvic cavity
    d. Cranial cavity

WORKPLACE APPLICATIONS

1. Daniela is learning suffixes. List ten suffixes that mean "pertaining to." ____________________

   ____

   ____

   ____

2. Daniela has floated to cardiology. Using the word parts in this chapter, create five medical terms for diseases a person might hear if working in a cardiology department.

   ____

   ____

   ____

3. Daniela was discussing directional terms with a peer in her class. She was explaining the importance of using directional terms in healthcare. Describe why directional terms are useful when documenting healthcare information.

   ____

   ____

   ____

   ____

4. Describe the organizational structure of the body from simple to complex.______________________

____

____

____

____

____

____

____

INTERNET ACTIVITIES

1. Using a reliable internet site, research healthcare related acronyms. Make a list of five acronyms.
2. Using a reliable internet site, identify 10 diseases that can be broken down into word parts. Make a list of the disease, then break down each disease name into word parts. Label each word part (e.g., prefix, suffix, root, combining vowel, and combining form). Define each word part.
3. Select one of the causes of disease (e.g., genetics, infectious pathogen). Using online resources, find four diseases that are caused by it. Research each disease and the cause of the disease. Create a paper, poster presentation, PowerPoint presentation, or storyboard based on your research.
4. Using online resources, research grading and staging of cancers. Create a short paper or PowerPoint presentation describing the difference between grading and staging.

Student Name________________________________ Date________________

chapter 7
Patient Coaching

CAAHEP Competencies	Assessments
V.C.5. Identify challenges in communication with different age groups	Skills and Concepts – C. 10-16
V.C.6. Identify techniques for coaching a patient related to specific needs	Skills and Concepts – C. 10-16; D. 1-6
V.C.10. Identify the role of the medical assistant as a patient navigator	Skills and Concepts – K. 4-5
V.C.13.b. Identify the basic concepts of the following theories: Erikson	Skills and Concepts – C. 2-9; Certification Preparation – 6; Workplace Applications – 1a-h.
V.C.13.c. Identify the basic concepts of the following theories: Kübler-Ross	Skills and Concepts – A. 1-10; Certification Preparation – 4
V.P.3.b. Coach patients regarding: medical encounters	Procedure 7.1
V.P.7. Use a list of community resources to facilitate referrals.	Procedure 7.2
X.P.3. Document patient care accurately in the medical record	Procedures 7.1, 7.2
A.4. Demonstrate active listening.	Procedure 7.1

ABHES Competencies	Assessments
5. Human Relations b. 3) List organizations and support groups that can assist patients and family members of patients experiencing terminal illnesses	Procedure 7.2
5.d. Adapt care to address the developmental stages of life	Procedure 7.1
8.h. Teach self-examination, disease management and health promotion	Procedure 7.1
8.i. Identify community resources and Complementary and Alternative Medicine practices (CAM)	Procedure 7.2
8.j. Make adaptations for patients with special needs (psychological or physical limitations)	Procedure 7.1
8.k. Make adaptations to care for patients across their lifespan	Procedure 7.1

VOCABULARY REVIEW

Using the word pool on the right, find the correct word to match the definition. Write the word on the line after the definition.

1. The act of sticking to something ____________________
2. The process of gaining new knowledge or skills through instruction, experience, or study ____________________
3. Patients are taking the right dose at the right times as prescribed by the provider ____________________
4. Bringing to an end ____________________
5. Provides personalized patient- and family-centered care in a team-based environment ____________________
6. The act of following through on a request or demand ____________________
7. The inability to feel or experience pleasure during a pleasurable activity ____________________
8. A person who identifies patients' barriers, works closely with the healthcare team and patients, and guides the patients through the healthcare system ____________________
9. The set of behaviors, ideas, and customs shared by a specific group of people, which distinguishes the members from other people ____________________
10. Focuses on the interrelationship among the physical, mental, social, and spiritual aspects of the person's life ____________________

Word Pool

- adherence
- anhedonia
- care coordination
- cessation
- compliance
- culture
- holistic approach
- learning
- medication adherence
- patient navigator

ABBREVIATIONS

Write out what each of the following abbreviations stands for.

1. Td ____________________
2. RZV ____________________
3. PCV13 ____________________
4. Tdap ____________________
5. PPSV23 ____________________
6. BSE ____________________
7. TSE ____________________
8. UV ____________________
9. PSA ____________________
10. DRE ____________________
11. AAA ____________________
12. PHQ-9 ____________________

13. NIH ______________________________

14. CDC ______________________________

15. ADA ______________________________

16. AHA ______________________________

17. HPV ______________________________

18. DEA ______________________________

19. FDA ______________________________

20. gFOBT ______________________________

21. FIT ______________________________

SKILLS AND CONCEPTS

Answer the following questions.

A. Making Changes for Health

Match the description and adaptive interactions with the correct stage of Kübler-Ross's theory. Answers can be used more than once.

1. _____ Person feels sad, fearful, and uncertain. They may grieve the loss of their health or independence.
2. _____ Refuse to accept the fact. May refuse to discuss the diagnosis.
3. _____ Has come to terms with situation.
4. _____ This emotion can be directed at self or others and surface at unrelated times.
5. _____ Attempts to negotiate with the higher power the person believes in (e.g., God).
6. _____ For this stage, provide handouts that explain the disease and treatment and encourage family support.
7. _____ For this stage, provide coaching on aspects of the disease and self-care management.
8. _____ For this stage, use therapeutic communication techniques to acknowledge the patient's feeling about the issue.
9. _____ For this stage, work with the healthcare team regarding the patient's requests.
10. _____ For this stage, encourage the patient to use the community and healthcare resources to help ease the change process.

a. denial
b. anger
c. bargaining
d. depression
e. acceptance

Select the correct answer.

11. The health belief model
    a. deals with a person's perception of their chance of developing a disease.
    b. deals with a person's perception of the severity of the disease.
    c. focuses on whether the person will take preventive action.
    d. all of the above

B. Domains of Learning

Match the domain of learning with the description of the domain. Answers can be used more than once.

1. _____ The "doing" domain
2. _____ The "feeling" domain
3. _____ Involves the mental processes of recall, application, and evaluation

a. cognitive domain
b. psychomotor domain
c. affective domain

Match the domain of learning with the tips that a medical assistant can use. Answers can be used more than once.

4. _____ Make sure that you address any barriers (e.g., pain) prior to educating a patient.
5. _____ Have the patient teach back the skill or do a return demonstration to check for accuracy.
6. _____ Have a family member present during the teaching.
7. _____ Present the information at an appropriate level for the patient.
8. _____ Present information in small chunks in a clear, well-organized manner.
9. _____ Build on the patient's prior knowledge about the topic.
10. _____ Repeated practice doing the skill helps with recall and retention of the steps.
11. _____ Provide the information in two different ways.
12. _____ Make sure to use the equipment and supplies the patient will be using at home.

a. cognitive domain
b. psychomotor domain
c. affective domain

Match the domain of learning with barriers to the domain and the strategies for adapting to barriers. Answers can be used more than once.

13. _____ Barriers include memory or cognitive issues.
14. _____ Barriers include anxiety, denial, fatigue, and stress.
15. _____ Barriers include cultural customs and previous experience.
16. _____ Barriers include language barriers.
17. _____ Barriers include tremors and paralysis.
18. _____ Barriers include visual and hearing impairments.
19. _____ Use adaptive equipment.
20. _____ Use an interpreter and provide handouts in the patient's primary language.

a. cognitive domain
b. psychomotor domain
c. affective domain

C. The Medical Assistant's Role in Coaching

1. When a medical assistant coaches a patient, it is important to
   a. recognize the patient is an individual.
   b. remember the patient has unique concerns.
   c. consider the barriers to learning.
   d. all of the above

Match the goal of the stage with the correct psychosocial developmental stages.

2. _____ Encourage to try new activities. Must assume responsibilities and learn new skills.
3. _____ To know who you are as a person and how you fit into the world around you. Creates a meaningful self-image.
4. _____ Must develop trust, with the ability to mistrust should the need arise.
5. _____ Must seek to finish tasks. Recognition for accomplishments is important.
6. _____ Must explore and manipulate things in their "world" to develop autonomy and self-esteem.
7. _____ Develops friendships; takes on commitments.
8. _____ Reflect on one's life and come to terms with it, instead of regretting the past.
9. _____ Achieve a balance between the concern for the next generation (having a family) and being self-absorbed.

a. Trust versus Mistrust
b. Autonomy versus Shame and Doubt
c. Initiative versus Guilt
d. Industry versus Inferiority
e. Identity versus Role Confusion
f. Intimacy versus Isolation
g. Generativity versus Stagnation
h. Ego Integrity versus Despair

Match the age group with the coaching strategies to use.

10. _____ Use engaging simple tools to communicate information.
11. _____ Provide privacy and independence. Promote responsible decision making and an honest discussion on lifestyle issues.
12. _____ Use a calm, soothing voice and hold patient securely.
13. _____ Use familiar words and simple explanations and demonstrations. Explain how the patient would sense the procedure.
14. _____ Use simple, familiar words, allow the patient to handle equipment, and make choices.
15. _____ Important to identify the patient's motivating factor to learn the new content.
16. _____ Communicate with dignity and respect; speak clearly and allow time for the patient to respond.

a. infants
b. toddlers
c. preschoolers
d. school-age children
e. adolescents
f. young and middle adults
g. older adults

D. Adapting Coaching for Communication Barriers

Match the communication barriers with the coaching strategies to use.

1. _____ Use a low-pitched voice and speak clearly, slowly, and distinctly. Pause between sentences or phrases. Speak naturally; do not shout.
2. _____ Use an interpreter or an interpretation service. Focus on the patient and not on the interpreter.
3. _____ Use translated materials.
4. _____ Face the patient directly. Make eye contact, if culturally appropriate. Use a normal tone of voice.
5. _____ Speak louder if you are wearing a mask.
6. _____ Provide the patient with large-print directions or brochures.

a. impaired vision
b. impaired hearing
c. language barriers

E. Cultural Diversity

1. What are factors affected by a person's culture that can impact healthcare?
   a. Role of the family and community
   b. Religion and beliefs regarding sexuality, fertility, and childbirth
   c. Views on health, wellness, death, dying, and complementary therapies
   d. All of the above
2. ______________________ involves applying suction to the skin, which can leave marks.
3. ______________________ involves applying firm pressure on specific points on the body.
4. ______________________ involves inserting fine needles into specific sites on the body.

F. Teaching-Learning Process

Match the steps in coaching a patient relevant to an individual patient's need with the description. Answers can be used more than once.

1. _____ First step in the teaching-learning process.
2. _____ Second step in the teaching-learning process.
3. _____ Third step in the teaching-learning process.
4. _____ Fourth step in the teaching-learning process.
5. _____ Fifth step in the teaching-learning process.
6. _____ Summarize the coaching provided in the patient's health record.
7. _____ Start with the basics and build from there. Keep the information simple and focused.
8. _____ After coaching on the topic, have the patient summarize what was stated. Obtain feedback from the patient during the coaching to determine if they understand the content.
9. _____ Consider the patient's individual needs and identify strategies to overcome issues that may impact the coaching.
10. _____ Identify what the patient needs to learn, the patient's motivation and concerns, and the patient's learning styles.

a. evaluating the patient's learning
b. identifying barriers to learning
c. identifying the patient's educational needs
d. documenting the coaching
e. coaching the patient on the topic

G. Coaching on Disease Prevention

1. Tetanus and diphtheria (Td) is given every ________ years.

2. Recombinant zoster vaccine schedule includes ________ doses for adults age 50 or older.

3. 13-valent pneumococcal conjugate vaccine (PCV13) involves ______ dose(s) usually after age 65 unless given before based on the patient's health.

4. What is incorrect regarding the CDC's respiratory hygiene/cough etiquette?
   a. Cover your mouth and nose with your sleeve when coughing or sneezing.
   b. Discard any tissues used in the nearest waste container.
   c. Wash your hands or use hand sanitizer.
   d. All of the above

5. ________________________ is the most reliable way to prevent STIs.

6. ________________________ tobacco includes chewing tobacco, moist snuff, snus, and moist powder tobacco.

7. Which statement is incorrect regarding nicotine?
   a. Nicotine is readily absorbed into the blood.
   b. Nicotine triggers the release of epinephrine, which stimulates the central nervous system.
   c. Epinephrine will lower the blood pressure and respiration and pulse rates.
   d. Nicotine increases the level of dopamine in the brain, helping the person feel happy and focused.

8. ________________________ causes lung cancer, strokes, low-birth-weight babies, and heart disease.

9. ________________________ is the residue or chemicals from the smoke that gets on skin, clothing, furniture, carpeting, and so on.

H. Coaching on Self-Exams for Health Maintenance and Wellness

1. Women with an average risk of breast cancer should have yearly mammograms between age _______ and _______.

2. ________________________ is the most dangerous type of skin cancer.

3. What is *not* a risk factor for skin cancer?
   a. Family or personal history of skin cancer
   b. Exposure to sun through work or play
   c. Brown eyes
   d. Skin that is lighter than normal color with freckles

4. What is not a sign or symptom of oral cancer?
   a. White or red patches in the mouth or on the gums
   b. Numbness or pain in the mouth
   c. Short-term hoarseness or sore throat
   d. Swelling in the jaw area or constant earache

I. Coaching on Screening for Health Maintenance and Wellness

1. People age 18-39 years should have a blood pressure check every _______ to _______ years.

2. Adults with no history of high cholesterol should have it checked every _______ to _______ years.
3. Adults 45 years and older with normal risk should have a fecal stool test (e.g., gFOBT) every _______ or a stool DNA test (Cologuard) every _______ years.
4. Adults 45 years and older with normal risk should have a colonoscopy every _______ years.
5. A dental exam and cleaning are recommended _______________________.
6. For women ages 30-65, a Pap test is recommended every 5 years if the _______________________ test is also done.
7. Type 2 diabetes mellitus screening should be done every _______ years starting at age 18.
8. What is *not* a risk factor for hepatitis C?
   a. Born between 1935 and 1965
   b. History of a blood transfusion or organ transplantation before 1992
   c. Use of injected illegal drugs
   d. Chronic liver disease, HIV, or AIDS
9. An alcoholic drink is classified as a(n) _______________________ of beer, a(n) _______________________ of wine, or a(n) _______________________ of liquor.
10. What is correct regarding intimate partner violence?
   a. Male and females can be victims of domestic abuse.
   b. Substance abuse, obesity, and depression can come from violence.
   c. Intimate partner violence includes controlling behaviors, physical abuse, and sexual abuse.
   d. All of the above

Match the type of elder abuse and neglect with the signs.

11. _____ Leaving the person in a public place
12. _____ Malnutrition, dehydration, lack of proper living conditions, and failing to treat health problems
13. _____ Unexplained sexually transmitted infections, bruising in the genital region, and reports from the older person
14. _____ Stealing from the older person, forging signatures on financial transactions, and any other illegal action that represents a financial loss for the older person
15. _____ Fractures, rope marks, cuts, bruising, dislocations, broken glasses, giving too little or too much medication, bleeding, and sudden changes in the person's personality or behavior
16. _____ Not communicating, withdrawn, agitated, and symptoms that mimic dementia

a. physical abuse
b. sexual abuse
c. emotional abuse
d. neglect
e. abandonment
f. financial abuse

J. Coaching on Diagnostic Tests and Treatment Plans

Match the procedure with the description.

1. _____ Uses x-rays to create pictures of cross-sections of the body. May require IV or oral contrast medium.
2. _____ Uses low-dose x-ray test that measures calcium and other minerals in the bone.
3. _____ An x-ray picture of the breasts used to find tumors.
4. _____ Uses powerful magnets and radio waves to create images of the body.
5. _____ Imaging test that uses an IV radioactive substance (tracer) to identify disease in the organs and tissues.
6. _____ Detects electrical activity in the brain using electrodes that are placed on the scalp.

a. mammography
b. MRI
c. EEG
d. PET
e. CT scan
f. bone density scan

Match the medical laboratory test with the common patient preparations. Answers may be used more than once.

7. _____ No preparation required.
8. _____ May need to fast overnight. May need to refrain from eating meat for a period of time.
9. _____ May require NPO (except for water) prior to the test.
10. _____ Two days prior to the test, refrain from sexual intercourse.
11. _____ Specimen is collected by the patient and returned to a specific medical laboratory for testing.
12. _____ Two days prior to the test, the patient should not douche or use vaginal medications or spermicidal products.

a. creatinine
b. lipid profile
c. Pap test
d. Cologuard stool DNA test

Select the correct answer.

13. When coaching patients on treatments to do at home, a medical assistant may need to discuss
    a. ways to remember to take medications.
    b. safely discarding used needles.
    c. safely discarding expired or unwanted medications.
    d. all of the above.

14. Which of the following should *not* be done when a patient is monitoring their blood pressure at home?
    a. Relax for 5 minutes before taking a blood pressure reading.
    b. Avoid caffeine and exercise for 15 minutes before the reading.
    c. Use the same area for the BP reading.
    d. Avoid smoking for 30 minutes before the reading.

15. Which of the following should be done when a patient is monitoring their blood pressure at home?
    a. Keep legs uncrossed and support the back and feet.
    b. Empty a full bladder and refrain from talking during the procedure.
    c. Use the correct cuff size and place the cuff on a bare arm.
    d. All of the above.

K. Care Coordinator

1. What is an advantage of care coordination?
   a. Greater efficiency in providing patient care
   b. Reduced cost and better patient care
   c. Encourages patients to focus on goals and self-management
   d. All of the above

2. The care coordinator communicates between the ______________________ and the ______________________.

3. A patient navigator has been described as a type of ______________________.

4. Which of the following is a role for the medical assistant as a patient navigator/care coordinator?
   a. Provide patients with resources based on their needs and barriers.
   b. Schedule and sequence appointments.
   c. Discuss special needs patients have with their healthcare team.
   d. All of the above.

5. Which of the following is a role for the medical assistant as a patient navigator/care coordinator?
   a. Interview patients to identify their needs and barriers to wellness and healthcare.
   b. Make sure the required information is communicated to and from specialty departments.
   c. Identify community resources for the patient.
   d. All of the above.

CERTIFICATION PREPARATION

Circle the correct answer.

1. Coaching provides patients with
   a. skills.
   b. knowledge.
   c. support and confidence.
   d. all of the above.

2. Providing patients with information on routine screenings and showing patients how to do self-exams is what type of coaching?
   a. Disease prevention
   b. Health maintenance
   c. Diagnostic tests
   d. Specific needs

3. Providing patients with information on respiratory hygiene practices, recommended vaccines, and nicotine cessation is what type of coaching?
   a. Disease prevention
   b. Health maintenance
   c. Diagnostic tests
   d. Specific needs

4. When a patient is experiencing sadness and uncertainty when grieving, what stage of Kübler-Ross' theory is the person in?
   a. Denial
   b. Anger
   c. Bargaining
   d. Depression

5. Language barriers are barriers to learning in the ________ domain.
   a. psychomotor
   b. affective
   c. cognitive
   d. a and c

6. According to Erikson's theory, an adolescent is in which stage?
   a. Identity versus Role Confusion
   b. Intimacy versus Isolation
   c. Industry versus Inferiority
   d. Generativity versus Stagnation

7. What colorectal cancer screening test requires no patient preparation and consists of a computer analysis that checks the stool for cancer and precancerous cells?
   a. gFOBT
   b. FIT
   c. PET
   d. Cologuard stool DNA test

8. Which imaging procedure uses x-rays to create pictures of cross-sections of the patient's body?
   a. X-ray
   b. Computed tomography scan
   c. Magnetic resonance imaging
   d. Mammography

9. What diagnostic test provides an x-ray picture of the breasts and is used to find tumors?
   a. X-ray
   b. Computed tomography scan
   c. Magnetic resonance imaging
   d. Mammography

10. What diagnostic test uses high-frequency sound waves to create an image of the organs and structures?
    a. Ultrasound
    b. Computed tomography scan
    c. Magnetic resonance imaging
    d. Mammography

WORKPLACE APPLICATIONS

1. Working in family medicine, Suzanne works with people of all ages. Describe tips to remember when coaching/working with patients of the following ages.
   a. 1-year-old ____________________
   ____
   b. 2-year-old ____________________
   ____
   c. 5-year-old ____________________
   ____
   d. 8-year-old ____________________
   ____
   e. 14-year-old ____________________
   ____
   f. 30-year-old ____________________
   ____
   g. 72-year-old ____________________
   ____
   ____

2. Suzanne is coaching a patient about the early warning signs of malignant melanoma. Describe the ABCDE rule.

____

____

____

____

INTERNET ACTIVITIES

1. Using the FDA website (https://www.fda.gov/), research "disposal of unused medications" in the home environment. Create a poster, PowerPoint, or paper summarizing your research. Focus on these areas:
   a. Using authorized collectors for disposal (e.g., take-back programs)
   b. Disposal in household trash
   c. Disposing of fentanyl patches
2. Using the CDC website (https://www.cdc.gov/), research recommended immunizations for children. Create a poster, PowerPoint, or paper summarizing your research. Focus on five recommended childhood immunizations and address the following for each:
   a. Name of immunization
   b. Why is it recommended or what does it prevent?
   c. Schedule of the vaccine (or the ages when a child should receive the immunization)
   d. Side effects of the vaccine
3. Using the CDC website (https://www.cdc.gov/), research recommended immunizations. Create a poster, PowerPoint, or paper summarizing your research. Focus on immunizations prior to, during, and after pregnancy.
   a. What is recommended? Why is it recommended?
   b. What is not recommended?

Procedure 7.1 Coach a Patient on Disease Prevention

Name ______________________ **Date** __________ **Score** __________

Tasks: Coach a patient on the recommended vaccinations for their age. Adapt the coaching for any communication barrier and the patient's developmental life stage. Document the coaching in the patient's health record.

Scenario: You are working with Dr. David Kahn. You need to room Charles Johnson (date of birth [DOB] 03/03/19XX), and his record indicates he has not been seen in several years. Charles has significant hearing loss, and he communicates by signing. His wife interprets for him. You look in his health record and see that he is due for influenza, Td, and recombinant zoster (shingles) vaccines. Per the provider's standing order, you need to coach adult patients on potential vaccines they are due for during the initial rooming process.

Directions: Role-play this scenario with two peers, who will play Charles and his wife. You are the medical assistant.

Equipment and Supplies:
- Vaccine Information Statements (VIS) (available at https://www.immunize.org/vis/)
- Patient's health record

Standard: Complete the procedure and all critical steps in _______ minutes with a minimum score of 85% within two attempts (*or as indicated by the instructor*).

Scoring: Divide the points earned by the total possible points. Failure to perform a critical step, indicated by an asterisk (*), results in grade no higher than an 84% (*or as indicated by the instructor*).

Time: Began_________ Ended_________ Total minutes: _________

Steps:	**Point Value**	**Attempt 1**	**Attempt 2**
1. Wash hands or use hand sanitizer.	**5**		
2. Greet the patient. Identify yourself. Verify the patient's identity with full name and date of birth. Explain what you will be doing.	**10**		
3. Arrange the chairs so the patient can see both you and the person signing. Speak slowly. Pause as needed to allow person signing to finish with the last statement. Look at the patient when communicating.	**15**		
4. Use simpler language when talking. Speak clearly and respectfully, while maintaining the patient's dignity. Allow time for the patient to respond. Listen to the patient's concerns. Use active listening skills. Use appropriate eye contact. Focus on the patient and avoid distractions. (*Refer to the Affective Behaviors Checklist – Respect and Active Listening and the Grading Rubric*)	**15***		
5. Ask the patient if he has received vaccines somewhere else over the past few years.	**5**		
Scenario update: Patient has not seen any healthcare providers over the last few years. The only vaccines received were given in this facility. 6. Describe the vaccines that are due. Use the VIS for each vaccine as you coach the patient on the purpose of the vaccine.	**15***		

Scenario update: The patient knows the shingles vaccine is not covered and costs more than $200. He refuses the shingles vaccine, and he does not believe in getting the influenza vaccine. He is interested in getting the Td vaccine. 7. Ask the patient which vaccines he is interested in getting. If he refuses, be respectful of his choice. Any reason he gives for the refusal should be communicated to the provider.	**15**		
8. Document the coaching in the patient's health record. Include the provider's name, what was taught, how the patient responded, and any vaccines refused.	**20**		
Total Points	**100**		

Affective Behavior	**Affective Behaviors Checklist** ***Directions:*** *Check behaviors observed during the role-play.*					
Respect	**Negative, Unprofessional Behaviors**	**Attempt 1**	**Attempt 2**	**Positive, Professional Behaviors**	**Attempt 1**	**Attempt 2**
	Rude, unkind, fake/false attitude, disrespectful, impolite, unwelcoming			Courteous, sincere, polite, welcoming		
	Unconcerned with person's dignity; brief, abrupt			Maintained person's dignity; took time with person		
	Unprofessional verbal communication; inappropriate questions			Professional verbal communication		
	Negative nonverbal behaviors, poor eye contact			Positive nonverbal behaviors, proper eye contact		
	Other:			Other:		
Active Listening	Biased, offensive			Remained neutral		
	Interrupted			Refrained from interrupting		
	Did not allow for silence or pauses			Allowed for periods of silence		
	Negative nonverbal behaviors (rolled eyes, yawned, frowned, avoided eye contact)			Positive nonverbal behaviors (smiled, nodded head, appropriate eye contact)		
	Distracted (looked at watch, phone)			Focused on patient, avoided distractions		
	Other:			Other:		

Grading Rubric for the Affective Behaviors Checklist **Directions:** *Based on checklist results, identify the points received for the procedure checklist. Indicate how the behaviors demonstrated met the expectations.*		**Points for Procedure Checklist**	**Attempt 1**	**Attempt 2**
Does not meet Expectation	• Response lacked respect or active listening. • Student demonstrated more than 2 negative, unprofessional behaviors during the interaction.	0		
Needs Improvement	• Response lacked respect or active listening. • Student demonstrated 1 or 2 negative, unprofessional behaviors during the interaction.	0		
Meets Expectation	• Response was respectful. Demonstrated active listening.. No negative, unprofessional behaviors observed. • More practice is needed for behavior to appear natural and for student to appear comfortable and at ease.	15		
Occasionally Exceeds Expectation	• Response was respectful. Demonstrated active listening, professional nonverbal communication. No negative, unprofessional behaviors observed. • At times student appeared comfortable and at ease; but more practice is needed for behavior to become natural and consistent with a professional medical assistant.	15		
Always Exceeds Expectation	• Response was respectful. Demonstrated active listening, professional nonverbal communication. No negative, unprofessional behaviors observed. • Student's behaviors appeared natural and comfortable. Behaviors are consistent with a professional medical assistant.	15		

Documentation

Comments

CAAHEP Competencies	Step(s)
V.P.3.b. Coach patients regarding: medical encounters	Entire procedure
X.P.3. Document patient care accurately in the medical record	8
A.4. Demonstrate active listening.	4
ABHES Competencies	**Step(s)**
5.d. Adapt care to address the developmental stages of life	4
8.h. Teach self-examination, disease management and health promotion	6
8.j. Make adaptations for patients with special needs (psychological or physical limitations)	3, 4
8.k. Make adaptations to care for patients across their lifespan	4

Procedure 7.2 Develop a List of Community Resources and Facilitate Referrals

Name ______________________ **Date** __________ **Score** __________

Tasks: As a patient navigator, develop a current list of community resources that meet the patient's health-care needs. Discuss the resources with the patient and facilitate referrals to the chosen resources.

Scenario 1: Robert Caudill (DOB 10/31/19XX) was just diagnosed with dementia. He currently lives with his daughter, Ruby, who works full time. Ruby is feeling overwhelmed with being his only caregiver and realizes that she needs to find someone to care for her father while she is working.

Scenario 2: Leslie Green (DOB 08/03/20XX) just tested positive for pregnancy. She does not feel that she has a support system to help her make decisions.

Scenario 3: Ella Rainwater's husband of 30 years died suddenly 1 month ago. Ella (DOB 07/11/19XX) stated that she feels alone and has no one to talk to. Her daughter feels that Ella needs the support of others who have gone through the same thing.

Directions: The instructor will assign each student a scenario. For steps 1 and 2, research resources for the scenario. For the remaining steps, role-play the scenario with two peers.

Equipment and Supplies:
- Computer with Internet or a telephone book
- Paper and pen
- Community Resource Referral Form (Work Product 7.1) or referral form
- Patient's health record

Standard: Complete the procedure and all critical steps in _______ minutes with a minimum score of 85% within two attempts (*or as indicated by the instructor*).

Scoring: Divide the points earned by the total possible points. Failure to perform a critical step, indicated by an asterisk (*), results in grade no higher than an 84% (*or as indicated by the instructor*).

Time: Began_________ Ended_________ Total minutes: _________

Steps:	**Point Value**	**Attempt 1**	**Attempt 2**
1. Using the assigned scenario, identify the possible types of community resources that would assist the patient or family. Identify three different types of resources (e.g., medical equipment, support group) that would meet the patient's needs.	**5**		
2. Using the Internet or the phone book, identify two local resources for each of the three kinds of resources (i.e., find two assisted living resources, two medical equipment suppliers, and so on). Make a list of six resources for the patient and family. Include the following: a. Organization's name b. Address and contact information c. Summary of the services provided d. Cost and other relevant information	**30**		
Scenario update: Role-play the scenario indicated by the instructor. 3. Provide the patient or family member with the list of six resources. Describe the services offered and any costs.	**15***		

4. Allow the patient or family member time to review the services. Answer any questions.	**10**		
5. Use professional, tactful verbal and nonverbal communication as you work with the patient or family member.	**10***		
6. Role-play making the community referrals. Have the patient or family member decide on two or more services they are interested in. Complete the referral document. Have the patient provide any additional information required on the form. Call the community resource agency and provide the referral information to the representative (a peer).	**20***		
7. Document the patient education and the referrals in the health record.	**10**		
Total Points	**100**		

Documentation

Comments

CAAHEP Competencies	Step(s)
V.P.7. Use a list of community resources to facilitate referrals.	3-6
X.P.3. Document patient care accurately in the medical record	7
ABHES Competencies	**Step(s)**
5. Human Relations b.3) List organizations and support groups that can assist patients and family members of patients experiencing terminal illnesses	1, 2
8.i. Identify community resources and Complementary and Alternative Medicine practices (CAM)	1, 2

Work Product 7.1 Community Resource Referral Form

To be used with Procedure 7.2.

Name ______________________ **Date** __________ **Score** __________

Patient's Name: Date of Birth:

Community Resource Information:

Agency: ____________ Contact Name: ____________

Address: ____________ Phone number: ____________

____________ Website: ____________

Services Provided:

Agency: ____________ Contact Name: ____________

Address: ____________ Phone number: ____________

____________ Website: ____________

Services Provided:

Agency: ____________ Contact Name: ____________

Address: ____________ Phone number: ____________

____________ Website: ____________

Services Provided:

Agency: ____________ Contact Name: ____________

Address: ____________ Phone number: ____________

____________ Website: ____________

Services Provided:

Student Name______________________________ Date______________

Technology

chapter 8

CAAHEP Competencies	Assessment
V.C.15. Identify the medical assistant's role in telehealth	Skills and Concepts – I. 19
VI.C.5. Identify the importance of data back-up	Skills and Concepts – J. 6-7
VI.C.6. Identify the components of an Electronic Medical Record, Electronic Health Record, and Practice Management System	Skills and Concepts – I. 10-17; Certification Preparation – 4-5
XII.C.7.b. Identify principles of: ergonomics	Skills and Concepts – H. 1-8

ABHES Competencies	Assessment
7. Administrative Procedure h. Perform basic computer skills	Procedure 8.2
8. Clinical Procedures a. Practice standard precautions and perform disinfection/sterilization techniques	Procedure 8.1

VOCABULARY REVIEW

Using the word pool on the right, find the correct word to match the definition. Write the word on the line after the definition.

Group A

1. Any peripheral hardware that allows the user to provide data to the computer ______________________
2. A set of electronic instructions to operate and perform different computer tasks ______________________
3. A pen-shaped device with a variety of tips that is used on touchscreens to write, draw, or enter commands ______________________
4. An electronic record that conforms to nationally recognized standards and contains health-related information about a specific patient; can be created, managed, and consulted by authorized clinicians and staff from more than one healthcare organization ______________________

Word Pool

- electronic health record (EHR)
- hardware
- input device
- optical character recognition
- output device
- patient portal
- secondary storage devices
- software
- stylus
- telemedicine

5. Computer hardware that displays the processed data from the computer (e.g., monitors and printers) ______________________
6. The remote diagnosis and treatment of patients using technology ______________________
7. A secure online website that gives patients 24-hour access to personal health information using a username and password ______________________
8. Scanners convert images to digital text through this process ______________________
9. Media (e.g., jump drive, flash drive, hard drive) capable of permanently storing data until they are replaced or deleted by the user ______________________
10. Physical equipment of the computer system required for communication and data processing functions ______________________

Group B

1. A computer application that allows the user to enter demographic information, schedule appointments, maintain lists of insurance payers, perform billing tasks, and generate reports ______________________
2. A system that links personal computers and peripheral devices to share information and resources ______________________
3. Peripheral computer hardware that connects to the router to provide internet access to the network or computer ______________________
4. A personal computer that doesn't contain a hard drive and allows the user only limited functions including access to software, the network, or the internet ______________________
5. Files are copied onto many servers in various locations ______________________
6. Computer hardware and software that perform data analysis, storage, and archiving; also called a *database server* ______________________
7. A private computer network that can only be accessed by authorized people ______________________
8. A collection of data or program records stored as a unit with a specific name ______________________
9. Used to allow multiple devices to be on the same network to send and receive information ______________________
10. A communication system for connecting several computers so information can be shared ______________________

Word Pool

- computer network
- data server
- downtime
- dumb terminal
- electronic medical record (EMR)
- ethernet
- file
- intranet
- modem
- practice management software (PMS)
- protected health information
- redundancy
- router

11. An electronic record of health-related information about an individual that can be created, gathered, managed, and accessed by authorized clinicians and staff members within a single healthcare organization; also called *EMR* ______________________

12. The interval of time during which something, such as hardware or software, is not functioning ______________________

13. Individually identifiable health information stored or transmitted by covered entities or business associates. Includes verbal, paper, or electronic information ______________________

ABBREVIATIONS

Write out what each of the following abbreviations stands for.

1. EHR ______________________
2. PC ______________________
3. ADF ______________________
4. NPP ______________________
5. LCD ______________________
6. CPU ______________________
7. ROM ______________________
8. RAM ______________________
9. HDD ______________________
10. USB ______________________
11. RW ______________________
12. TB ______________________
13. LAN ______________________
14. WAN ______________________
15. ISP ______________________
16. DSL ______________________

SKILLS AND CONCEPTS

Answer the following questions. Write your answer on the line or in the space provided.

A. Computers

Match the type of computer to the description.

1. _____ Large tower computers that are used by large organizations to store large quantities of information
2. _____ Smaller computers that have their own central processing unit (CPU)
3. _____ Expensive, very large computers that have incredibly fast processing speeds
4. _____ Large multiprocessing machines that support about 200 users at a time
5. _____ Computers that can be carried, such as laptops, netbooks, tablets, and smartphones

a. mobile computer
b. personal computer
c. minicomputer
d. mainframe computer
e. supercomputer

Fill in the blank.

6. A server can also be a(n) ____________________.
7. The personal computer is a(n) ____________________, or the primary computer equipment and all other forms of physical equipment used with the PC are called ____________________.

B. Input Devices

1. Which is *not* an input device?
   a. Printer and monitor
   b. Keyboard and mouse
   c. Touchscreen and signature pad
   d. Webcam and microphone

Fill in the blank.

2. For a radiofrequency connection to work, a(n) ____________________ must be plugged into the Universal Serial Bus (USB) drive on the device.
3. ____________________ uses shortwave radio frequencies to interconnect wireless electronic devices.
4. A touchscreen allows a person to interact with the computer by touching the display screen with a finger or ____________________.
5. A(n) ____________________ or smart pen is a battery-operated device that looks like and functions like a regular pen but can also digitally capture handwriting or drawing.
6. The remote diagnosis and treatment of patients using technology is called ____________________, a form of telehealth.
7. Scanners convert images to digital text through a process called ____________________.

C. Output Devices

1. Which of the following is an output device?
   a. Monitor
   b. Speakers
   c. Printer
   d. All of the above

Fill in the blank.

2. Images are created on monitors using ______________________; the ______________________ the number, the sharper the image.

3. A laser printer uses a(n) ______________________, ______________________, and ______________________ to produce images on paper.

D. Internal Computer Components

Fill in the blank.

1. The ______________________ is the "brain" of the computer and it sits on the ______________________.

2. The hard drive, ______________________ of the computer, contains the operating system and the related system fields.

Match the primary memory with the correct description.

3. _____ Main working memory; lost if power is turned off
4. _____ Provides temporary use of information; contains data and instructions for opened programs
5. _____ Contains memory that has hardwire instructions. Not lost if power is cut, since a small long-life battery supports it
6. _____ Used for loading and running programs
7. _____ Allows programs to operate more quickly and efficiently
8. _____ Used to boot a computer or start the system diagnostic checks

a. read-only memory (ROM)
b. cache memory
c. random access memory (RAM)

E. Secondary Storage Devices and Cloud Storage

1. A(n) ______________________ is usually considered a character, such as a number, letter, or symbol.

2. Put these data storage capacities in order from smallest to largest: MB, GB, TB, KB__________________

____

3. ______________________, also called file sharing or online storage; allows computer files to be stored using the internet and a third-party service.

4. The advantage of having the healthcare facility's computer environment on the cloud is
   a. the user can access the healthcare facility's computer environment from any location with web access and through a wired or wireless connection.
   b. Access can occur at any time of the day.
   c. All of the above

F. Network and Internet Access Devices

1. The intranet allows the employers to ______________________ with each other and share ______________________.

2. Only ______________________ can access the intranet or network in a healthcare facility.

3. A(n) ______________________ must be used to allow multiple devices to be on the same network.

4. For a healthcare facility's computer network to access the internet, they need to subscribe to a(n) ______________________ and to have its router connected to a(n) ______________________.

G. Maintaining Computer Hardware

1. What is a way to prevent computer problems?
   a. Hardware should be located on a stable, even surface, away from heat sources.
   b. Ventilation slots should be clear, allowing air to flow into the device to cool the components.
   c. Cables and electric cords should be securely plugged in.
   d. Liquids and food should be kept away from the hardware.
   e. All of the above

2. How should the hardware's casing be cleaned?
   a. Use a damp lint-free cloth to wipe the hardware's casing to remove the grime and dirt.
   b. Wipe clean all vents and air holes.
   c. All of the above

3. What is an infection control practice for technological devices in the ambulatory care facility?
   a. Disinfect keyboards daily.
   b. Healthcare professionals should sanitize hands before and after using keyboards.
   c. Gloves should not be worn during computer use.
   d. Touchscreen computer monitors and signature pads should be cleaned and disinfected daily per the manufacturer's guidelines.
   e. All of the above

H. Computer Workstation Ergonomics

1. ______________________ is the field of study that involves reducing strain and injuries by improving workstation design.

2. The ______________________ should help support the upper body and the backrest lumbar support area should be fitted to the small of the back

3. The ______________________ should support the forearms with the shoulders in a relaxed position.

4. The torso and neck should be ______________________ and ______________________.

5. The feet need to be ________________________ on the floor or a footrest.

6. The monitor should be directly in front of the person with the ________________________ of the monitor at or just below eye level.

7. The work surface and mouse should be at ________________________ for typing.

8. The wrist should be supported by a foam ________________________.

I. Software Used in Ambulatory Care

1. ________________________ is a collection of programs that operate and control the computer.

2. The ________________________ loads on the computer and operates in the background while application software is used.

3. ________________________ allows the user or other applications to perform specific tasks.

Match the description with the correct application software. Answers can be used more than once.

4. _____ Microsoft Access and EHR software
5. _____ Microsoft Excel and Google Sheets
6. _____ Microsoft Word and Google Docs
7. _____ PMS
8. _____ Corel WordPerfect

a. word processing software
b. spreadsheet software
c. database software

Select the correct answer.

9. What task is done with PMS?
   a. Scheduling appointments
   b. Patient registration
   c. Billing and coding medical charges
   d. Managing finances
   e. All of the above

10. Which of the following is a component of PMS?
    a. Claim denial management and electronic claim submission
    b. Financial and management reporting
    c. Scheduler and insurance eligibility verification
    d. Medical coding or encoder
    e. All of the above

Match the description with the correct PMS features.

11. _____ Used to detect errors on insurance claims before they are electronically submitted
12. _____ Used to verify patients' insurance benefits quickly
13. _____ Used to create customized business reports to show the amount of revenue the provider brought into the business
14. _____ Used to select diagnostic and procedural codes during the billing process
15. _____ Used to manage the provider's schedule and to schedule patient appointments

a. claim denial management and electronic claim submission
b. financial and management reporting
c. scheduler
d. medical coding or encoder
e. insurance eligibility verification

Select the correct answer or fill in the blank.

16. The ________________________ is a digital version of the paper medical record and contains limited information usually related to medical treatment for one healthcare facility.

17. What is a component of the EHR?
    a. Patient's past medical history and family history
    b. Visit information
    c. Laboratory and diagnostic imaging reports
    d. Hospital documents and consultation reports
    e. All of the above

18. A(n) ________________________ is a secure website that allows a patient 24-hour access to their health information

19. What is the medical assistant's role in virtual visits (telehealth)?
    a. Scheduling the visit for the patient
    b. Providing patients directions on how to access the software
    c. Explain the virtual visit process to the patient
    d. Update the patient's information during the visit
    e. All of the above

J. Computer Network Privacy and Security

1. The ________________________ include administrative policies, procedures, and actions to manage the security measures to protect electronic health information.

2. ________________________ involves identifying potential computer network breach threats and the likelihood that they will occur.

3. ________________________ include the physical measures, policies, and procedures used to protect the computer network and related buildings and equipment from hazards and unauthorized access.

4. ________________________ include technology, policies, and procedures that protect the ePHI and access to it.

5. ________________________ is software used to encode or change the information into nonreadable or encrypted data and the reader will need to enter a password for decryption to occur and to make the text readable again.

6. ______________________ is a process in which the network files are copied using an external hard drive, a server, or an online backup system.

7. What is the importance of data backup?
   a. It protects the data from a disaster in the medical facility.
   b. The data backup file can be used if the facility's data is compromised by errors, natural causes, or human causes.
   c. All of the above

8. ______________________ are devices that attach to the monitor that allow visualization of the screen contents only if the user is directly in front of the screen; also called monitor filters or privacy screens.

9. A(n) ______________________ is a record of computer activity used to monitor users' actions within software, including additions, deletions, and viewing of electronic records.

10. ______________________ means that each employee with network access must log in using a unique password.

11. A(n) ______________________ is a program or hardware device that acts as a barrier or filter between the network and the internet.

K. Recognizing and Preventing Phishing Attacks

1. ______________________ is defined as a generic cyberattack toward many individuals or organizations with the intent to steal confidential data or install malware on the users' devices.

2. ______________________ is defined as a customized cyberattack toward an individual or organization with the intent to steal confidential data or install malware on the user's device.

3. ______________________ is to assume or mimic the identity of another user to gain access to a computer system.

4. ______________________ is malicious software that can infiltrate the computer system and any network.

5. How can a person protect against phishing attacks?
   a. Use virus protection software.
   b. Do not respond to any text or email that asks for your username or password.
   c. Do not click on anything in unsolicited email or text messages.
   d. Be careful of the information shared online and on social media.
   e. All of the above

L. Continual Technologic Advances in Healthcare

Match the description with the correct term.

1. _____ The use of electronic software to communicate with pharmacies and send prescribing information
2. _____ Something designed to be used at or near where the patient is seen
3. _____ A method used to gather patient data outside of the traditional healthcare environment by using technologic devices

a. remote patient monitoring
b. point-of-care
c. e-prescribing

CERTIFICATION PREPARATION

Circle the correct answer.

1. What is one kilobyte equivalent to?
   a. 1024 bytes
   b. 1024 MB
   c. 1024 GB
   d. 1024 TB

2. Which software protects computers against viruses?
   a. Database software
   b. Presentation software
   c. Anti-malware software
   d. Spreadsheet software

3. What is a physical safeguard that is used over monitors to prevent others from seeing the information?
   a. Firewalls
   b. Screen savers
   c. Authentication
   d. Privacy filters

4. Which is a type of software that allows the user to enter demographic information, schedule appointments, maintain lists of insurance payers, perform billing tasks, and generate reports?
   a. EHR
   b. EMR
   c. PMS
   d. Microsoft Word and Excel

5. What is an electronic version of a patient's paper record?
   a. EHR
   b. EMR
   c. PMS
   d. a and b

6. What are records of computer activity used to monitor users' actions within software, including additions, deletions, and viewing of electronic records?
   a. Automatic log-off
   b. Authentication
   c. Firewalls
   d. Audit trails

7. What is malicious software designed to damage or disrupt a system (e.g., a virus)?
   a. Decryption
   b. Ethernet
   c. Hacker
   d. Malware

8. What means potential threats to the computer system security are identified, the likelihood of such occurrence is determined, and additional safeguards are implemented?
   a. Firewalls
   b. Security risk analysis
   c. Authentication
   d. Privacy filters

9. What makes a strong password?
   a. Using a person's name
   b. Consisting of eight or more characters
   c. A random combination of upper- and lowercase letters, numbers, and symbols
   d. b and c

10. Which is the computer memory used for loading and running programs?
    a. ROM
    b. RAM
    c. Cache
    d. Hard drive

WORKPLACE APPLICATIONS

1. As part of her role, Christiana is learning about security measures to keep the network secure and confidential. Identify the security measures described.

   a. Records of computer activity used to monitor users' actions within software, including additions, deletions, and viewing of electronic records.

   ____

b. A program or hardware device that acts as a barrier or filter between the network and the internet.

____

c. After a period of inactivity, the workstation logs off. ______________________________

____

d. Potential threats of network breaches are identified and action plans are instituted to prevent the breaches.

____

e. Used to encode or change the information into nonreadable or encrypted data. ______________

____

2. Christiana is evaluating the scanners in the reception area and the health information management department, which handles scanning documents into EHRs. Discuss types of scanners that might be used in both of these areas.

____

____

____

3. Christiana would like to have a computer with internet access available for patients to use in the reception area. What are things that she will need to consider?

____

____

INTERNET ACTIVITIES

1. Review the content of one of the patient education websites listed in the chapter. Create a poster presentation, a PowerPoint presentation, or write a paper summarizing your research.
2. Select a disease. Find two reputable patient education websites that provide information on the disease, diagnostic tests, and treatments. One of your websites must be different than those listed in the chapter. Create a poster presentation, a PowerPoint presentation, or write a paper summarizing your research and include the websites used.
3. You need to purchase a printer for your department. Research a business-sized laser printer and an inkjet printer. Create a poster presentation, a PowerPoint presentation, or write a paper summarizing your research and include the websites used. Include the following points for each printer:
   a. Name and model number of the printer
   b. Cost of the printer
   c. Cost of a new printer cartridge
   d. Speed of the printer
   e. Additional features of the printer that would be useful in a business setting

Procedure 8.1 Prepare a Workstation

Name ______________________________ **Date** __________ **Score** __________

Tasks: Perform infection control procedures and create an ergonomically friendly workstation.

Equipment and Supplies:
- Nonabrasive disinfectant (hospital grade) wipes or specially made wipes for computer hardware or as indicated by the keyboard manufacturer
- Gloves (if required for using wipes)
- User guide for keyboard or facility's infection control procedure for computer hardware
- Desktop computer with adjustable monitor
- Office chair with an adjustable seat, armrest, and backrest
- Footrest (if needed)
- Foam wrist rest
- Document holder (optional)
- Hand sanitizer (optional)

Standard: Complete the procedure and all critical steps in _______ minutes with a minimum score of 85% within two attempts (*or as indicated by the instructor*).

Scoring: Divide the points earned by the total possible points. Failure to perform a critical step, indicated by an asterisk (*), results in grade no higher than an 84% (*or as indicated by the instructor*).

Time: Began_________ Ended_________ Total minutes: _________

Steps:	Point Value	Attempt 1	Attempt 2
1. While sitting in the chair, adjust the backrest so it supports the upper body and the lumbar support area fits to the small of the back. Adjust the seat pan height so the feet are flat on the floor or footrest. Adjust the armrest to support the forearms with the shoulders in a relaxed position.	20		
2. Adjust the monitor so it is directly in front of the person and the top of the monitor is at or just below the eye level. If using a document holder, position it so it is at the same distance and height as the monitor.	20		
3. Place the keyboard at a height and an angle to allow the wrists to be in a neutral position. Position the mouse so it is at elbow level for typing. Support the wrists with a foam wrist rest.	20		
4. While sitting with your torso and neck vertically and in line, identify if everything is positioned correctly and comfortably. Make any adjustments as needed.	10		
5. Using the keyboard user guide or the facilities' infection control procedure for computer hardware, determine the product to use to disinfect the keyboard. Don gloves if needed. Using a disinfectant wipe, clean the surface using friction for 5 seconds in each area. Discard gloves if worn.	20*		
6. Wash hands or use hand sanitizer before using the keyboard.	10*		
Total Points	**100**		

Comments

ABHES Competencies	Step(s)
8. Clinical Procedures a. Practice standard precautions and perform disinfection/ sterilization techniques	5

Procedure 8.2 Identify a Reliable Patient Education Website

Name ______________________________ **Date** ____________ **Score** __________

Tasks: Research a disease or condition and evaluate a patient education website.

Equipment and Supplies:
- Computer with internet access, word processing software, and printer

Standard: Complete the procedure and all critical steps in ______ minutes with a minimum score of 85% within two attempts (*or as indicated by the instructor*).

Scoring: Divide the points earned by the total possible points. Failure to perform a critical step, indicated by an asterisk (*), results in grade no higher than an 84% (*or as indicated by the instructor*).

Time: Began________ Ended________ Total minutes: ________

Steps:	Point Value	Attempt 1	Attempt 2
1. Select a disease or condition. Using the internet, find a website with information about the disease or condition. Do not use a website listed in this chapter.	10*		
2. Identify the mission or purpose of the website, who supports or runs the website, and whether there is advertising present on the page. If advertising is present, is the advertising mixed in with the content or text?	20		
3. Determine if the information is current or less than 3 years old.	10		
4. Identify the author(s) and the person's background. Does a panel of healthcare experts review the content?	20		
5. Identify if a person needs to enter personal information to view pages of the website. If so, what does the website's host do with the personal information?	20		
6. Compose a one-page paper on your findings. Use double line spacing and a 12-point font size. Include the website you used. Discuss if the website is reliable and if the content is updated. Proofread and spell-check your document prior to printing it.	20		
Total Points	**100**		

Comments

ABHES Competencies	Step(s)
7. Administrative Procedure h. Perform basic computer skills	Entire procedure

Student Name______________________________ Date______________

Written Communication

chapter **9**

CAAHEP Competencies	Assessment
V.C.7. Identify different types of electronic technology used in professional communication	Skills and Concepts – E. 1; H. 1
V.P.6. Using technology, compose clear and correct correspondence	Procedures 9.1, 9.2, 9.3, 9.4, 9.5

ABHES Competencies	Assessment
7. Administrative Procedures g. Display professionalism through written and verbal communications	Procedures 9.1, 9.2, 9.3, 9.4, 9.5, 9.6
h. Perform basic computer skills	Procedures 9.1, 9.2, 9.3, 9.4, 9.5

VOCABULARY REVIEW

Using the word pool on the right, find the correct word to match the definition. Write the word on the line after the definition.

Group A

1. Types of communication ______________________
2. A word or group of words that describes a noun or pronoun ______________________
3. A word or group of words that answers *how, where, when,* or *to what extent*, thus further describing a verb, adjective, or adverbs ______________________
4. Often begin with words such as *although, since, when, because,* and *if;* needs a subject and verb to be a complete sentence ______________________
5. A word that indicates a relationship or location between a noun or pronoun and the rest of the sentence ______________________
6. A group of words without a subject or verb ______________________

Word Pool

- adjective
- adverb
- copy notation
- dependent clauses
- media
- phrase
- practice management software
- preposition
- reference notation
- template

7. Notes the initials of the person who composed the letter in uppercase followed by the initials of the person who keyed (typed) the letter in lowercase ____________________
8. Used to notify the letter's recipient who else received a copy of the letter ____________________
9. A type of software that allows the user to enter demographic information, schedule appointments, maintain lists of insurance payers, perform billing tasks, and generate reports ____________________
10. A document or file that has a preset format ____________________

Group B

1. A person who has written documentation that he or she can accept a shipment for another individual ____________________
2. An electronic record that conforms to nationally recognized standards and contains health-related information about a specific patient ____________________
3. The most common layout for a printed page; the height of the paper is greater than its width ____________________
4. Documents sent to a patient explaining that the provider is ending the physician-patient relationship and the patient needs to see another provider ____________________
5. The measurement around something; when referring to mail, it is the measurement around the middle of the package that is being shipped ____________________
6. A region or geographic area used for shipping ____________________
7. A term describing employees for whom an employer has obtained a fidelity bond from an insurance company that will cover losses from any dishonest acts (e.g., embezzlement, theft) committed by those employees ____________________

Word Pool

- authorized agent
- bonded
- electronic health record
- girth
- portrait orientation
- termination letters
- zone

SKILLS AND CONCEPTS

Answer the following questions either by filling in the blank or selecting the correct answer.

A. Parts of Speech

1. A(n) ____________________ is a word or phrase for a person, place, thing, or idea.
2. A(n) ____________________ is a word or a phrase that shows action or a state of being.
3. A(n) ____________________ is a phrase without a main clause and is a major error in writing.
4. A(n) ____________________ is a word or group of words that describes a noun or pronoun; may come before or after the noun or pronoun it describes.

5. A(n) ____________________ is a word or group of words that answers *how, where, when,* or *to what extent,* thus further describing a verb, adjective, or other adverbs.

6. A(n) ____________________ is a word that indicates a relationship or location between a noun or pronoun and the rest of the sentence.

B. Common Communication Errors

1. ____________________ are words that sound alike.

2. Which of the following statements contains a noun and pronoun mismatch?
   a. The providers see patients in the exam room.
   b. The receptionists asks patients for their updated insurance cards.
   c. The medical assistants room patients and obtain their vital signs.
   d. All of the above

3. Which statement is grammatically *incorrect*?
   a. Sally works as a receptionist at the dental clinic.
   b. The affect of the bad weather, patients arrived late.
   c. "Your good at your job," stated the patient.
   d. b and c

4. Which statement is grammatically correct?
   a. Tom went to room the patient.
   b. Jess was late, too.
   c. Two patients were left in the reception area.
   d. All of the above
   e. a and c

5. Which statement is grammatically *incorrect*?
   a. There were three exam rooms opened.
   b. Their provider was running late after doing hospital rounds.
   c. They're out to lunch.
   d. Their are two providers off today.

C. Punctuation

Fill in the blank.

1. Use a(n) ____________________ for a sentence that makes a statement.

2. Use a(n) ____________________ after a direct question.

3. Use a(n) ____________________ for sentences that express strong emotion.

4. A(n) ____________________ is a common punctuation mark used in professional letters and documentation.

5. A(n) ____________________ is used to introduce a series of items either in the sentence or a bulleted list.

6. ____________________ are used to set off direct quotes.

7. A(n) ____________________ is used to show ownership.

Match the error in the statement with the correct answers. Answers can be used more than once.

8. _____ Zac the receptionist greeted the patients when they arrived.
9. _____ My retirement is set for March 30 2027.
10. _____ Marie and I arrived early at the medical office
11. _____ Yes I will need your new insurance card.
12. _____ Thank you Katie for all your hard work.

a. missing a comma
b. missing two commas
c. missing a period

D. Capitalizations and Number

1. Which is a situation where capitalization is needed?
   a. The first letter of the first word in a sentence or question
   b. The pronoun "I"
   c. The first letter of proper nouns
   d. All of the above

2. Spell out all numbers at the __________________ of a sentence.

E. Written Correspondence

1. How does the medical assistant use electronic technology in professional communication?
   a. They may communicate with vendors or supply companies.
   b. They may also need to send written communication to patients and other providers.
   c. They will compose letters and emails.
   d. All of the above

2. Professional letters use __________________ paper or letterhead paper.

3. The letter typically has __________________ margins on all four sides, although shorter letters may use larger margins.

4. The entire letter should be written using __________________ line spacing.

5. What information is found in the sender's address?
   a. Facility's name, street address, or post office box
   b. City, state, and ZIP code
   c. May also include phone numbers, website address, and an email address
   d. All of the above

6. What is the correct format for the date in a professional letter?
   a. January 6, 2027
   b. January 6th 2027
   c. 01/06/2027
   d. January 6 2027

7. What punctuation mark is used after the greeting in a professional letter?
   a. Period
   b. Colon
   c. Semicolon
   d. Comma

8. How is the reference notation keyed if Kayla Smith typed the letter for Dr. James Martin?
   a. KS/JM
   b. JM/ks
   c. JM:ks
   d. JM:KS
   e. b and c

9. ____________________ is used to notify the letter's recipient who else received a copy of the letter.

10. ____________________ is used if the sender does not want the recipient to know a copy was sent to another person.

11. What should be on a continuation page?
    a. Recipient's name
    b. Page number
    c. Date
    d. All of the above

F. Business Letter Formats

1. Professional letters use "____________________" punctuation, meaning all parts of the letter use punctuation marks.

2. Informal letters sometimes use "open" punctuation, which means the only punctuation used is found in the ____________________ of the letter.

3. With a full block letter format, all lines start flush with the ____________________ margin.

4. The semi-block format ____________________ the paragraphs in the body of the letter.

G. Memoranda

1. Letters and memos use ________________________ orientation.

2. Which of the following headings is *not* used in a memorandum?
   a. To
   b. Sender
   c. Date
   d. Subject

3. The headings are ________________________ justified with a blank line between each header.

4. The headings in a memorandum are
   a. keyed in bold font.
   b. keyed in capital letters.
   c. followed by a colon.
   d. all of the above

H. Professional Emails

1. Why do medical assistants need to know how to compose a professional email?
   a. Professional emails are used to communicate with providers and other staff members.
   b. Professional emails are now used more often to communicate with patients.
   c. All of the above

2. What is *not* an appropriate greeting for a professional email?
   a. "Good morning, Mr. Jones,"
   b. "Dear Mr. Jones,"
   c. "Hey Mr. Jones,"

3. You are sending an email to Mr. Black and Dr. Martin asked that you blind-copy him on the email. To do this, you would add Dr. Martin's name to ______________________ address line.

4. Refrain from using all ______________________ letters, since the reader may feel you are shouting at them.

5. When sending an email to several people, separate each email address by a(n) ______________________.

6. Add an email address to the ______________________ line if another person needs to receive a courtesy copy of the email.

7. How do you end a professional email?
   a. "Kind regards"
   b. "Thank you"
   c. "Sincerely"
   d. All of the above

I. Faxed Communications

1. When sending a fax regarding a patient, which federal law does *not* apply?
   a. HIPAA
   b. HITECH
   c. Confidentiality Act
   d. a and c

2. What information is included on a typical fax face sheet?
   a. Sender's name and phone number
   b. Receiver's name, company, fax number, and phone number
   c. Number of pages, date, and subject
   d. All of the above

3. When sending a fax, the medical assistant should
   a. include the fax cover sheet in the page count.
   b. fax the cover sheet last.
   c. All of the above

J. Preparing Mail

1. Business letters should be enclosed in standard ______________________ envelopes, which measure ______________________.

2. An automated mail processing machine reads the address on an envelope
   a. top line (the person's name) first.
   b. second address line (the street address) first.
   c. bottom line (i.e., city, state, and ZIP code) first.

3. When addressing mail, the medical assistant should
   a. use a simple black font of at least 10-point size.
   b. use all uppercase letters and no punctuation marks.
   c. left-justify the address.
   d. use only approved abbreviations.
   e. all of the above

4. When addressing mail, what should *not* be done?
   a. Use the # sign.
   b. Put one space between the city and state and two spaces between the state and ZIP code.
   c. Use the ZIP+4 code.
   d. Include an attention line below the last line of the delivery address.

K. Outgoing and Incoming Mail

1. Which factor affects the postage rate of mail?
   a. Weight and size of the item
   b. Urgency for arrival
   c. Delivery zone
   d. Services required
   e. All of the above

2. A(n) ________________________ shows the date when the item was mailed and additional information on when the delivery occurred and the recipient's signature.

3. Termination letters are sent by ________________________.

4. ________________________ is an optional mail service that protects against loss or damage and the cost is based on the declared value of the item.

5. ________________________ is an optional mail service that requires the addressee or authorized agent to verify identity when signing for the delivery.

6. ________________________ is an optional mail service that requires the recipient to pay for the merchandise and shipping when the package is received.

CERTIFICATION PREPARATION

Circle the correct answer.

1. Which is a word or group of words that describes a noun or pronoun?
   a. Adverb
   b. Adjective
   c. Verb
   d. Noun

2. Which needs to be capitalized?
   a. The first letter of the first word in a sentence or question
   b. The first letter of proper nouns
   c. The pronoun "I"
   d. All of the above

3. When should a comma be used?
   a. Before a coordinator (and, but, yet, nor, for, or, so) that links two main clauses
   b. To separate items in a list of three or more things
   c. After certain words (e.g., yes, no) at the start of a sentence
   d. All of the above

4. What punctuation is used at the end of the salutation in a professional letter?
   a. Colon
   b. Semicolon
   c. Comma
   d. Period

5. What includes the initials of the person who composed the letter?
   a. Enclosure notation
   b. Reference notation
   c. Copy notation
   d. Attachment notation

6. Which type of business letter format has the sender's and inside addresses and paragraphs left-justified and the date, closing, and signature block starts at the center point?
   a. Semi-block
   b. Memo
   c. Modified block
   d. Full block

7. Which is the most common mail service used for envelopes weighing up to 13 ounces, and provides delivery in 3 days or less?
   a. Priority Mail
   b. Priority Mail Express
   c. First-Class Mail
   d. Media Mail

8. Which optional mail service is used to protect expensive items, a mailing receipt is provided, and upon request, an electronic verification of delivery or delivery attempt can be sent?
   a. Registered Mail
   b. Standard Insurance
   c. Certified Mail
   d. Return Receipt

9. Dr. James Smith composed a letter and Cathy Black keyed the letter. What is the correct format for the notation in the letter?
   a. cb:JS
   b. JS:cb
   c. CB:js
   d. js:CB

10. Which is *not* a header in a memo?
    a. TO
    b. FROM
    c. DEPARTMENT
    d. SUBJECT

Workplace Applications

1. Christiana is composing the following letters. Indicate the name that should appear in the signature block.

   a. A letter from her to the office supply company. ______________________________

   b. A letter to Mrs. White from Dr. James Martin. ______________________________

   c. A referral letter about a patient from Dr. James Martin to Dr. Robert Black. ____________

   ____

2. When Christiana Zwellen is composing a letter for Dr. James Martin, indicate two ways she can create the reference notation.

   ____

   ____

3. Christiana needs to fold a letter for a #10 envelope. Describe how this is done. ______________________

____

____

____

INTERNET ACTIVITIES

1. Research professional email etiquette. Describe five ways you can improve your written communication with patients and professionals.

____

____

____

2. Research the two-letter postal abbreviations for the states. Write each address provided as it should appear on an envelope. Use only approved U.S. Postal Service standard street abbreviations and the two-letter postal abbreviation for states.

   a. Walden-Martin Family Medical Clinic, 1234 Any Street, Anytown, Alabama 14453 ________________

   ____

   ____

   b. John Smith, 383 E. Center, Anytown, Nebraska 13333-2232 ______________________________

   ____

   ____

   c. Sally Black, 39291 S. Parkway, Anytown, Wisconsin 54334-6443 ____________________________

   ____

   ____

   d. Jeff Jones, 454 Boulevard, Anytown, Minnesota 49932-1234 ______________________________

   ____

   ____

   e. Sam House, 599 State Highway, Anytown, Illinois 69532-1651 ____________________________

   ____

   ____

3. Use the ZIP code look-up tool on www.usps.com to find the ZIP codes for the following cities. Write the ZIP code on the line to the right of the city.

   a. Chicken, AK ______________________

   b. Rabbit Hash, KY ______________________

   c. Oatmeal, TX ______________________

   d. Turkey, TX ______________________

   e. Popcorn, IN ______________________

   f. Toast, NC ______________________

   g. Corn, OK ______________________

   h. Cucumber, WV ______________________

   i. Chili, WI ______________________

   j. Cream, WI ______________________

Procedure 9.1 Compose a Professional Business Letter Using the Full Block Letter Format

Name ______________________________ **Date** ____________ **Score** __________

Tasks: Compose a professional letter using technology. Use the full block letter format and closed punctuation. Address the envelope and fold the letter.

Scenario: Jean Burke, NP (nurse practitioner), has requested that you compose a letter to the parent (Lisa Parker) of Johnny Parker (date of birth [DOB]: 06/15/20XX) to let her know that Johnny's throat culture from last Wednesday was negative. If he is not improving or if she has any questions, she should call the office. Lisa Parker's address is 91 Poplar Street, Anytown, AL 12345-1234. You are working at Walden-Martin Family Medical Clinic. The healthcare facility's address is 1234 Anystreet, Anytown, AL 12345. The phone number is 123-123-1234 and the fax number is 123-123-5678.

Equipment and Supplies:
- Patient's health record
- Computer with word processing software and printer
- Paper
- #10 envelope

Standard: Complete the procedure and all critical steps with a minimum score of 85% within two attempts *(or as indicated by the instructor).*

Scoring: Divide the points earned by the total possible points. Failure to perform a critical step, indicated by an asterisk (*), results in grade no higher than an 84% *(or as indicated by the instructor).*

Steps:	Point Value	Attempt 1	Attempt 2
1. Obtain the intended recipient's contact information and determine the message you want to convey. Using the computer and word processing software, compose the letter using the full block letter format. Use 1-inch margins on all four sides, portrait orientation, and single line spacing throughout the letter. Use an easy-to-read font (e.g., Times New Roman or Calibri) in a 10- or 12-point size.	5		
2. Create a letterhead in the header of the document. Include the clinic's name, street address or post office box, city, state, and ZIP code.	10		
3. Key (type) the date starting at the left margin. Have one blank line between the date line and the last line of the letterhead.	10		
4. Key the inside address starting at the left margin and use the correct spelling and punctuation. Leave one to nine blank lines between the date and the inside address to center the body of the letter on the page.	10*		
5. Key the salutation starting at the left margin and use the correct spelling and punctuation. Leave one blank line between the inside address and the salutation.	10		
6. Use your critical thinking skills to compose a concise, accurate message. Type the message in the body of the letter starting at the left margin. Leave one blank line between the salutation and the first line of the body and then between each paragraph of the body. The message should be clear, concise, and professional. Use proper grammar, punctuation, capitalization, and sentence structure.	10		
7. Key a proper closing starting at the left margin and use correct spelling and punctuation. Leave one blank line between the last line of the body and the closing.	10		

8. Key the signature block starting at the left margin and use the correct spelling and punctuation. Leave four blank lines between the closing and the signature block. If you are preparing the letter for a provider, you must include a reference notation.	**10**		
9. Spell-check and proofread the document. Check for the proper tone, grammar, punctuation, capitalization, and sentence structure. Check for proper spacing between the parts of the letter. Make any final corrections. Print the document.	**5**		
10. Address the envelope, using either the computer and word processing software or a pen and following the correct format.	**10**		
11. When using a #10 envelope, fold the letter by pulling up the bottom end until it reaches just below the inside address or two-thirds of the way up the letter. Crease at the fold. Then, fold the top of the letter down so that it is flush with the bottom fold and crease the paper.	**5**		
12. File a copy of the letter in the paper medical record or upload an electronic copy of the letter to the electronic health record (EHR).	**5**		
Total Points	**100**		

Comments

CAAHEP Competencies	Step(s)
V.P.6. Using technology, compose clear and correct correspondence	Entire procedure
ABHES Competencies	**Step(s)**
7. Administrative Procedures g. Display professionalism through written and verbal communications	Entire procedure
7.h. Perform basic computer skills	Entire procedure

Procedure 9.2 Compose a Professional Business Letter Using the Modified Block Letter Format

Name ______________________________ **Date** ____________ **Score** __________

Tasks: Compose a professional letter using technology. Use the modified block letter format (with the center point option). Address the envelope (if needed) and fold the letter.

Scenario: Julie Walden, MD, has requested that you compose a letter to Carl C. Bowden (DOB: 04/05/19XX) to let him know that his hepatitis C laboratory test was negative. If he has any questions, he should call the office. His address is 19 Beale Street, Anytown, AL 12345-1234. You are working at Walden-Martin Family Medical Clinic. The healthcare facility's address is 1234 Anystreet, Anytown, AL 12345. The phone number is 123-123-1234 and the fax number is 123-123-5678.

Equipment and Supplies:
- Patient's health record
- Computer with word processing software and printer
- Paper
- #10 envelope or window business envelope

Standard: Complete the procedure and all critical steps with a minimum score of 85% within two attempts *(or as indicated by the instructor).*

Scoring: Divide the points earned by the total possible points. Failure to perform a critical step, indicated by an asterisk (*), results in grade no higher than an 84% *(or as indicated by the instructor).*

Steps:	Point Value	Attempt 1	Attempt 2
1. Obtain the intended recipient's contact information and determine the message you want to convey. Using the computer and word processing software, compose the letter using the modified block letter format. Use 1-inch margins on all four sides, portrait orientation, and single line spacing throughout the letter. Use an easy-to-read font (e.g., Times New Roman or Calibri) in a 10- or 12-point size.	5		
2. Create a letterhead in the header of the document. Include the clinic's name, street address or post office box, city, state, and ZIP code.	10		
3. Key (type) the date starting at the center point of the line, which is usually about 3.25 inches from the margin. Have one blank line between the date line and the last line of the letterhead.	10		
4. Key the inside address starting at the left margin and use the correct spelling and punctuation. Leave one to nine blank lines between the date and the inside address to center the body of the letter on the page. If using a window business envelope, adjust the address position to fit the window.	10*		
5. Key the salutation starting at the left margin and use the correct spelling and punctuation. Leave one blank line between the inside address and the salutation.	10		

6. Use your critical thinking skills to compose a concise, accurate message. Type the message in the body of the letter starting at the left margin. Leave one blank line between the salutation and the first line of the body and then between each paragraph of the body. The message should be clear, concise, and professional. Use proper grammar, punctuation, capitalization, and sentence structure.	**10**		
7. Key a proper closing. Start the closing at the center point of the line. (The first letter of the closing should align vertically with the first letter of the date.) Use correct spelling and punctuation. Leave one blank line between the last line of the body and the closing.	**10**		
8. Key the signature block. Start the signature block at the center point of the line. (The first letter of the signature block should align vertically with the first letter of the date and closing.) Use the correct spelling and punctuation. Leave four blank lines between the closing and the signature block. If you are preparing the letter for a provider, you must include a reference notation.	**10**		
9. Spell-check and proofread the document. Check for the proper tone, grammar, punctuation, capitalization, and sentence structure. Check for proper spacing between the parts of the letter. Make any final corrections. Print the document. If needed, address the envelope, using either the computer and word processing software or a pen and following the correct format.	**10**		
10. When using a #10 envelope, fold the letter by pulling up the bottom end until it reaches just below the inside address or two-thirds of the way up the letter. Crease at the fold. Then, fold the top of the letter down so that it is flush with the bottom fold and crease the paper. For window business envelopes, have the letter's print side facing up and place the envelope over the top third of the letter. Fold the bottom edge of the paper up to the bottom edge of the envelope and crease at the fold. Then, remove the envelope and flip the letter over and fold the top of the letter down to the prior crease line and crease at the fold. Place the letter in the envelope so that the recipient's address shows through the window.	**10**		
11. File a copy of the letter in the paper medical record or upload an electronic copy of the letter to the electronic health record (EHR).	**5**		
Total Points	**100**		

Comments

CAAHEP Competencies	Step(s)
V.P.6. Using technology, compose clear and correct correspondence	Entire procedure
ABHES Competencies	**Step(s)**
7. Administrative Procedures g. Display professionalism through written and verbal communications	Entire procedure
7.h. Perform basic computer skills	Entire procedure

Procedure 9.3 Compose a Professional Business Letter Using the Semi-Block Letter Format

Name ______________________________ **Date** ____________ **Score** ____________

Tasks: Compose a professional letter using technology. Use the semi-block letter format (with the center point option). Address the envelope and fold the letter.

Scenario: Julie Walden, MD, has requested that you compose a letter to Amma Patel (DOB: 01/14/19XX) to let her know that her thyroid test was normal, but her vitamin D level was low. Dr. Walden would like Amma to take 15 mcg of vitamin D each morning. She can purchase this over the counter. She needs to have her vitamin D rechecked in 6 months. She can call to schedule a blood test closer to that time. If she has any questions, she should call the office. Her address is 1346 Charity Lane, Anytown, AL 12345-1234. You are working at Walden-Martin Family Medical Clinic. The healthcare facility's address is 1234 Anystreet, Anytown, AL 12345. The phone number is 123-123-1234 and the fax number is 123-123-5678.

Equipment and Supplies:
- Patient's health record
- Computer with word processing software and printer
- Paper
- #10 envelope or #6¾ envelope

Standard: Complete the procedure and all critical steps with a minimum score of 85% within two attempts *(or as indicated by the instructor).*

Scoring: Divide the points earned by the total possible points. Failure to perform a critical step, indicated by an asterisk (*), results in grade no higher than an 84% *(or as indicated by the instructor).*

Steps:	Point Value	Attempt 1	Attempt 2
1. Obtain the intended recipient's contact information and determine the message you want to convey. Using the computer and word processing software, compose the letter using the semi-block letter format. Use 1-inch margins on all four sides, portrait orientation, and single line spacing throughout the letter. Use an easy-to-read font (e.g., Times New Roman or Calibri) in a 10- or 12-point size.	5		
2. Create a letterhead in the header of the document. Include the clinic's name, street address or post office box, city, state, and ZIP code.	10		
3. Key (type) the date starting at the center point of the line, which is usually about 3.25 inches from the margin. Have one blank line between the date line and the last line of the letterhead.	10		
4. Key the inside address starting at the left margin and use the correct spelling and punctuation. Leave one to nine blank lines between the date and the inside address to center the body of the letter on the page.	10*		
5. Key the salutation starting at the left margin and use the correct spelling and punctuation. Leave one blank line between the inside address and the salutation.	10		

6. Use your critical thinking skills to compose a concise, accurate message. Type the message in the body of the letter starting at the left margin. Leave one blank line between the salutation and the first line of the body and then between each paragraph of the body. Each paragraph should be indented five spaces. The message should be clear, concise, and professional. Use proper grammar, punctuation, capitalization, and sentence structure.	**10**		
7. Key a proper closing. Start the closing at the center point of the line. (The first letter of the closing should align vertically with the first letter of the date.) Use correct spelling and punctuation. Leave one blank line between the last line of the body and the closing.	**10**		
8. Key the signature block. Start the signature block at the center point of the line. (The first letter of the signature block should align vertically with the first letter of the date and closing.) Use the correct spelling and punctuation. Leave four blank lines between the closing and the signature block. If you are preparing the letter for a provider, you must include a reference notation.	**10**		
9. Spell-check and proofread the document. Check for the proper tone, grammar, punctuation, capitalization, and sentence structure. Check for proper spacing between the parts of the letter. Make any final corrections. Print the document.	**5**		
10. Address the envelope, using either the computer and word processing software or a pen and following the correct format.	**10**		
11. When using a #10 envelope, fold the letter by pulling up the bottom end until it reaches just below the inside address or two-thirds of the way up the letter. Crease at the fold. Then, fold the top of the letter down so that it is flush with the bottom fold and crease the paper. When using a #6{3/4} envelope, pull the bottom edge of the letter up until it is 1/2 inch from the top edge of the document and crease at the fold. Bring the right edge two-thirds of the way across the width of the document and crease the paper. Then bring the left edge to the right edge and crease at the fold. Flip the document so the left edge is on the bottom and insert the letter into the envelope.	**5**		
12. File a copy of the letter in the paper medical record or upload an electronic copy of the letter to the electronic health record (EHR).	**5**		
Total Points	**100**		

Comments

CAAHEP Competencies	**Step(s)**
V.P.6. Using technology, compose clear and correct correspondence	Entire procedure
ABHES Competencies	**Step(s)**
7. Administrative Procedures g. Display professionalism through written and verbal communications	Entire procedure
7.h. Perform basic computer skills	Entire procedure

Procedure 9.4 Compose a Memorandum

Name ______________________________ **Date** ____________ **Score** __________

Task: Compose a professional memorandum.

Scenario: You are asked by the supervisor to compose a memo that can be posted in the department. You are to remind the staff about the department meeting next Tuesday at noon in the conference room. Staff can bring their lunches and beverages will be provided.

Equipment and Supplies:
- Computer with word processing software and printer
- Paper

Standard: Complete the procedure and all critical steps with a minimum score of 85% within two attempts *(or as indicated by the instructor).*

Scoring: Divide the points earned by the total possible points. Failure to perform a critical step, indicated by an asterisk (*), results in grade no higher than an 84% *(or as indicated by the instructor).*

Steps:	**Point Value**	**Attempt 1**	**Attempt 2**
1. Determine the message you want to convey. Using the computer and word processing software, compose the memo. Use 1-inch margins on all four sides, portrait orientation, and single line spacing throughout the memo. Use an easy to read font (e.g., Times New Roman or Calibri) in a 10- or 12-point size.	15		
2. Left-justify the headers and use boldface and capital letters, followed by a colon. Headers include TO, FROM, DATE, and SUBJECT. Leave one blank line between each header.	15		
3. Key (type) the information following the headers in regular font, using a mix of capital and lowercase letters. Using the tab tool, align the information vertically down the page. Key the date as indicated for professional letters.	15		
4. Add a centered black line between the headers and the body (optional). Leave two to three blank lines between the headers and the body of the memo.	15		
5. Key the message in the body of the memo. Left-justify the content in the body and use single line spacing. Use proper grammar and correct spelling and punctuation. With multiple paragraphs, skip a single line between paragraphs.	15		
6. Write the content of the message in the body of the memo clearly, concisely, and accurately. Add special notations as needed.	15		
7. Spell-check and proofread the document. Check for the proper tone, grammar, punctuation, capitalization, and sentence structure. Check for proper spacing between the parts of the memo. Make any final corrections. Print the document.	10		
Total Points	**100**		

Comments

CAAHEP Competencies	Step(s)
V.P.6. Using technology, compose clear and correct correspondence	Entire procedure
ABHES Competencies	**Step(s)**
7. Administrative Procedures g. Display professionalism through written and verbal communications	Entire procedure
7.h. Perform basic computer skills	Entire procedure

Procedure 9.5 Compose a Professional Email

Name ______________________________ **Date** ____________ **Score** __________

Task: Compose a professional email that conveys the message to the reader clearly, concisely, and accurately.

Scenario: Aaron Jackson (DOB: 10/17/20XX) has an appointment at 11 a.m. next Thursday. Send his guardian an appointment reminder via email. Aaron will be seeing David Kahn, MD. The guardian should bring in any medications Aaron is currently taking. You are working at Walden-Martin Family Medical Clinic. The healthcare facility's address is: 1234 Anystreet, Anytown, AL 12345. The phone number is 123-123-1234 and the fax number is 123-123-5678. Your instructor will supply you with the guardian's name and email address.

Equipment and Supplies:
- Patient's health record
- Computer with email software

Standard: Complete the procedure and all critical steps with a minimum score of 85% within two attempts *(or as indicated by the instructor).*

Scoring: Divide the points earned by the total possible points. Failure to perform a critical step, indicated by an asterisk (*), results in grade no higher than an 84% *(or as indicated by the instructor).*

Steps:	Point Value	Attempt 1	Attempt 2
1. Obtain the intended recipient's contact information and determine the message you want to convey.	5		
2. Using the computer and email software, key (type) the recipient's email address. If the email has two recipients, use a semicolon (;) after the name of the first recipient. Double-check the email addresses for accuracy.	5*		
3. Key a subject, keeping it simple but focused on the contents of the email.	10		
4. Key a formal greeting, using correct punctuation.	10		
5. Key the message in the body of the email using proper grammar, spelling, punctuation, capitalization, and sentence structure. Avoid abbreviations. The message should be clear, concise, and professional.	20		
6. Finish the email with closing remarks.	10		
7. Key a closing, followed by your name and title on the next line. Include the clinic's name and contact information below your name.	10		
8. Spell-check and proofread the email. Check for proper tone, grammar, punctuation, capitalization, and sentence structure. Check for proper spacing between the parts of the email.	10		
9. Make any final revisions, select any features to apply to the email, and then send it.	10		
10. Print a copy of the email to be filed in the paper medical record or upload an electronic copy of the email to the patient's electronic health record (EHR).	10		
Total Points	**100**		

Comments

CAAHEP Competencies	**Step(s)**
V.P.6. Using technology, compose clear and correct correspondence	Entire procedure
ABHES Competencies	**Step(s)**
7. Administrative Procedures g. Display professionalism through written and verbal communications	Entire procedure
7.h. Perform basic computer skills	Entire procedure

Procedure 9.6 Complete a Fax Cover Sheet

Name ______________________________ **Date** ____________ **Score** __________

Task: Complete a fax cover sheet clearly and accurately.

Scenario: Lisa Parker, mother of Johnny Parker (DOB: 06/15/20XX), requested his immunization history to be sent to Anytown School, attention: Susie Payne. The school's phone number is 123-123-5784, and the fax number will be supplied by your instructor. The release of medical records has been completed and signed by Lisa, Johnny's guardian/mother. Your phone number is the main clinic number listed on the header of the fax cover sheet.

Equipment and Supplies:
- Document to be faxed (optional)
- Fax machine and fax number (optional)
- Pen
- Fax cover sheet (Work Product 9.1, HIPAA-Compliant Fax Cover Sheet)

Standard: Complete the procedure and all critical steps with a minimum score of 85% within two attempts *(or as indicated by the instructor).*

Scoring: Divide the points earned by the total possible points. Failure to perform a critical step, indicated by an asterisk (*), results in grade no higher than an 84% *(or as indicated by the instructor).*

Steps:	**Point Value**	**Attempt 1**	**Attempt 2**
1. Using a pen and the fax cover sheet, clearly and accurately write your name, phone number, and the date.	**20**		
2. Clearly and accurately write the name of the person receiving the fax. Also include the company, fax number, and phone number.	**20**		
3. Write the number of pages. The cover sheet must be counted in the total.	**20**		
4. Complete Re: by indicating the subject of the fax. Be general with the subject and refrain from including anything confidential.	**20**		
5. Proofread the fax cover sheet. Verify the name, agency, and contact information of the recipient. Verify the document(s) being sent are correct. Optional: organize the documents so the coversheet is on top and fax to the recipient.	**20**		
Total Points	**100**		

Comments

ABHES Competencies	**Step(s)**
7. Administrative Procedures g. Display professionalism through written and verbal communications	Entire procedure

Work Product 9.1 HIPAA-Compliant Fax Cover Sheet

To be used with Procedure 9.6.

Name ______________________________ Date __________ Score __________

WALDEN-MARTIN
FAMILY MEDICAL CLINIC
1234 ANYSTREET | ANYTOWN, ANYSTATE 12345
PHONE 123-123-1234 | FAX 123-123-5678

Fax

To: ____________	From: ____________
Company: ____________	Phone: ____________
Fax: ____________	Date: ____________
Phone: ____________	
Pages: ____________	
Re: ____________	

CONFIDENTIAL NOTICE

The material enclosed with this facsimile transmission is confidential and private. The material is the property of the sender and some or all of the information may be protected by the Health Insurance Portability & Accountability Act (HIPAA). This information is intended exclusively for the addressed person or agency indicated above. If you are not the intended individual or entity of this information, you are hereby notified that any use, duplication, circulation, or transmission of the information is strictly prohibited under state and federal law. Please notify the sender immediate using the telephone number indicated above.

Student Name______________________________ Date______________

chapter **10**

Telephone Techniques

CAAHEP Competencies	Assessments
V.P.4. Demonstrate professional telephone techniques	Procedure 10.1
V.P.5. Document telephone messages accurately	Procedure 10.2
X.P.2.a. Apply HIPAA rules in regard to: privacy	Procedure 10.1
X.P.3. Document patient care accurately in the medical record	Procedures 10.1, 10.2
A.1 Demonstrate critical thinking skills	Procedure 10.2

ABHES Competencies	Assessments
7. Administrative Procedures g. Display professionalism through written and verbal communications	Procedures 10.1, 10.2

VOCABULARY REVIEW

Using the word pool on the right, find the correct word to match the definition. Write the word on the line after the definition.

Group A

1. A commercial service that answers telephone calls for its clients ______________________
2. An unexpected, life-threatening situation that requires immediate action ______________________
3. A business telephone system that allows more than one telephone line ______________________
4. A feature that states who the caller is and displays the telephone numbers of incoming calls made to a particular line ______________________
5. The depth of a tone or sound; a distinctive quality of sound ______________________
6. A telephone feature that allows calls made to one number to be sent to another specified number ______________________

Word Pool

- multiple line telephone system
- ergonomics
- speakerphone
- caller ID
- voice mail
- emergency
- call forwarding
- answering service
- intercom
- provider
- speed dialing
- pitch

7. An applied science concerned with designing and arranging things needed to do a job in an efficient and safe way ______________________
8. An individual or company that supplies medical care and services to a patient or the public ______________________
9. A telephone with a loudspeaker and a microphone; it can be used without having to pick up and hold the handset ______________________
10. A telephone function in which a selected stored number can be dialed by pressing only one key ______________________
11. An electronic system that allows messages from telephone callers to be recorded and stored ______________________
12. A two-way communication system with a microphone and loudspeaker at each station; often a feature of business telephones ______________________

Group B

1. Ability to communicate effectively in two languages ______________________
2. A physician or other healthcare provider who enters into a contract with a specific insurance company or program and by doing so agrees to abide by certain rules and regulations set forth by that third-party payer ______________________
3. A set dollar amount that the patient must pay for each visit ______________________
4. A system that distributes incoming calls to a specific group or person based on customer need; for example, the customer presses 1 for appointments, 2 for billing questions, and so on ______________________
5. A succession of syllables, words, or sentences spoken in an unvaried key or pitch ______________________
6. The use of articulate, clear sounds when speaking ______________________
7. The quality of having a sense of what to do or say to maintain good relations with others or to prevent offense ______________________
8. The vocabulary of a particular profession as opposed to common, everyday terms ______________________
9. A system for examining and separating into different groups; in the healthcare facility, it means determining the severity of illness that patients experience and prioritizing appointments based on that severity ______________________
10. The process of assigning degrees of urgency to patients' conditions ______________________
11. An acute situation that requires immediate attention but is not life-threatening ______________________
12. The medical abbreviation for the Latin term *statum*, meaning immediately; at this moment ______________________

Word Pool

- monotone
- enunciation
- tactful
- jargon
- screen
- triage
- urgent
- copayment (copay)
- participating provider
- STAT
- bilingual
- automatic call routing

SKILLS AND CONCEPTS

Answer the following questions. Write your answer on the line or in the space provided.

A. Telephone Equipment

1. Give an example of when the following telephone features would be used.

Speakerphone: ______________________________

Conference calls: ______________________________

Voice mail: ______________________________

Call forwarding: ______________________________

Intercom: ______________________________

B. Effective Use of the Telephone

1. List three things involved in active listening.

   a. ______________________________

   b. ______________________________

   c. ______________________________

2. If you are speaking clearly and distinctly, you are using good ____________.

3. It is important to make sure that patients understand what we are saying to them. In healthcare, medical terminology or ____________ can make things more difficult for patients to understand.

C. Managing Telephone Calls

1. List the supplies needed to be prepared to answer incoming telephone calls. ____________

   ____

   ____

   ____

   ____

2. How should a second incoming call be handled when you are already answering another call?

   ____

   ____

   ____

   ____

3. How should callers who refuse to identify themselves be handled? ____________

   ____

   ____

   ____

   ____

   ____

4. List the conditions and/or symptoms that would be considered an emergency call. ____________

   ____

   ____

   ____

   ____

5. What questions should be asked of the patient who calls the healthcare facility to give the provider the information that they need?

____

____

____

____

D. Typical Incoming Calls

1. When a patient calls requesting a medication refill, what information is needed? ____________

____

____

____

____

____

____

2. How should requests for directions be handled? ______________________

____

____

____

____

3. When a patient calls and asks for a referral to another provider, what should the medical assistant do?

____

____

____

____

____

E. Special Incoming Calls

1. If a patient refuses to discuss their symptoms over the phone with the medical assistant and the provider is not able to take the call, what should the medical assistant suggest the patient do?

____

____

2. What is the best policy when a patient calls for test results that are abnormal? ______________________

3. What documentation should be in place before a medical assistant can give information to a third party?

4. How should a caller with a complaint be handled? ______________________

F. Handling Difficult Calls

Indicate how you would handle the following calls.

1. Angry callers ______________________

2. Aggressive callers ______________________

3. Unauthorized inquiry calls ______________________

4. Sales calls ______________________

5. Callers who speak foreign languages or have heavy accents: ______________________________

____

____

____

____

G. Typical Outgoing Calls

1. Use Figure 10.4 in the textbook to answer the following questions.
   a. You are in the Central time zone and need to call an insurance carrier in the Pacific time zone. It is 9:00 AM in your location. What time is it in the Pacific time zone?

   ____

   b. You are in the Pacific time zone and your provider has asked you to contact another provider in the Eastern time zone. It is 10:00 AM in your time zone. What time is it in the Eastern time zone?

   ____

   c. You are in the Eastern time zone and need to contact a patient who is vacationing in the Mountain time zone. It is 3:00 PM in your time zone. What time is it in the Mountain time zone?

   ____

H. Using Directory Assistance

1. List options for locating a telephone number. ______________________________

____

____

____

____

____

I. Telephone Services

1. Explain the difference between an answering machine and answering service. ______________________________

____

____

____

____

____

CERTIFICATION PREPARATION

Circle the correct answer.

1. Which best describes the primary goal of "screening" telephone calls?
   a. Preventing calls from reaching the provider
   b. Handling calls at the lowest level possible
   c. Selecting which calls should be forwarded to which staff members through an understanding of the purpose of the call
   d. Determining whether the calls are emergencies

2. Active listening involves
   a. giving the same attention to a person on the telephone as would be given to a person face to face.
   b. concentrating on the conversation at hand.
   c. discovering vital information.
   d. all of the above.

3. The medical assistant should be extremely careful when using a speakerphone because
   a. the service is expensive.
   b. it is distracting.
   c. the call can be traced.
   d. confidentiality can be violated.

4. Which term would be considered jargon?
   a. Encephalalgia
   b. Rash
   c. Dizziness
   d. Headache

5. The medical assistant may help an angry caller calm down by
   a. getting angry in return.
   b. speaking in a lower tone of voice.
   c. referring the situation to the office manager immediately.
   d. calling the provider into the situation.

6. If your office is in New York and you need to contact a supplier in Seattle, which New York time would be the earliest that you should call to place an order, assuming that the supplier opens at 8 AM?
   a. 8:00 AM
   b. 9:00 AM
   c. 10:00 AM
   d. 11:00 AM

7. Which types of calls should be limited in the professional setting?
   a. Local
   b. Long distance
   c. Toll free
   d. Personal

8. Enunciation is
   a. the choice of words.
   b. the highness or lowness of sound.
   c. articulation of clear sounds.
   d. a change in pitch.

9. Which is *not* required when a telephone message is taken?
   a. The caller's name and phone number
   b. The time and date
   c. The name of the person to whom the call is directed
   d. The caller's account number

10. When placing callers on hold, how often should you check back to make sure the caller still wants to remain on hold?
    a. No longer than 1 minute
    b. Every 2 minutes
    c. Until time is available to talk
    d. It is not necessary to check back; patients will hold until you return to the call

WORKPLACE APPLICATIONS

1. Mr. Ken Thomas calls to get his prescription for Ambien refilled. His pharmacy is Wolfe Drug, and the drugstore phone number is 214-555-4523. Mr. Thomas is allergic to penicillin. His phone number is 214-555-2377. Mr. Thomas' message was received on July 23 at 10:15 AM.

   a. Who should receive this message? ______________________________

   ____

   b. Questions to ask the patient: ______________________________

   ____

   ____

   c. What action should be taken after speaking with the patient? ______________________________

   ____

   ____

   ____

   ____

2. Message retrieved from the answering machine, "This is Sarah at AnyTown Lab with a STAT laboratory report. It is 9:35 AM on November 16. The patient's name is Noemi Rodriguez, date of birth November 4, 19XX and her WBC count is 18,000. Please notify Dr. Walden immediately. The laboratory phone number is 800-555-3333 and my extension is 255. If she has any questions, please have her give me a call. Thanks."

   a. Who should receive this message? ______________________________

   ____

   b. Questions to ask Sarah: ______________________________

   ____

   ____

   c. What action should be taken? ______________________________

   ____

   ____

   ____

   ____

   ____

3. Denise has been the receptionist for a moderately large clinic for the past 3 months. She replaced Dorothy, who retired. Denise has been overwhelmed with the calls to the clinic, and the office manager has spoken to her twice about missing calls. Denise insists that she is constantly on the phone answering and transferring calls. She is beginning to lose faith in herself, but as she considers why she is failing at her job, she realizes that two new physicians have joined the practice since Dorothy left, and numerous calls come to the clinic for those two providers. Denise wants to suggest to the office manager that perhaps the time has come for a second receptionist, but she is unsure how to broach the subject. How can Denise begin her conversation with the office manager? What should she not do or say?

____

____

____

____

____

____

INTERNET ACTIVITIES

1. Using online resources, locate the following telephone numbers for your city or community.
   a. Nonemergency number for the police department ______________________
   b. Local social security office ______________________
   c. American Red Cross office ______________________
   d. Acute care hospital ______________________
   e. Meals on Wheels ______________________
   f. American Cancer Society ______________________
   g. Local senior center ______________________
   h. Local food bank ______________________
   i. Poison control ______________________
   j. Local child protective services ______________________

Procedure 10.1 Demonstrate Professional Telephone Techniques

Name ______________________________ **Date** ____________ **Score** __________

Task: To answer the telephone in a provider's office in a professional manner and respond to a request for action.

Scenario: Charles Johnson, DOB 3/3/19XX, an established patient of Dr. Martin, has called to schedule an appointment to have his blood pressure checked. This will be a follow-up appointment that is 15 minutes long. He is requesting that the appointment be on a Friday during his lunchtime between 11:00 and 12:00.

Equipment and Supplies:
- Telephone
- Pen or pencil
- Computer
- Notepad

Standard: Complete the procedure and all critical steps in _______ minutes with a minimum score of 85% within two attempts (*or as indicated by the instructor*).

Scoring: Divide the points earned by the total possible points. Failure to perform a critical step, indicated by an asterisk (*), results in grade no higher than an 84% (*or as indicated by the instructor*).

Time: Began_________ Ended_________ Total minutes: _________

Steps:	**Point Value**	**Attempt 1**	**Attempt 2**
1. Demonstrate telephone techniques by answering the telephone by the third ring.	**10**		
2. Speak distinctly with a pleasant tone and expression, at a moderate rate, and with sufficient volume for the person to understand every word.	**15***		
3. Identify the office and/or provider and yourself.	**10**		
4. Verify the identity of the caller, and if using an electronic health record, bring the patient's health record to the active screen of the computer.	**15***		
5. Screen the call if necessary.	**10**		
6. Apply active listening skills to assess whether the caller is distressed or agitated and to determine the concern to be addressed.	**10***		
7. Determine the needs of the caller and provide the requested information or service if possible. Provide the caller with excellent customer service. Be as helpful as possible. Check the appointment schedule and determine the first Friday that would have an open appointment between 11:00 and 12:00.	**10**		
8. Obtain sufficient patient information to schedule the appointment, including the patient's full name, DOB, insurance information, and preferred contact method. Repeat the date and time of the appointment to ensure that the patient has the correct information.	**10**		
9. Terminate the call in a pleasant manner and replace the receiver gently, always allowing the caller to hang up first.	**10**		
Total Points	**100**		

Comments

CAAHEP Competencies	Step(s)
V.P.4. Demonstrate professional telephone techniques	Entire procedure
X.P.2.a Apply HIPAA rules in regard to: privacy	4
X.P.3. Document patient care accurately in the medical record	Entire procedure
ABHES Competencies	**Step(s)**
7. Administrative Procedures g. Display professionalism through written and verbal communications	Entire procedure

Procedure 10.2 Document Telephone Messages and Report Relevant Information Concisely and Accurately

Name ______________________________ **Date** __________ **Score** __________

Tasks: To take an accurate telephone message and follow up on the requests made by the caller.

Scenario: Norma Washington, DOB 8/1/19XX, an established patient of Dr. Martin, has called to report her blood pressure readings that she has been taking at home. Dr. Martin had made a recent change in her medication and wanted her to monitor her BP at home for 3 days and call in with the results. She has taken her blood pressure in the morning and in the evening for the past 3 days, with the following results: (Role play this scenario with a peer who is the patient.)

- Day 1: 144/92 in the AM, 156/94 in the PM
- Day 2: 136/84 in the AM, 142/86 in the PM
- Day 3: 132/80 in the AM, 138/82 in the PM

Equipment and Supplies:

- Telephone
- Computer or message pad
- Pen or pencil
- Health record

Standard: Complete the procedure and all critical steps in _______ minutes with a minimum score of 85% within two attempts (*or as indicated by the instructor*).

Scoring: Divide the points earned by the total possible points. Failure to perform a critical step, indicated by an asterisk (*), results in grade no higher than an 84% (*or as indicated by the instructor*).

Time: Began________ Ended________ Total minutes: ________

Steps:	**Point Value**	**Attempt 1**	**Attempt 2**
1. Demonstrate telephone techniques by answering the telephone using the guidelines in Procedure 10.1.	**15**		
2. Using a message pad or the computer, take the phone message (either on paper or by data entry into the computer) and obtain the following information: • Name of the person to whom the call is directed • Name of the person calling • Caller's telephone number • Reason for the call, using critical thinking skills to ask the appropriate questions (Refer to the Checklist for Affective Behaviors) • Action to be taken, using critical thinking skills to determine the correct action to be taken (Refer to the Checklist for Affective Behaviors) • Date and time of the call • Initials of the person taking the call	**15***		
3. Apply active listening skills and repeat the information back to the caller after recording the message.	**10**		
4. End the call and wait for the caller to hang up first.	**10**		

5. Document the telephone call with all pertinent information in the patient's health record.	**10***		
6. Deliver the phone message to the appropriate person.	**10**		
7. Follow up on important messages.	**10**		
8. If using paper messaging, keep old message books for future reference. Carbonless copies allow the facility to keep a permanent record of phone messages. If using an electronic system, the message will be saved to the patient's record automatically.	**10**		
9. File pertinent phone messages in the patient's health record. Make sure the computer record is closed after the documentation has been done.	**10**		
Total Points	**100**		

Checklist for Affective Behaviors

Affective Behavior	**Directions:** *Check behaviors observed during the role-play.*					
Critical Thinking	**Negative, Unprofessional Behaviors**	**Attempt 1**	**Attempt 2**	**Positive, Professional Behaviors**	**Attempt 1**	**Attempt 2**
	Coached or told of an issue or problem			Independently identified the problem or issue		
	Failed to ask relevant questions related to the condition			Asked appropriate questions to obtain the information required		
	Failed to consider alternatives; failed to ask questions that demonstrate understanding of principles/concepts			Willing to consider other alternatives; asked appropriate questions that showed understanding of principles/concepts		
	Failed to make an educated, logical judgment/decision; actions or lack of actions demonstrated unsafe practices and/or do not follow the protocol			Made an educated, logical judgment/decision based on the protocol; actions reflected principles of safe practice		
	Other:			Other:		

Grading for Affective Behaviors		Point Value	Attempt 1	Attempt 2
Does not meet Expectation	• Response fails to show critical thinking. • Student demonstrated more than 2 negative, unprofessional behaviors during the interaction.	0		
Needs Improvement	• Response fails to show critical thinking. • Student demonstrated 1 or 2 negative, unprofessional behaviors during the interaction.	0		
Meets Expectation	• Response demonstrates critical thinking; no negative, unprofessional behaviors observed. • More practice is needed for behavior to appear natural and for student to appear comfortable and at ease.	15		
Occasionally Exceeds Expectation	• Response demonstrates critical thinking; no negative, unprofessional behaviors observed. • At times student appeared comfortable and at ease; but more practice is needed for behavior to become natural and consistent with a professional medical assistant.	15		
Always Exceeds Expectation	• Response demonstrates critical thinking; no negative, unprofessional behaviors observed. • Student's behaviors appeared natural and comfortable. Behaviors are consistent with a professional medical assistant.	15		

Comments

CAAHEP Competencies	Step(s)
V.P.4. Demonstrate professional telephone techniques	1, 3, 4
V.P.5. Document telephone messages accurately	2, 5
A.1 Demonstrate critical thinking skills	2
X.P.3. Document patient care accurately in the medical record	Entire procedure
ABHES Competencies	**Step(s)**
7. Administrative Procedures g. Display professionalism through written and verbal communications	Entire procedure

Student Name_______________________________________ Date_______________________

chapter 11

Scheduling Appointments and Patient Processing

CAAHEP Competencies	Assessments
VI.C.1. Identify different types of appointment scheduling methods	Skills and Concepts – C. 1-3
VI.C.2. Identify critical information required for scheduling patient procedures	Skills and Concepts – G. 1
VI.P.1. Manage appointment schedule using established priorities	Procedures 11.1, 11.2, 11.4
VI.P.2. Schedule a patient procedure	Procedure 11.5
VII.P.2. Input accurate patient billing information in Practice Management System (PMS)	Procedure 11.2
V.P.3.a. Coach patients regarding: office policies	Procedure 11.3
A.1. Demonstrate critical thinking skills	Procedures 11.2, 11.5
A.3. Demonstrate empathy for patients' concerns	Procedure 11.2
ABHES Competencies	**Assessments**
7. Administrative Procedures e. Apply scheduling principles	Procedures 11.1, 11.2, 11.4, 11.5

VOCABULARY REVIEW

Using the word pool on the right, find the correct word to match the definition. Write the word on the line after the definition.

Group A

1. Documentation in the medical record to track the patient's condition and progress ______________________
2. Space of time between events ______________________
3. An unexpected event that throws a plan into disorder; an interruption that prevents a system or process from continuing as usual or as expected ______________________
4. Skilled as a result of training or practice ______________________
5. A rule that controls how something should be done; guidelines or boundaries ______________________
6. An appointment type used when a patient needs to see the provider after a condition should have been resolved or to monitor an ongoing condition ______________________
7. The environment where something is created or takes shape; a base on which to build ______________________
8. Statistical data of a population; in healthcare, this includes patient name, address, date of birth, employment, and other details ______________________
9. A type of software that allows the user to enter demographic information, schedule appointments, maintain lists of insurance payers, perform billing tasks, and generate reports ______________________
10. Essential; being an indispensable part of a whole ______________________

Word Pool

- parameters
- demographics
- integral
- intervals
- matrix
- follow-up appointment
- proficiency
- practice management software
- progress notes
- disruption

Group B

1. A means of achieving a particular end, as in a situation requiring urgency or caution ______________________
2. The process of confirming health insurance coverage for the patient ______________________
3. A written document describing the healthcare facility's privacy practices ______________________
4. A system for examining and separating into different groups; in the healthcare facility, it means determining the severity of illness that patients experience and prioritizing appointments based on that severity ______________________
5. The process of determining if a procedure or service is covered by the insurance plan and what the reimbursement is for that procedure or service ______________________

Word Pool

- Notice of Privacy Practices
- preauthorization
- precertification
- established patients
- screening
- no-show
- expediency
- triage
- patient portal
- verification of eligibility

6. To sort out and classify the injured; used in the military and emergency settings to determine the priority of a patient to be treated ______________________
7. A patient who has been treated previously by the healthcare provider within the past 3 years ______________________
8. A secure online website that gives patients 24-hour access to personal health information using a username and password ______________________
9. When a patient fails to keep an appointment without giving advance notice ______________________
10. The process of determining if a procedure or service is covered by the insurance plan and what the reimbursement is for that procedure or service ______________________

ABBREVIATIONS

Write out what each of the following abbreviations stands for.

1. ECG______________________
2. NPP______________________
3. MRI______________________
4. CT______________________
5. EMT______________________
6. EHR______________________
7. HIPAA______________________
8. CDC______________________

SKILLS AND CONCEPTS

Answer the following questions. Write your answer on the line or in the space provided.

Scheduling Appointments

A. Establishing the Appointment Schedule

1. When developing an appointment schedule, ______________________ and ______________________ must be considered.

2. ______________________ information includes the patient's address, insurance information, and email address.

B. Creating the Appointment Matrix

1. Time would be blocked out in the schedule for what four reasons when setting up the appointment matrix?

   a. ______________________________

   b. ______________________________

   c. ______________________________

   d. ______________________________

2. How can the medical assistant handle a provider who habitually spends more than the allotted time with patients?

   ____

   ____

   ____

   ____

3. Using the appointment schedule page that follows, schedule these appointments, blocking out the appropriate amount of time:

   Recheck appointment 15 minutes

   Complete physical examination (PE) 45 minutes

   a. Jana Green; recheck appointment, prefers Wednesdays
   b. Pedro Gomez; complete physical examination, prefers Tuesdays
   c. Truong Tran; recheck, prefers Thursdays after 9:00 AM
   d. Walter Biller; complete physical examination, prefers Mondays as early as possible
   e. Reuven Ahmad; complete physical examination, prefers Fridays

	Monday	Tuesday	Wednesday	Thursday	Friday
8:00					
8:15					
8:30					
8:45					
9:00					
9:15					
9:30					
9:45					
10:00					

C. Methods of Scheduling Appointments

1. The two most common methods of appointment scheduling are ____________________ and ____________________.

2. Computerized scheduling utilizes ____________________ software.

3. The type of computerized scheduling that allows the patient to use secure links to find and select appointments is called ________________________.

D. Types of Appointment Scheduling

Briefly describe each type of scheduling and list one advantage and one disadvantage of each.

1. Time-specified (stream) scheduling ____

2. Open office hours ____

3. Wave scheduling ____

4. Modified wave scheduling ____

5. Double booking ____________________

6. Grouping procedures ____________________

E. Telephone Scheduling

1. When scheduling an appointment over the telephone, what options are available to remind patients of the appointment?

____

F. Scheduling Appointments for New Patients

1. To determine how much time to allow for an appointment, the medical assistant needs to obtain information about the ____________________.
2. New patients should be asked to arrive ____________________ minutes early to complete necessary paperwork.
3. An ideal tool to provide new patients with information is a(n) ____________________.

G. Scheduling Other Types of Appointments

1. Identify critical information required for scheduling patient procedures. ____________________

2. Identify the special requests that a provider may have for inpatient surgeries. ______________________

____

____

____

____

H. Special Circumstances

1. What is the difference between an emergency appointment and an urgent appointment? ______________

____

____

____

____

2. How does the medical assistant handle a patient who arrives at the clinic to see the provider but does not have an appointment?

____

____

____

____

I. Increasing Appointment Show Rates

Practice completing appointment reminder cards on the forms provided. Students should be able to fill out the appointment cards with the information provided without difficulty.

1. Tai Yan has an appointment for August 23, 20XX, at 3:00 PM with Dr. Martin.

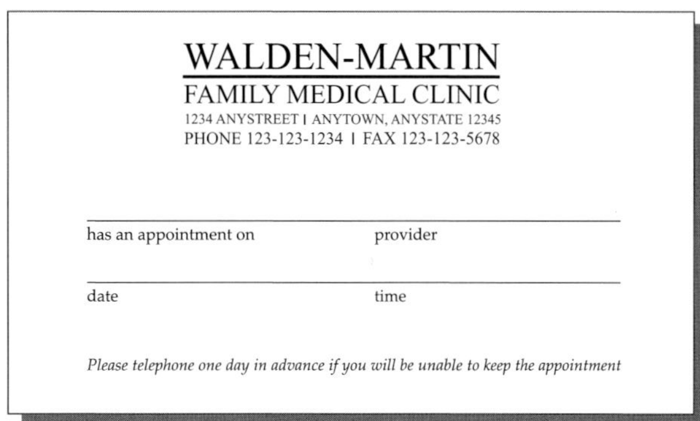
WALDEN-MARTIN
FAMILY MEDICAL CLINIC
1234 ANYSTREET | ANYTOWN, ANYSTATE 12345
PHONE 123-123-1234 | FAX 123-123-5678

has an appointment on ____________ provider ____________

date ____________ time ____________

Please telephone one day in advance if you will be unable to keep the appointment

2. Diego Lopez has an appointment for May 1, 20XX, at 9:00 AM with Dr. Walden.

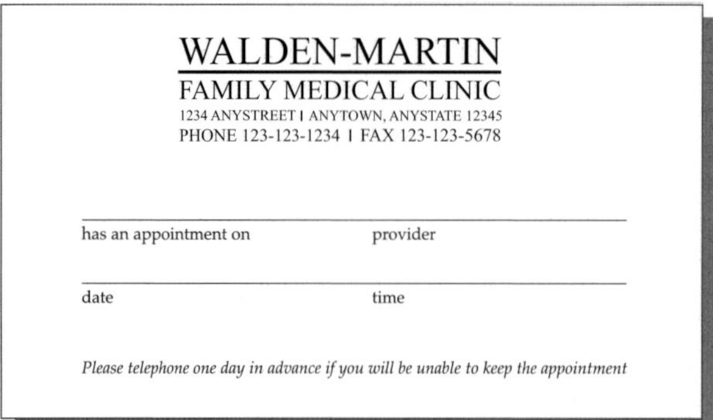
WALDEN-MARTIN
FAMILY MEDICAL CLINIC
1234 ANYSTREET | ANYTOWN, ANYSTATE 12345
PHONE 123-123-1234 | FAX 123-123-5678

has an appointment on provider

date time

Please telephone one day in advance if you will be unable to keep the appointment

3. Julia Berkley has an appointment for June 13, 20XX, at 11:45 AM with Dr. Walden.

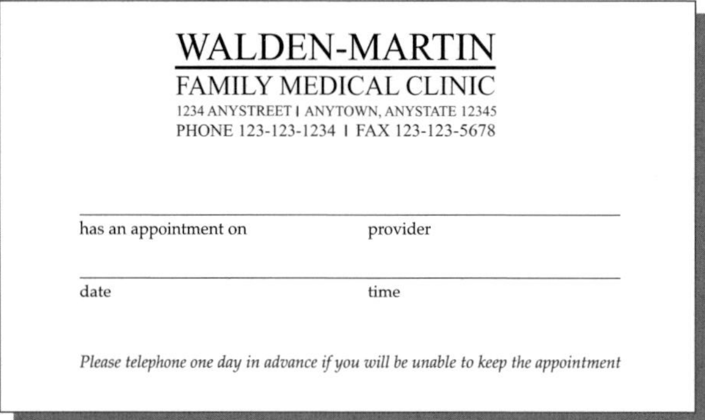
WALDEN-MARTIN
FAMILY MEDICAL CLINIC
1234 ANYSTREET | ANYTOWN, ANYSTATE 12345
PHONE 123-123-1234 | FAX 123-123-5678

has an appointment on provider

date time

Please telephone one day in advance if you will be unable to keep the appointment

4. Monique Jones has an appointment for September 12, 20XX, at 2:40 PM with Jean Burke, N.P.

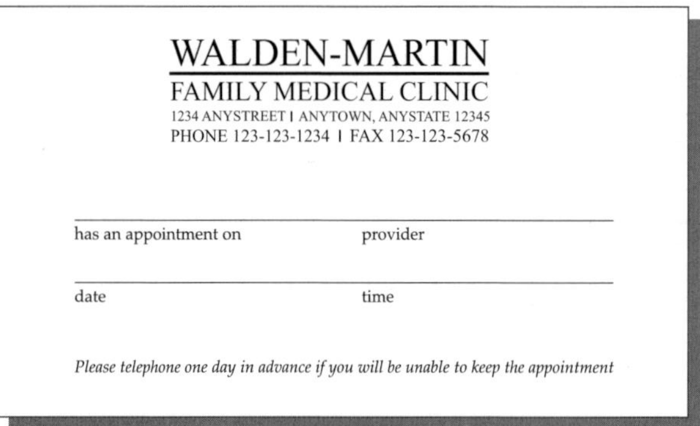
WALDEN-MARTIN
FAMILY MEDICAL CLINIC
1234 ANYSTREET | ANYTOWN, ANYSTATE 12345
PHONE 123-123-1234 | FAX 123-123-5678

has an appointment on provider

date time

Please telephone one day in advance if you will be unable to keep the appointment

5. Ken Thomas has an appointment for December 15, 20XX, at 4:30 PM with Dr. Martin.

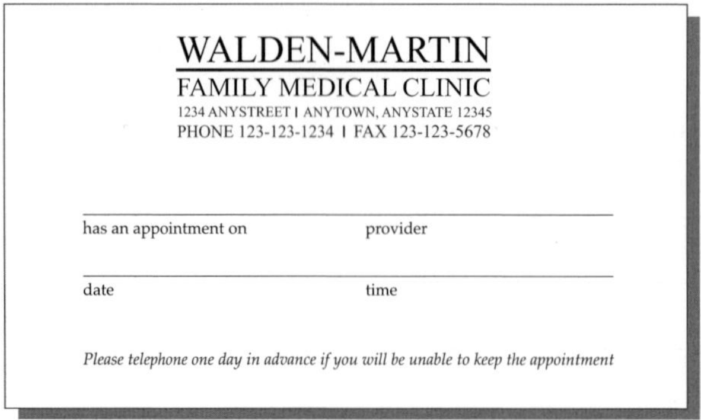
WALDEN-MARTIN
FAMILY MEDICAL CLINIC
1234 ANYSTREET | ANYTOWN, ANYSTATE 12345
PHONE 123-123-1234 | FAX 123-123-5678

has an appointment on provider

date time

Please telephone one day in advance if you will be unable to keep the appointment

Patient Processing Tasks

1. When screening patients at the reception desk, what patient conditions require immediate action by the medical assistant?

2. What action should the medical assistant take when patients have emergent conditions?

3. If a medical assistant is unable to greet a patient at the reception desk, what actions can help acknowledge the person?

4. List six features of a HIPAA-appropriate sign-in register.

5. List three features that would cause a HIPAA violation with sign-in registers.

6. How does a medical assistant take steps to protect other patients in the reception area?

7. What must occur if a patient refuses to sign the NPP form? ______________________

8. How should a medical assistant review a new patient brochure with a new patient? ______________________

9. During the check-in process, what three things must the medical assistant do for all patients? ______________________

10. If the provider is delayed, what should the medical assistant do with the patients who are waiting?

11. How should a medical assistant handle a situation when a patient is angry? ______________________

12. What occurs during the checkout process? ______________________

CERTIFICATION PREPARATION

Circle the correct answer.

1. The medical assistant may help an angry caller to calm down by
   a. getting angry in return.
   b. speaking in a lower tone of voice.
   c. referring the situation to the office manager immediately.
   d. calling the provider into the situation.

2. Why is it necessary to include a note in the patient's chart when the person does not show up for a scheduled appointment?
   a. To bill the patient for the time
   b. To keep count of the number of no-shows for a possible drop in the future
   c. To be prepared for future legal consequences regarding the patient's care
   d. To provide the medical assistant with a reminder to call and reschedule

3. What is the appointment-setting method by which a patient logs onto the internet and views a facility's schedule to set his or her own appointment?
   a. Flexible office hours
   b. Self-scheduling
   c. Grouping procedures
   d. Advance booking

4. An obstetrician who devotes two afternoons a week to seeing pregnant patients is using an appointment scheduling method called
   a. wave scheduling.
   b. advance booking.
   c. grouping procedures.
   d. modified wave scheduling.

5. Which type of scheduling is an attempt to create short-term flexibility within each hour?
   a. Time-specified scheduling
   b. Wave scheduling
   c. Stream scheduling
   d. Modified wave scheduling

6. All patients want to be kept informed about how long they should expect to wait to see the provider. Any delay longer than _____ minutes should be explained.
   a. 15
   b. 20
   c. 30
   d. No explanation is necessary

7. When screening patients at the reception desk, which patient has an emergent condition and requires immediate care?
   a. Chest pain
   b. Sore throat
   c. Tick bite
   d. Ankle injury

8. When calling a patient from the reception room to escort him to an exam room, how should the medical assistant call the patient?
   a. "James Brown, Dr. Walden is ready for you."
   b. "James Brown with the sore throat"
   c. "James Brown with a birthdate of June 6"
   d. "James Brown"

9. The statistical characteristics of human populations are called
   a. numbers.
   b. perceptions.
   c. demographics.
   d. phonetics.

10. An effective way to deal with patients who are always late for appointments is to
    a. refuse to schedule them after this happens several times.
    b. have them wait until it is convenient for the physician.
    c. advise them that they disrupt the office schedule.
    d. give them the last appointment of the day.

WORKPLACE APPLICATIONS

1. Janie Haynes consistently arrives at the clinic between 15 and 45 minutes late. She always has a "good" excuse, but she could make her appointments on time if she had better time management skills. The office manager has mentioned to Paula, the receptionist, that Janie is to be scheduled at 4:45 PM and if she is late, she will not be seen by the provider. Paula books Janie's next three appointments at that time, and Janie actually arrives early. However, on the fourth appointment, Janie arrives at 5:50 PM, and Paula knows that it is her responsibility to tell Janie that she cannot see the provider. How does Paula handle this task? What are the options for Paula?

2. Jill is the receptionist for Drs. Boles and Bailey, who are psychiatrists. Each week, Sara Ables comes to her appointments but brings her two children, Joey and Julie, ages 8 and 6 years, respectively. When Sara goes back for her appointment, the children are almost uncontrollable in the reception area. Although there are never more than two patients waiting, the kids are a serious disruption in the clinic. When Jill mentioned the problem to Dr. Boles, he said that Sara really needs the sessions and that Jill should try to work with Sara on this issue. What can Jill do to remedy the situation?

INTERNET ACTIVITIES

1. Using online resources, research group appointments. Create a poster presentation, a PowerPoint presentation, or write a paper summarizing your research. Include the following points in your project:
   a. Description of a group appointment
   b. List the types of conditions that are best suited for group appointments
   c. Explain whose confidentiality is maintained with group appointments
   d. List the benefits for patients and providers when group appointments are used

Procedure 11.1 Establish the Appointment Matrix

Name ______________________________ **Date** ____________ **Score** __________

Task: To establish the matrix of the appointment schedule.

Scenario: You have been asked to set up the schedule matrix for Dr. Julie Walden, Dr. James Martin, and Dr. Angela Perez. Block off the following times in the appointment schedule:

Dr. Julie Walden:
- Lunch; daily from 11:30 AM to 12:30 PM
- Hospital Rounds; Mondays and Wednesday from 8:00 AM to 9:00 AM

Dr. James Martin:
- Lunch; daily from 12:00 PM to 1:00 PM
- Hospital Rounds; Tuesdays and Thursday from 8:00 AM to 9:00 AM

Dr. Angela Perez:
- Lunch; daily from 12:30 PM to 1:30 PM
- Hospital Rounds; Fridays from 8:00 AM to 9:00 AM

Equipment and Supplies:
- Appointment book or computer with scheduling software
- Office procedure manual (optional)
- Black pen, pencil, and highlighters
- Calendar

Standard: Complete the procedure and all critical steps in _______ minutes with a minimum score of 85% within two attempts (*or as indicated by the instructor*).

Scoring: Divide the points earned by the total possible points. Failure to perform a critical step, indicated by an asterisk (*), results in grade no higher than an 84% (*or as indicated by the instructor*).

Time: Began_________ Ended_________ Total minutes: _________

Steps:	**Point Value**	**Attempt 1**	**Attempt 2**
1. Using the calendar, determine when the office is not open (e.g., holidays, weekends, evenings). If using the appointment book and a black pen, draw an *X* through the times the office is not open. If using the scheduling software, block the times the office is not open.	25*		
2. Identify the times each provider is not available. If using the appointment book, write in the providers' names on each column and then draw an *X* through their unavailable times. If using the scheduling software, select each provider and block the times the provider is unavailable.	25*		
3. Using the office procedure manual or providers' preferences, determine when each provider performs certain types of examinations. In the appointment book, indicate these examinations either by writing the examination time or by highlighting the examination times. Follow the office's procedure on indicating these examination times in the appointment book. When using scheduling software, set up the times for the examinations or use the highlighting feature if available.	25*		

4. Using the office procedure manual or the list of providers' preferences and availability, identify other times to block on the scheduling matrix. Some providers require catch-up times and these time slots are blocked. Some medical facilities save appointment times for same-day appointments. When saving time blocks for same-day appointments, make sure to use pencil so it can be erased and the patient's information entered on the day of the appointment. For the scheduling software, block those times when patients cannot be booked and indicate the times for the same-day appointments.	**25***		
Total Points	**100**		

Comments

CAAHEP Competencies	Step(s)
VI.P.1. Manage appointment schedule using established priorities	Entire procedure
ABHES Competencies	**Step(s)**
7. Administrative Procedures e. Apply scheduling principles	Entire procedure

Procedure 11.2 Schedule a New Patient

Name ____________________ **Date** __________ **Score** __________

Task: To schedule a new patient for a first office visit and identify the urgency of the visit using established priorities.

Scenario: Patricia Black, a new patient, calls. She just moved to the area and her asthma has flared up over the last 24 hours, but her albuterol inhaler is empty, and she needs a new prescription for it. She states that she is doing okay, but without the albuterol she knows it will get worse within the next few days. According to your screening guidelines, she needs to be seen today and scheduling guidelines indicate she needs a 45-minute appointment.

Equipment and Supplies:

- Appointment book or computer with scheduling software
- Scheduling and screening guidelines
- Pencil

Standard: Complete the procedure and all critical steps in _______ minutes with a minimum score of 85% within two attempts (*or as indicated by the instructor*).

Scoring: Divide the points earned by the total possible points. Failure to perform a critical step, indicated by an asterisk (*), results in grade no higher than an 84% (*or as indicated by the instructor*).

Time: Began_________ Ended_________ Total minutes: _________

Steps:	**Point Value**	**Attempt 1**	**Attempt 2**
1. Obtain the patient's demographic information (e.g., full name, birth date, address, and telephone number). Write this information down or enter it into the scheduling software. Verify the information.	**15***		
2. Determine whether the patient was referred by another provider.	**10**		
3. Determine the patient's chief complaint and when the first symptoms occurred. Utilize the scheduling and screening guidelines as needed. *(Refer to the Checklist for Affective Behaviors)*	**15***		
4. Search the appointment book or scheduling software for the first suitable appointment time and an alternate time. Offer the patient a choice of these dates and times. Be open to alternative times if the patient cannot make the initial options you gave. Provide additional appointment options as needed.	**10***		
5. Enter the mutually agreeable time into the schedule. Enter the patient's name, telephone number, and add *NP* for new patient.	**10**		
6. Obtain the patient's insurance information. If new patients are expected to pay at the time of the visit, explain this financial arrangement when the appointment is made.	**15***		
7. Provide the patient with directions to the healthcare facility and parking instructions if needed.	**10**		
8. Before ending the call, ask if the patient has any questions. Reinforce the date and time of the appointment. Politely and professionally end the call, making sure to thank the patient for calling. *(Refer to the Checklist for Affective Behaviors)*	**15**		
Total Points	**100**		

Checklist for Affective Behaviors

Affective Behavior	***Directions:*** *Check behaviors observed during the role-play.*					
	Negative, Unprofessional Behaviors	**Attempt 1**	**Attempt 2**	**Positive, Professional Behaviors**	**Attempt 1**	**Attempt 2**
Critical Thinking	Coached or told of an issue or problem			Independently identified the problem or issue		
	Failed to ask relevant questions related to the condition			Asked appropriate questions to obtain the information required		
	Failed to consider alternatives; failed to ask questions that demonstrated understanding of principles/concepts			Willing to consider other alternatives; asked appropriate questions that showed understanding of principles/concepts		
	Failed to make an educated, logical judgment/decision; actions or lack of actions demonstrated unsafe practices and/or did not follow the protocol			Made an educated, logical judgment/decision based on the protocol; actions reflected principles of safe practice		
	Other:			Other:		
Empathy	Distracted; not focused on the other person			Focused full attention on the other person		
	Judgmental attitude; not accepting attitude			Nonjudgmental, accepting attitude		
	Failed to clarify what the person verbally or nonverbally communicated			Used summarizing or paraphrasing to clarify what the person verbally or nonverbally communicated		
	Failed to acknowledge what the person communicated			Acknowledged what the person communicated		
	Rude, discourteous			Pleasant and courteous		
	Disregarded the person's dignity and rights			Maintained the person's dignity and rights		
	Other:			Other:		

Grading for Affective Behaviors		Point Value	Attempt 1	Attempt 2
Does not meet Expectation	• Response was disrespectful and/or insensitive. • Student demonstrated more than 2 negative, unprofessional behaviors during the interaction.	0		
Needs Improvement	• Response was disrespectful and/or insensitive. • Student demonstrated 1 or 2 negative, unprofessional behaviors during the interaction.	0		
Meets Expectation	• Response was respectful and sensitive; no negative, unprofessional behaviors observed. • More practice is needed for behavior to appear natural and for student to appear comfortable and at ease.	15		
Occasionally Exceeds Expectation	• Response was respectful and sensitive; no negative, unprofessional behaviors observed. • At times student appeared comfortable and at ease; but more practice is needed for behavior to become natural and consistent with a professional medical assistant.	15		
Always Exceeds Expectation	• Response was respectful and sensitive; no negative, unprofessional behaviors observed. • Student's behaviors appeared natural and comfortable. Behaviors are consistent with a professional medical assistant.	15		

Comments

CAAHEP Competencies	**Step(s)**
VI.P.1. Manage appointment schedule using established priorities	1-7
VI.A.1. Display sensitivity when managing appointments	3, 8
VII.P.2. Obtain accurate patient billing information	6
A.1 Demonstrate critical thinking skills	3
A.3 Demonstrate empathy for patients' concerns	8
ABHES Competencies	**Step(s)**
7. Administrative Procedures e. Apply scheduling principles	1-7

Procedure 11.3 Coach Patients Regarding Office Policies

Name ______________________________ **Date** ____________ **Score** __________

Tasks: Create a new patient brochure and then role-play ways to coach patients regarding office policies.

Scenario: You work at Walden-Martin Family Medical Clinic. Your supervisor asks you to create a new patient brochure for the clinic. The healthcare facility's information is listed here. After you complete the brochure, you coach the following patients regarding office procedures:

- Mr. Charles Johnson (he has a question regarding the payment policy)
- Ms. Monique Jones (she has a question regarding the medication refill procedure)

Healthcare Facility	Providers
Walden-Martin Family Medical Clinic 1234 Anystreet Anytown, Anystate 12345 Phone: 123-123-1234 Fax: 123-123-5678	Julie Walden, M.D. James Martin, M.D. Angela Perez, M.D. David Kahn, M.D. Jean Burke, N.P.

Equipment and Supplies:

- Computer with word processing software and printer
- Office procedure manual (optional)

Standard: Complete the procedure and all critical steps with a minimum score of 85% within two attempts (*or as indicated by the instructor*).

Scoring: Divide the points earned by the total possible points. Failure to perform a critical step, indicated by an asterisk (*), results in grade no higher than an 84% (*or as indicated by the instructor*).

Steps:	Point Value	Attempt 1	Attempt 2
1. Using word processing software, design an informational brochure for patients that provides information about the healthcare facility and describes practice procedures. At a minimum, the information should include the following: a. Description of the healthcare facility (e.g., type of practice, mission statement) b. Location or a map of the facility c. Contact information (i.e., telephone numbers, emails, and website addresses) d. Providers' names and credentials e. Services offered f. Hours of operation g. How appointments can be scheduled h. Healthcare facility's policies and procedures (e.g., payment policies, appointment cancellations, medication refills, assistance after hours) i. Insurance plans accepted	55		
2. Proofread the brochure. Revise as needed. Print the brochure.	5		
3. Using the scenario for the first patient, give a brief summary of the different parts of the brochure. Use words the patient will understand.	10*		

4. Ask if the patient has any questions. Actively listen to the patient's concerns. Address those concerns.	**10***		
5. Using the scenario for the second patient, give a brief summary of the different parts of the brochure. Use words that the patient understands.	**10***		
6. Ask if the patient has any questions. Actively listen to the patient's concerns. Address those concerns.	**10***		
Total Points	**100**		

Comments

CAAHEP Competencies	Step(s)
V.P.3.a. Coach patients regarding: office policies	3-6

Procedure 11.4 Schedule an Established Patient

Name ____ **Date** ____________ **Score** __________

Task: To manage the provider's schedule by scheduling appointments for an established patient and handling rescheduling and a no-show appointment.

Scenario: Celia Tapia has just finished seeing Dr. Martin and is checking out at your desk. You see that she needs to schedule a follow-up appointment in 2 weeks. The scheduling guidelines indicate a follow-up appointment is 15 minutes long.

Equipment and Supplies:
- Appointment book or computer with scheduling software
- Scheduling guidelines
- Pencil, red pen
- Reminder card
- Patient's health record

Standard: Complete the procedure and all critical steps in ______ minutes with a minimum score of 85% within two attempts (*or as indicated by the instructor*).

Scoring: Divide the points earned by the total possible points. Failure to perform a critical step, indicated by an asterisk (*), results in grade no higher than an 84% (*or as indicated by the instructor*).

Time: Began________ Ended________ Total minutes: ________

Steps:	**Point Value**	**Attempt 1**	**Attempt 2**
1. Obtain the patient's name and information, purpose of the visit, the provider to be seen, and any scheduling preferences. If using the scheduling software, enter the patient's name and date of birth (DOB). Verify the correct patient is selected.	**15**		
2. Identify the length of the appointment by using the scheduling guidelines.	**15***		
3. Search the appointment book or scheduling software for the first suitable appointment time and an alternate time. Offer the patient a choice of these dates and times. Be open to alternative times if the patient cannot make the initial options you gave. Provide additional appointment options as needed.	**15**		
4. Using a pencil, write the patient's name and phone number in the appointment book and block out the correct amount of time. Add in any other relevant information per the facility's procedures. If using the scheduling software, create the appointment per the facility's guidelines.	**15***		
5. Complete the appointment reminder card and ensure the date and time on the card matches the appointment time. Give the card to the patient.	**10**		
Scenario continues: Later that day, Celica Tapia calls and needs to reschedule her appointment for the next day at the same time.			
6. When a patient calls to reschedule an appointment, follow steps #1 through #4. When the new appointment is made, make sure to erase the old appointment from the appointment log. With the scheduling software, ensure the old appointment time is removed from the schedule. Repeat the appointment date and time to the patient.	**15**		

Scenario continues: Celia Tapia no-shows for her follow-up appointment.			
7. In the appointment book, using red pen, indicate the patient no-showed. Using the patient's health record, document that the patient failed to show for the follow-up examination with the provider. In an electronic system, change the appointment status to no-show and ensure that it is documented in the health record.	**15**		
Total Points	**100**		

Comments

CAAHEP Competencies	**Step(s)**
VI.P.1. Manage appointment schedule using established priorities	All
ABHES Competencies	**Step(s)**
7. Administrative Procedures e. Apply scheduling principles	All

Procedure 11.5 Schedule a Patient Procedure

Name ____ **Date** _____________ **Score** ___________

Task: To schedule a patient for a procedure within the time frame needed by the provider, confirm with the patient, and issue all required instructions.

Scenario: Monique Jones has just completed seeing Dr. Walden and is checking out at your desk. She gives you an order from the provider that states she needs to have a magnetic resonance image (MRI) of her left ankle within a week. The radiology department in your facility performs MRIs.

Equipment and Supplies:
- Provider's order detailing the procedure required
- Computer with order entry software (optional)
- Name, address, and telephone number of facility where procedure will take place
- Patient's demographic and insurance information
- Patient's health record
- Procedure preparation instructions
- Telephone
- Consent form (if required for procedure)

Standard: Complete the procedure and all critical steps in _______ minutes with a minimum score of 85% within two attempts (*or as indicated by the instructor*).

Scoring: Divide the points earned by the total possible points. Failure to perform a critical step, indicated by an asterisk (*), results in grade no higher than an 84% (*or as indicated by the instructor*).

Time: Began_________ Ended_________ Total minutes: _________

Steps:	**Point Value**	**Attempt 1**	**Attempt 2**
1. Obtain an oral or written order from the provider for the exact procedure to be performed.	**15**		
2. Gather the patient's demographic and insurance information. If using an electronic health record, verify you have the correct patient. *(Refer to the Checklist for Affective Behaviors)*	**15**		
3. Determine the patient's availability within the time frame provided by the provider for the procedure.	**15**		
4. Contact the diagnostic facility and schedule the patient's procedure. If you are using a computerized provider order entry (CPOE) system and your facility performs the procedure, you also need to enter the order using the CPOE system. • Provide the patient's diagnosis and provider's exact order, including the name of procedure and time frame. • Establish the date and time for the procedure. • Give the patient's name, age, address, telephone number, and insurance information (i.e., insurance policy numbers, precertification information, and addresses for filing claims). • Determine any special instructions for the patient or special anesthesia requirements. • Notify the facility of any urgency for test results.	**20***		

5. If a consent form is required for the procedure, ensure the provider has reviewed the form with the patient and the patient has signed the consent form. A copy of the consent form may be required by the diagnostic facility before the procedure. The consent form should be scanned and uploaded into the electronic health record or placed in the paper record.	**15**		
6. Document the details of the scheduled procedure in the patient's health record. If applicable, create a reminder to check on the procedure results after the appointment date.	**20***		
Total Points	**100**		

Checklist for Affective Behaviors

Affective Behavior	***Directions:*** *Check behaviors observed during the role-play.*					
Critical Thinking	**Negative, Unprofessional Behaviors**	**Attempt**		**Positive, Professional Behaviors**	**Attempt**	
		1	**2**		**1**	**2**
	Coached or told of an issue or problem			Independently identified the problem or issue		
	Failed to ask relevant questions related to the condition			Asked appropriate questions to obtain the information required		
	Failed to consider alternatives; failed to ask questions that demonstrated understanding of principles/concepts			Willing to consider other alternatives; asked appropriate questions that showed understanding of principles/concepts		
	Failed to make an educated, logical judgment/decision; actions or lack of actions demonstrated unsafe practices and/or did not follow the protocol			Made an educated, logical judgment/decision based on the protocol; actions reflected principles of safe practice		
	Other:			Other:		

Grading for Affective Behaviors		**Point Value**	**Attempt 1**	**Attempt 2**
Does not meet Expectation	• Response was disrespectful and/or insensitive. • Student demonstrated more than 2 negative, unprofessional behaviors during the interaction.	0		
Needs Improvement	• Response was disrespectful and/or insensitive. • Student demonstrated 1 or 2 negative, unprofessional behaviors during the interaction.	0		
Meets Expectation	• Response was respectful and sensitive; no negative, unprofessional behaviors observed. • More practice is needed for behavior to appear natural and for student to appear comfortable and at ease.	15		
Occasionally Exceeds Expectation	• Response was respectful and sensitive; no negative, unprofessional behaviors observed. • At times student appeared comfortable and at ease; but more practice is needed for behavior to become natural and consistent with a professional medical assistant.	15		
Always Exceeds Expectation	• Response was respectful and sensitive; no negative, unprofessional behaviors observed. • Student's behaviors appeared natural and comfortable. Behaviors are consistent with a professional medical assistant.	15		

Comments

CAAHEP Competencies	**Step(s)**
VI.P.2. Schedule a patient procedure	All
A.1 Demonstrate critical thinking skills	2
ABHES Competencies	**Step(s)**
7. Administrative Procedures e. Apply scheduling principles	All

Student Name____________________________ Date______________

chapter 12

Health Records

CAAHEP Competencies	Assessment
V.C.12. Identify subjective and objective information	Skills and Concepts – B. 7-16
VI.C.5. Identify the importance of data back-up	Skills and Concepts – C. 8.
VI.C.6. Identify the components of an Electronic Medical Record, Electronic Health Record, and Practice Management System	Skills and Concepts – A. 2-6
VI.P.3. Input patient data using an electronic system	Procedures 12.1, 12.2

ABHES Competencies	Assessment
1. General Orientation d. List the general responsibilities and skills of the medical assistant	Skills and Concepts – B. 17
4. Medical Law and Ethics a. Follow documentation guidelines	Skills and Concepts – C. 3-7
4. Medical Law and Ethics b. Institute federal and state guidelines when: 1) Releasing medical records or information 2) Entering orders in and utilizing electronic health records	Procedures 12.1, 12.2
7. Administrative Procedures a. Gather and process documents	Procedures 12.2, 12.5, 12.6
7. Administrative Procedures b. Navigate electronic health records systems and practice management software	Procedures 12.1, 12.2

VOCABULARY REVIEW

Using the word pool on the right, find the correct word to match the definition. Write the word on the line after the definition.

Group A

1. Data or information obtained from the patient ____________________
2. A process to ensure the reliability of test results ____________________
3. A computerized record that conforms to nationally recognized standards and contains health-related information about a specific patient ____________________
4. Data obtained through physical examination, laboratory and diagnostic testing, and measurable information ____________________
5. The likely outcome of a disease including chance of recovery ____________________
6. The ability to work with other systems ____________________
7. A rule that controls how something should be done; guidelines or boundaries ____________________
8. An interconnection between systems ____________________
9. A secure online website that gives patients 24-hour access to personal health information using a username and password ____________________
10. Meeting the standards and regulations of the practice's established policies and procedures ____________________

Word Pool

- electronic health record (EHR)
- quality control
- interoperability
- patient portal
- parameters
- interface
- compliance
- subjective information
- objective information
- prognosis

Group B

1. Occurring later or after ____________________
2. Granted or endowed with a particular authority, right, or property; to have a special interest in ____________________
3. Using as few words as possible to express the message ____________________
4. A temporary diagnosis made before all test results have been received ____________________
5. The smooth continuation of care from one provider to another that allows the patient to receive the most benefit and no interruption or duplication of care ____________________
6. Passed from parents to offspring through the genes ____________________
7. How often something happens ____________________
8. To remove or destroy all traces of; do away with ____________________
9. The most recent item is on top and oldest item is last ____________________
10. Pertaining to the measurement of the size and proportions of the human body ____________________

Word Pool

- continuity of care
- incidence
- hereditary
- concise
- anthropometric
- provisional diagnosis
- subsequent
- vested
- reverse chronologic order
- obliteration

Group C

1. The age at which a person is recognized by law to be an adult; it varies by state ______________________
2. A heading, title, or subtitle under which records are filed ______________________
3. To say something aloud for another person to write down ______________________
4. A chronologic file used as a reminder that something must be dealt with on a certain date ______________________
5. The filing of records, correspondence, or cards by number ______________________
6. To make a written copy of dictated material ______________________
7. A sturdy cardboard or plastic file-sized card used to replace a folder temporarily removed from the filing space ______________________
8. A system made up of combinations of the letters and numbers ______________________
9. A filing system where materials can be located without consulting another source of reference ______________________
10. Any system that arranges names or topics according to the sequence of the letters in the alphabet ______________________
11. A method or plan for retaining or keeping health records and for their movement from active to inactive to closed ______________________

Word Pool

- transcription
- dictation
- retention schedule
- age of majority
- out guides
- caption
- alphabetic filing
- direct filing system
- numeric filing
- alphanumeric
- tickler file

ABBREVIATIONS

Write out what each of the following abbreviations stands for.

1. AMA ______________________
2. CPT ______________________
3. EHR ______________________
4. HHS ______________________
5. HIE ______________________
6. HIPAA ______________________
7. HIV ______________________
8. ICD ______________________
9. NPP ______________________
10. ONC ______________________
11. PCP ______________________
12. PHI ______________________

13. PHR ______________________________

14. POR ______________________________

15. SOR ______________________________

16. TPR ______________________________

SKILLS AND CONCEPTS

Answer the following questions. Write your answer on the line or in the space provided.

A. Electronic Records

1. A(n) ____________________ is used to document patient care that is provided.

2. The health care facility's billing and accounting systems are part of the ____________________.

3. A(n) ____________________ can be accessed by more than one healthcare organization, while a(n) ____________________ can only be utilized by the healthcare organization that created it.

4. The legislation that provided financial incentives for providers to use an EHR in a meaningful way is
   a. HIPAA.
   b. ACA.
   c. HITECH.
   d. CMS.

5. The Promoting Interoperability program has _____ objectives that focus on patient health data access and interoperability.

B. Contents of the Health Record

1. Which of the following is a reason for having accurate health records?
   a. To provide legal protection for those who provided care to the patient
   b. To provide critical information for others
   c. To provide statistical information that is helpful to researchers
   d. To provide the best possible medical care for the patient
   e. All of the above

2. Patient's full name, email address, name of employer, and health insurance information are all examples of ________________________.

3. Previous illnesses, hospitalizations, and surgeries are considered ________________________.

4. The ________________________ contains health information about the patient's parents and siblings.

5. Lifestyle factors such as tobacco use, employment, and alcohol use are part of the ________________________.

6. The ________________________ is where information about the nature, location, frequency, and duration of pain of the patient's current condition are documented.

Match the description with the type of information. Answers can be used more than once.

7. _____ Patient's address
8. _____ Yellowed eyes
9. _____ Patient's email address
10. _____ Insurance information
11. _____ Elevated blood pressure
12. _____ Bloated stomach
13. _____ Complaint of headache
14. _____ Weight of 143 pounds
15. _____ Bruises on upper arms
16. _____ Patient's phone number

a. subjective
b. objective

17. Which of the following are the medical assistant's responsibilities when documenting in the health record?
    a. Ensure patient privacy.
    b. Use good interviewing techniques to obtain information.
    c. Document only in the EHR.
    d. All of the above
    e. a and b

C. Working with Health Records

1. Which of the following is considered a category used for organizing information in a POR system?
    a. Database
    b. Problem list
    c. Treatment plan
    d. Progress notes
    e. All of the above

2. Which of the following is an example category used in an SOR system?
    a. Progress notes
    b. Laboratory
    c. Database
    d. Radiology
    e. a, b, and d

Correct the following entries as would be done in the health record. Then rewrite the entries correctly. Handwritten corrections are acceptable on these exercises.

3. The correct date of the appointment below was October 12, 20XX.

    10-21-20XX 1330 Patient did not arrive for scheduled appointment. P. Smith, RMA

    ____

    ____

    ____

    ____

4. The patient stated that the chest pain began 2 weeks ago.

   1-31-20XX 10:00 AM Patient complained of chest pain for the past 2 months. No pain noted in arms. No nausea. Desires ECG and bloodwork to check for heart problems. R. Smithee, CMA (AAMA)

   ____

   ____

   ____

   ____

Document the following exercises.

5. Eric Robertson canceled his surgical follow-up appointment today for the third time. Document this information.

   ____

   ____

   ____

   ____

6. Angela Adams called to report that she was not feeling any better since her office visit on Monday. She wants the doctor to call in a refill for her antibiotics. The chart says that she was to return to the clinic on Thursday if she was not feeling better. Today is Monday, and she says she cannot come into the clinic this week. The physician wants to see her before prescribing any other medication. Document this information.

   ____

   ____

   ____

   ____

   ____

   ____

7. Mary Elizabeth Smith called the physician's office to report redness around an injection site. She was in the office 3 hours ago and received an injection of penicillin. She says she also is itching quite a bit around the site and having trouble breathing. The doctor has left the office for the day. Office policy states that if the physician is out of the office and a patient presents or calls with an emergency, they are to be referred to the ER. Document the action that the medical assistant should take.

   ____

   ____

   ____

   ____

   ____

   ____

8. Explain the importance of data backup. ____

____

____

____

9. If there is no rule to specify how long to retain records, it is best to keep them for _______ years.

10. According to HIPAA, which of the following has to be included on a release of information form?
    a. Who is releasing the information
    b. To whom the information is being released
    c. What specific information is to be released
    d. An expiration date for the release
    e. All of the above

D. Creating an Efficient Paper Health Records Management System

1. A(n) _________________________ have door locks to protect the contents and allows several individuals to have access to files at the same time.

2. ____________________ are used to replace a folder that has been temporarily removed.

3. Describe the indexing rules for alphabetic filing. _________________________________

____

____

____

____

____

____

____

____

____

E. Filing Methods

1. Using alphabetic filing, place the names below in correct alphabetic order with the last name first.

Cassidy Kay Hale
Candace Cassidy LeGrand
Taylor Ann Jackson
Anton Douglas Conn
Mitchel Michael Gibson
Lorienda Gaye Robison
LaNelle Elva Crumley
Allison Gaile Yarbrough
Sarah Kay Haile
Marie Gracelia Stuart
Karry Madge Chapmann
Randi Ann Perez
Cecelia Gayle Raglan
Sarah Sue Ragland
Riley Americus Belk
Starr Ellen Beall
Mitchell Thomas Gibson
George Scott Turner
Winston Roger Murchison
Sara Suzelle Montgomery
Tamika Noelle Frazier
Alisa Jordan Williams
Alisha Dawn Chapman
Bentley James Adams
Montana Skye Kizer
Dakota Marie LaRose
Robbie Sue Metzger
Thomas Charles Bruin
Percival "Butch" Adams
Carlos Perez Santos

1. ____________________
2. ____________________
3. ____________________
4. ____________________
5. ____________________
6. ____________________
7. ____________________
8. ____________________
9. ____________________
10. ____________________
11. ____________________
12. ____________________
13. ____________________
14. ____________________
15. ____________________
16. ____________________
17. ____________________
18. ____________________
19. ____________________
20. ____________________
21. ____________________
22. ____________________
23. ____________________
24. ____________________
25. ____________________
26. ____________________
27. ____________________
28. ____________________
29. ____________________
30. ____________________

2. Using terminal filing, place the numbers below in the correct order.

01-61-22	a.	________________
72-55-20	b.	________________
44-41-20	c.	________________
17-41-20	d.	________________
56-42-21	e.	________________
91-88-21	f.	________________
15-24-22	g.	________________
82-49-20	h.	________________
08-94-21	i.	________________
24-42-22	j.	________________

F. Organization of Files

1. Correspondence related to the operation of the of the office is considered ________________________ correspondence.

2. A filing system designed to remind you of something that needs to be done or followed up is a ________________________ file.

CERTIFICATION PREPARATION

Circle the correct answer.

1. Information that is obtained by questioning the patient or taken from a form is called ______ information.
   a. confidential
   b. subjective
   c. necessary
   d. objective

2. How would you properly index the name "Amanda M. Stiles-Duncan" for filing?
   a. Stilesduncan Amanda M.
   b. Stiles Duncan Amanda M.
   c. Duncanstiles Amanda M.
   d. Duncan Amanda M. Stiles

3. Who is the legal owner of the information stored in a patient's record?
   a. The patient
   b. The provider or agency where services were provided
   c. The patient's insurance company
   d. Both the patient and the provider

4. Which is *not* objective information?
   a. Progress notes
   b. Family history
   c. Diagnosis
   d. Physical examination and findings

5. Many healthcare facilities now use voice recognition software for transcription. The system can be used to dictate which types of reports?
   a. Progress notes
   b. Letters
   c. Emails
   d. All of the above

6. Perhaps the most essential action for the medical assistant working with a patient and using an electronic record is to
   a. type in every word the patient says.
   b. make sure the patient is not hiding any part of the health history.
   c. make frequent eye contact with patient and smile.
   d. sit in a chair across from the patient so that the person cannot see the screen.

7. Which EHR system backup requires the least amount of hardware?
   a. Online backup system
   b. External hard drives
   c. Full server backup
   d. Thumb drive backup

8. The concise account of symptoms in the patient's own words is the ______.
   a. objective information
   b. provisional diagnosis
   c. chief complaint
   d. caption

9. To completely remove all traces of an entry in a health record is ______.
   a. interface
   b. obliteration
   c. dictation
   d. compliance

10. The process of electronic data entry of a provider's instructions for the treatment of patients is called ______.
    a. progress notes
    b. computerized physician/provider order entry
    c. direct filing system
    d. continuity of care

WORKPLACE APPLICATIONS

1. Dr. Martin wants to be sure the Walden-Martin Family Medical (WMFM) Clinic is meeting all of the requirements for Promoting Interoperability. He has asked Susan to put together a list of what WMFM Clinic should be doing to meet those requirements. What would be on Susan's list?

   ____

   ____

   ____

   ____

2. Susan has been learning about the various EHR systems available. She has also been learning about the need to back up to protect the information stored in the EHR. Susan has asked the office manager at WMFM Clinic how the EHR is backed up at their facility. The office manager states that they currently use an external hard drive, but would like to look closer at other options. She asks Susan to determine what other options are available. Write a brief description of each of the options below.

   a. External hard drive ____

   ____

   b. Full server backup ____

   ____

   c. Online backup system ____

   ____

INTERNET ACTIVITIES

1. Using online resources, research EHR systems. Choose the one you think would be the best option and create a poster presentation, a PowerPoint presentation, or write a paper summarizing your research. Include the following points in your project:
   a. Description of the EHR
   b. Description of the practice management functions
   c. Does it include backup features?
   d. How does it meet the meaningful use requirements?

2. Using online resources, research a voice recognition software. Create a poster presentation, a PowerPoint presentation, or write a paper summarizing your research. Include the following points in your project:
   a. Description voice recognition software
   b. List the uses for voice recognition software
   c. Compare three different products
   d. Determine which one would be the best product

Procedure 12.1 Upload Documents to the Electronic Health Record

Name ______________________________ **Date** ____________ **Score** __________

Task: Scan paper records and upload digital files to the EHR.

Scenario: A new patient brings in a laboratory report and a radiology report that he would like to have added to his EHR. You need to scan in the original documents and upload them to the EHR.

Equipment and Supplies:
- Scanner
- Computer with SimChart for the Medical Office or EHR software
- Patient's laboratory and radiology reports (Figures 12.1 and 12.2)

Standard: Complete the procedure and all critical steps in ______ minutes with a minimum score of 85% within two attempts (*or as indicated by the instructor*).

Scoring: Divide the points earned by the total possible points. Failure to perform a critical step, indicated by an asterisk (*), results in grade no higher than an 84% (*or as indicated by the instructor*).

Time: Began________ Ended________ Total minutes: ________

Steps:	**Point Value**	**Attempt 1**	**Attempt 2**
1. Obtain the patient's name and date of birth if not on the reports.	**10**		
2. Using a scanner that is connected to the computer, scan each document, creating an individual digital image for each.	**20**		
3. Locate the file of the two scanned images in the computer drive. Open the files to ensure the images are clear.	**15***		
4. To help ensure the integrity of the practice management and EHR systems, a search for the new patient's name must always be done. In the EHR, search for the patient, using the patient's last and first name. Verify the patient's date of birth.	**15***		
5. Locate the window to upload diagnostic/laboratory results and add a new result. Enter the date of the test. Select the correct type of result. Browse for the image file of the laboratory file and attach it. Save the information.	**15***		
6. Select the option to add a new result and repeat the steps to upload the second report.	**10***		
7. To help ensure the integrity of the EHR system, verify that the correct documents were uploaded and specific headers (titles) were given to the document.	**15***		
Total Points	**100**		

Comments

CAAHEP Competencies	Step(s)
VI.P.3. Input patient data using an electronic system	2-6
ABHES Competencies	**Step(s)**
7. Administrative Procedures a. Gather and process documents	2-5
7. Administrative Procedures b. Navigate electronic health records systems and practice management software	All

Figure 12.1 Laboratory Report

AnyTown Laboratory

Date Reported: 04/25/20XX **Date Received:** 04/25/20XX
Patient Name: Jonathan S. Scott **DOB:** 08/01/1990
Ordering Provider: George St. Cyr, MD
Date Collected: 04/15/20XX **Time Collected:** 0830
Test Requested: Lipid Panel **Fasting?:** Yes

Test	Result	Flag	Reference Range
Cholesterol, total	210	High	<200 mg/dL
HDL Cholesterol	26	Low	>40 mg/dL
LDL Cholesterol	142	High	<130 mg/dL
Triglycerides	236	High	<150 mg/dL
Total Cholesterol/HDL ratio	5.8	High	<4.5

Figure 12.2 Radiology Report

AnyTown Radiology

Date:	10/31/20XX	**Time:**	1430
Patient Name:	Jonathan S. Scott	**DOB:**	08/01/1990
Exam Type:	Chest x-ray 2 views	**Ordering Provider:**	George St. Cyr, MD

Final Report:
History: Cough and fever
Report: Frontal and lateral views of the chest
Comparison: None

Findings:
Lungs: The lungs are well inflated and clear. There is no evidence of pneumonia or pulmonary edema.
Pleura: There is no pleural effusion or pneumothorax.
Heart and mediastinum: The cardiomediastinal silhouette is normal.
Impression: Clear lungs without evidence of pneumonia.
Recommendation: None.
Provider: Bones, Seymore MD

Procedure 12.2 Register a New Patient in the Practice Management Software

Name ______________________________ **Date** ____________ **Score** __________

Task: Register a new patient in the practice management software, prepare a Notice of Privacy Practices (NPP) form and a Disclosure Authorization form for the new patient, and document this in the electronic health record (EHR).

Scenario: The patient received both documents and signed the Disclosure Authorization form.

Equipment and Supplies:
- Computer with SimChart for the Medical Office or practice management and EHR software
- Completed patient registration form (Figure 12.3)
- Scanner

Standard: Complete the procedure and all critical steps in _______ minutes with a minimum score of 85% within two attempts (*or as indicated by the instructor*).

Scoring: Divide the points earned by the total possible points. Failure to perform a critical step, indicated by an asterisk (*), results in grade no higher than an 84% (*or as indicated by the instructor*).

Time: Began_________ Ended_________ Total minutes: _________

Steps:	**Point Value**	**Attempt 1**	**Attempt 2**
1. Obtain the new patient's completed registration form. Log into the practice management software.	**10**		
2. To help ensure the integrity of the practice management and EHR systems, a search for the new patient's name must always be done before registering that patient. Using the patient's last and first names and date of birth, search the database for the patient. To help ensure the integrity of the practice management and EHR systems, a search for the new patient's name must always be done before registering that person. This prevents a double record from being created if the patient had been entered into the database earlier.	**15***		
3. If the database does not contain the patient's name, add a new patient and enter the patient's demographics from the completed registration form.	**10***		
4. Correctly spell the patient's name and accurately enter the patient's date of birth.	**15***		
5. Verify that the information entered is correct and that all fields are completed before saving the data.	**10**		
6. Using the EHR software, prepare and print a copy of the NPP and a Disclosure Authorization form for the new patient. The Disclosure Authorization form should indicate the disclosure will be to the patient's insurance company.	**15**		
Scenario Update: The patient received both documents and signed the Disclosure Authorization form.			
7. Using the EHR, document that the patient received a copy of the NPP and signed the Disclosure Authorization form. Scan the Disclosure Authorization form and upload it into the EHR.	**15***		
8. Log out of the software upon completion of the procedure.	**10**		
Total Points	**100**		

Comments

CAAHEP Competencies	Step(s)
VI.P.3. Input patient data using an electronic system	All
ABHES Competencies	**Step(s)**
7. Administrative Procedures a. Gather and process documents	All
7. Administrative Procedures b. Navigate electronic health records systems and practice management software	All

Figure 12.3 Patient Information Form

Patient Information:
Name: Jonathan S. Scott
Address: 922 Golf Road, Anytown, AK 12345
Date of Birth: 08/01/1990
Email: jscott16@anytown.mail
Sex: M
Home Phone: 123-123-3098
SSN: 987-66-1223
Emergency Contact Name: Callie Scott
Emergency Contact Phone: 123-123-0857

Guarantor Information:
Relationship of Guarantor to Patient: Self
Employer Name: Anytown Bank
Work Phone: 123-567-9012
Primary Provider: David Kahn, MD

Insurance Information:

Primary Insurance:

Insurance: Aetna
Name of Policyholder: Jonathan S. Scott
SSN of Policyholder: 987-66-1223
Policy/ID Number: JS8884910
Group Number: 66574W
Claims Address: 1234 Insurance Way, Anytown, AL 12345-1234
Claims Phone Number: 180-012-3222

Procedure 12.3 Protect the Integrity of the Medical Record

Name ______________________________________ **Date** ____________ **Score** __________

Tasks: Protect the integrity of the medical record.

Scenario: You are mentoring a medical assistant student who is in practicum. You notice the student routinely does not sign out of the electronic health record before leaving the desk. The facility's policy is to sign out or lock the computer before leaving it.

Directions: Role-play the scenario with a peer, who plays the student. You, the medical assistant, must explain to the "student" the facility's policy. Also address the hazards of not protecting the medical record. If the student does not change the behavior, you will need to address the situation with the department supervisor.

Standard: Complete the procedure and all critical steps in ______ minutes with a minimum score of 85% within two attempts (*or as indicated by the instructor*).

Scoring: Divide the points earned by the total possible points. Failure to perform a critical step, indicated by an asterisk (*), results in grade no higher than an 84% (*or as indicated by the instructor*).

Time: Began________ Ended________ Total minutes: ________

Steps:	Point Value	Attempt 1	Attempt 2
1. Professionally and respectfully discuss the situation with the student.	25		
2. Inform the student about the facility's policy and the hazards of not protecting the electronic health record.	25		
3. Provide the student with strategies to protect the electronic health record.	25		
4. Inform the student what will occur if they do not protect the electronic record.	25		
Total Points	**100**		

Comments

CAAHEP Competencies	Step(s)
A.1. Demonstrate critical thinking skills	Entire procedure

Procedure 12.4 Developing a Plan in the Event of Loss of EMR and PMS

Name ______________________________ **Date** ____________ **Score** __________

Task: To develop a plan to ensure information integrity and patient care when the access to the EMR and PMS is lost for more than 24 hours.

Scenario: Your supervisor at WMFM Clinic has asked you to develop a plan to protect patient information in case access is lost to the EHR and PMS.

Equipment and Supplies:
- Paper and pen, or word processing software

Standard: Complete the procedure and all critical steps in _______ minutes with a minimum score of 85% within two attempts (*or as indicated by the instructor*).

Scoring: Divide the points earned by the total possible points. Failure to perform a critical step, indicated by an asterisk (*), results in grade no higher than an 84% (*or as indicated by the instructor*).

Time: Began_________ Ended_________ Total minutes: _________

Steps:	**Point Value**	**Attempt 1**	**Attempt 2**
1. Using reliable internet resources, research ways to protect the information contained in the EMR and PMS.	25		
2. Develop a list of the top four options for protecting patient information and patient care.	20		
3. Develop a pros/cons list for each of the four options.	25		
4. Determine which option you would choose and create plan for implementing it at WMFM Clinic. Your plan should include how patients can still be seen and provided the same level of care.	30*		
Total Points	100		

Comments

CAAHEP Competencies	**Step(s)**
VI.C.5. Identify the importance of data back-up	All

Procedure 12.5 Create and Organize a Patient's Paper Health Record

Name ______________________ **Date** __________ **Score** __________

Task: Create a paper health record for a new patient. Organize health record documents in a paper health record.

Equipment and Supplies:
- End tab file folder
- Completed patient registration form
- Divider sheets with different color labels (4)
- Progress note sheet (1)
- Name label
- Color-coding labels (first two letters of the last name and first letter of the first name)
- Year label
- Allergy label
- Black pen or computer with word processing software to process labels
- Health record documents (i.e., prior records, laboratory reports)
- Hole puncher

Standard: Complete the procedure and all critical steps in _______ minutes with a minimum score of 85% within two attempts (*or as indicated by the instructor*).

Scoring: Divide the points earned by the total possible points. Failure to perform a critical step, indicated by an asterisk (*), results in grade no higher than an 84% (*or as indicated by the instructor*).

Time: Began_________ Ended_________ Total minutes: _________

Steps:	Point Value	Attempt 1	Attempt 2
1. Obtain the patient's first and last names.	10		
2. Neatly write or word-process the patient's name on the name label. Left-justify the last name, followed by a comma, the first name, middle initial, and a period (e.g., Smith, Mary J.).	15*		
3. Adhere the name label to the bottom-left side of the record tab. When you hold the record by the main fold in your left hand, the writing should be easy to read. (For directional purposes, assume the record main fold is on the left and the tab is at the bottom.)	10		
4. Put the color-coding labels on the bottom-right edge of the folder. Start by placing the first letter of the last name at the farthest-right edge. Working left, place the second letter of the last name, then the first letter of the first name, and lastly the year label. The year label should be close to the name label.	15*		
5. Place the allergy label on the front of the record. If allergies are known, clearly write the allergy on the label in red ink.	15*		
6. Place the divider labels on the record divider sheets if they come separately. Ensure the labels on the divider sheets are staggered so they do not overlap. Print the name of the section on the front and back of the label. The print should be easy to read when the record is held by the main fold.	15*		

7. Using the prongs on the left-hand side of the record, secure the registration form.	**10**		
8. Using the prongs on the right-hand side of the record, secure the index dividers with a progress note sheet under the progress note tab.	**10**		
Total Points	**100**		

Comments

ABHES Competencies	**Step(s)**
7. Administrative Procedures a. Gather and process documents	All

Procedure 12.6 File Patient Health Records

Name ______________________________ **Date** ____________ **Score** __________

Task: File patient health records using two different filing systems: the alphabetic system and the numeric system.

Scenario: The agency utilizes the alphabetic system. You need to file health records in the correct location.

Equipment and Supplies:
- Paper health records using the alphabetic filing system
- Paper health records using the numeric filing system
- File box(es) or file cabinet

Standard: Complete the procedure and all critical steps in _______ minutes with a minimum score of 85% within two attempts (*or as indicated by the instructor*).

Scoring: Divide the points earned by the total possible points. Failure to perform a critical step, indicated by an asterisk (*), results in grade no higher than an 84% (*or as indicated by the instructor*).

Time: Began_________ Ended_________ Total minutes: _________

Steps:	**Point Value**	**Attempt 1**	**Attempt 2**
1. Using alphabetic guidelines, place the records to be filed in alphabetic order.	**20**		
2. Using the file box or file cabinet, locate the correct spot for the first file.	**10**		
3. Place the health record in the correct location. Continue these filing steps until all the health records are filed.	**20***		
4. Using numeric guidelines, place the records to be filed in numeric order.	**20**		
5. Using the file box or file cabinet, locate the correct spot for the first file.	**10**		
6. Place the health record in the correct location. Continue these filing steps until all the health records are filed.	**20***		
Total Points	**100**		

Comments

ABHES Competencies	**Step(s)**
7. Administrative Procedures a. Gather and process documents	All

Student Name________________________________ Date________________

chapter 13 Daily Operations and Safety

CAAHEP Competencies	Assessment
VI.C.3. Recognize the purpose of routine maintenance of equipment	Skills and Concepts – C. 5; Certification Preparation – 5
VI.C.4. Identify steps involved in completing an inventory	Skills and Concepts – D. 7-9
XII.C.3. Identify fire safety issues in a healthcare environment	Skills and Concepts – J. 2-3
XII.C.4. Identify emergency practices for evacuation of a healthcare setting	Skills and Concepts – K. 9-18; Internet Activities – 3
XII.C.7.a. Identify principles of: body mechanics	Skills and Concepts – H. 2-3; Certification Preparation – 6; Workplace Application – 2
XII.C.8. Identify critical elements of an emergency plan for response to a natural disaster or other emergency	Skills and Concepts – K. 1-5; Certification Preparation – 8; Internet Activities – 3
XII.C.9. Identify the physical manifestations and emotional behaviors of persons involved in an emergency	Skills and Concepts – L. 3; Certification Preparation – 10; Procedure 13.5 (Step 6)
VI.P.4. Perform an inventory of supplies.	Procedure 13.3
XII.P.2.b. Demonstrate proper use of: fire extinguishers	Procedure 13.6
XII.P.3. Use proper body mechanics	Procedure 13.3
XII.P.4. Evaluate an environment to identify unsafe conditions	Procedure 13.4
A.8. Demonstrate self-awareness	Procedure 13.5

ABHES Competencies	Assessment
7. Administrative Procedures f. Maintain inventory of equipment and supplies	Procedures 13.1, 13.3

VOCABULARY REVIEW

Using the word pool on the right, find the correct word to match the definition. Write the word on the line after the definition.

1. Doors made of fire-resistant materials; close manually or automatically during a fire to prevent the spread of the fire ____________________
2. A lack of similarity between what is stated and what is found; for instance, the computer inventory count is different than the physical count ____________________
3. Unforeseen situations that threaten employees and visitors; they can disrupt services provided ____________________
4. A document that accompanies purchased merchandise and shows what is in the box or package ____________________
5. Unique number assigned by the ordering facility that allows the facility to track or reference the order ____________________
6. Assistance (i.e., service) that is provided by a healthcare provider and can be billed to the insurance company or patient ____________________
7. To diminish in value (e.g., the value of an item) over a period of time; a concept used for tax purposes ____________________
8. Refers to how often an item is purchased; this depends on how frequently the item is used and the storage space available for it ____________________
9. Companies that sell supplies, equipment, or services to other companies or individuals ____________________
10. Billing statements that list the amount owed for goods or services purchased ____________________
11. An order placed for an item that is temporarily out of stock and will be sent later ____________________
12. Money owed by a company to other companies for services and goods; pertains to paying the bills of the facility ____________________
13. Reducing the level or intensity; bring down a person's anger or elevated emotions ____________________

Word Pool

- accounts payable
- backordered
- billable service
- buying cycle
- de-escalating
- depreciate
- discrepancy
- fire doors
- invoices
- packing slip
- purchase order number
- vendors
- workplace emergencies

ABBREVIATIONS

Write out what each of the following abbreviations stands for.

1. EHR ____
2. GPOs ____
3. PBGs ____
4. PO ____
5. OSH Act ____

6. OSHA ______________________________

7. ADA ______________________________

8. GAS ______________________________

9. BTL ______________________________

10. BX ______________________________

11. CS ______________________________

12. EA ______________________________

13. PKG ______________________________

14. DDL ______________________________

15. PYMT ______________________________

16. QTY ______________________________

SKILLS AND CONCEPTS

Answer the following questions.

A. Opening Tasks for the Medical Assistant

Select the correct answer or fill in the blank.

1. Which is *not* an opening task for the clinical medical assistant?
   a. Preparing the exam rooms.
   b. Updating the voice mail message.
   c. Unlocking supply cabinets.
   d. Performing quality control tests on laboratory equipment.

2. The process to ensure the reliability of test results, often using manufactured samples with known values is called ______________________.

3. A commercial service that answers telephone calls for its clients is called a(n) ______________________.

4. Documentation in the medical record that can be used to track the patient's condition and progress is called the ______________________.

5. Which is *not* an opening task for the administrative medical assistant?
   a. Completing refrigerator and freezer temperature logs
   b. Checking the voice mail
   c. Turning on the computers
   d. Preparing the reception area
   e. Printing schedules of the day's appointments

6. For facilities with paper health records, what must the medical assistant do?
   a. Pull the paper health records, using a copy of the appointment schedule.
   b. Verify that the correct record was pulled for each patient.
   c. Check off the patient's name on the copy of the appointment schedule.
   d. All of the above

B. Closing Tasks for the Medical Assistant

Select the correct answer.

1. Which is *not* a closing task for the clinical medical assistant?
   a. Restock the rooms and organize any reading materials.
   b. Prepare the patient records and documents for the next day.
   c. Turn off computers and other devices.
   d. Sanitize, disinfect, or sterilize equipment and instruments.

2. Which is *not* a closing task for the administrative medical assistant?
   a. Turning off the computers, copy machine, and other office equipment.
   b. Lock supply and medication cabinets.
   c. Follow office procedures for handling money at the end of the day.
   d. Secure any confidential documents.

Match the description with the correct term.

3. _____ The ability to determine what needs to be done and take action on your own.
4. _____ The process of cleaning to destroy or prevent the growth of disease-causing microorganisms.
5. _____ The process of replacing the supplies that were used.
6. _____ The process of removing all microorganisms.
7. _____ Supplies and equipment stored in a cart and ready for an emergency.
8. _____ The process of cleaning equipment and instruments with detergent and water to remove debris and reduce the number of microorganisms.

a. Restock
b. Disinfect
c. Sanitize
d. Sterilize
e. Initiative
f. Crash cart

C. Equipment Management

Select the correct answer or fill in the blank.

1. A detailed list of equipment and supplies owned and stored is called a(n) ______________________.

2. A(n) ______________________ is the process of counting the supplies in stock.

3. How can an inventory be used?
   a. The information is used when preparing tax paperwork.
   b. The information is used to replace equipment lost in a disaster or theft.
   c. The information is used by the supervisors to identify equipment that needs to be replaced.
   d. All of the above

4. When creating an inventory list of equipment, what information is documented?
   a. Equipment name, manufacturer, and serial number
   b. Purchase date, cost, and supplier
   c. Warranty information
   d. All of the above

5. What is the purpose of routine maintenance of administrative and clinical equipment? ______________________

____

6. When performing routine maintenance, what must the medical assistant do?
   a. Check electrical cords on equipment for damage.
   b. Address any suspected overheating issues.
   c. Investigate any unusual noise or change in performance.
   d. Clean and maintain equipment routinely in accordance with the user's guide.
   e. All of the above

D. Supply Inventory

Select the correct answer or fill in the blank.

1. _______________________ involves ordering, tracking inventory, and identifying the quantity of product to purchase.

2. What is the goal of inventory management? ____

   ____

3. The amount of supplies that need to be ordered is called the _______________________.

4. The point at which low inventory requires the product to be ordered is called the _______________________.

5. Calculate the reorder point for this scenario. The practice uses 6 rolls of table paper per day. It takes 7 workdays to receive the order from the medical supply company. The medical practice wants 4 extra days' worth of supplies on hand to prevent issues related to running out of the item. What is the reorder point for the table paper rolls? _______________________

6. Calculate the reorder point for this scenario. The practice uses 12 vials of sterile normal saline per day. It takes 4 workdays to receive the order from the medical supply company. The medical practice wants 6 extra days' worth of supplies on hand to prevent issues related to running out of the item. What is the reorder point for the vials of sterile normal saline? _______________________

7. When a company uses an automated inventory control system:

   a. A hand-counted inventory must be done at least _______________________ a year.

   b. The hand inventory counts are compared to the computer counts and _______________________ are identified.

   c. The manual inventory procedure provides the company with information on the _______________________ of items in stock.

8. What type of information is found on a supply inventory list?
   a. Name, size, and quantity of the product
   b. Item number and supplier's name
   c. Cost, reorder point, and quantity to reorder
   d. All of the above

9. You have prepared supply inventory list and are ready to inventory the supplies in your department. Which of the following would be done when completing an inventory?
   a. Identify the correct item on the supply inventory list.
   b. Count the number of items and document the number on the supply inventory list.
   c. Neatly replace the supplies.
   d. Ensure the older supplies are in front of the new supplies.
   e. All of the above

E. Ordering Process

Fill in the blank.

1. Some medical facilities join ______________________, which combine orders from many different medical facilities and receive volume discounts.
2. ______________________ offer providers potential cost-saving pricing for vaccines.
3. Some medical facilities use ______________________, giving each order a unique reference number.
4. A(n) ______________________ is a preset borrowing limit.

F. Receiving Orders

Fill in the blank.

1. When an order arrives, the medical assistant must use the ______________________ and compare the items in the package to it.
2. The ______________________ stock should be placed in the front so it is used first.
3. Any items with expiration dates should be placed with the items ______________________ in front, so they are used first.
4. If you are removing expired stock, remember to ______________________ the quantity from the inventory system.

G. Vaccine Storage Requirements

Select the correct answer or fill in the blank.

1. How should vaccines be stored per the CDC?
   a. Each type of vaccine should be placed in its own tray.
   b. Allow space between the vials promote air circulation.
   c. Place newer vaccines behind older vaccines.
   d. Keep vaccine vials in their original boxes to prevent light exposure.
   e. All of the above

2. When storing vaccines, what is recommended by the CDC?
   a. The refrigerators should maintain temperatures between 36° F and 56° F.
   b. The freezer should maintain temperatures between -58° F and 25° F.
   c. Position vaccines and diluents 2 to 3 inches from the walls, ceiling, and floor.
   d. All of the above

3. All vaccine storage units must have a(n) ______________________, which should be placed in the center of the unit, with vaccines surrounding it.
4. The temperature of the refrigerator and freezer should be checked at the ______________________ of each workday.
5. The temperature monitoring log sheet should include which of the following?
   a. Date and time
   b. Current temperature or the maximum and minimum temperature record on the device
   c. Any action taken if the temperature is out of range
   d. Name or initials of person who checked and recorded the temperature
   e. All of the above

6. What do you do if the temperature log is missing a temperature check? ______________________________

____

____

7. What should the medical assistant do if the temperature is out of range?
   a. Notify the vaccine coordinator and the supervisor.
   b. The vaccines should be labeled "DO NOT USE."
   c. Place vaccines in a separate container.
   d. All of the above

H. Personal Safety and Body Mechanics

Select the correct answer or fill in the blank.

1. The provisions of the Occupational Safety and Health Act of 1970 are enforced by the ________________________.

2. Which is a principle of proper body mechanics?
   a. To lift an object, maintain a wide, stable base with your feet.
   b. Your feet should be shoulder-width apart, and you should have good footing.
   c. Bend at the knees, keeping your back straight.
   d. Lift smoothly, using the major muscles in your arms and legs.
   e. All of the above

3. Which is a principle of proper body mechanics?
   a. When lifting and carrying heavy items, keep the item directly in front of you to avoid rotating your spine.
   b. Carry the item close to your body.
   c. Keep your movements smooth.
   d. When you reach for an object, your feet should face the object.
   e. All of the above

I. Providing a Safe Environment

Answer the question, select the correct answer, or fill in the blank.

1. How should cash drawers be stored? ____

____

____

2. Narcotic medications should always be in a(n) ________________________ cabinet.

3. What is an increased risk factor for violence in healthcare?
   a. Working with patients or family members who have a history of violence and abuse alcohol or other substances.
   b. Poorly designed work environments.
   c. Lack of emergency communication and training of employees.
   d. High employee turnover.
   e. All of the above

4. What is a strategy to secure the workplace environment?
   a. Physical barriers
   b. Bright, effective lighting and accessible exits
   c. Closed-circuit video
   d. De-escalating areas for patients and visitors
   e. All of the above

J. Evaluating the Work Environment

Select the correct answer or fill in the blank.

1. Which is *not* a high-risk situation that can result in an accident?
   a. Standing water on the floor
   b. Rugs and mats that are smooth and flat
   c. Cords, cables, and boxes in the walkway
   d. Heavy objects placed on high shelves

2. Which is *not* a way to prevent injuries and fires?
   a. Checking electrical cords and plugs for damage
   b. Turning off equipment that appears to be overheating
   c. Storing potentially flammable chemicals and supplies according to the manufacturer's guidelines
   d. Ensuring power strips are overloaded
   e. Not using electricity near water

3. Oxygen, other gases, and combustible chemicals should not be in the room when ________________________ equipment is used.

K. Emergency Response Plan

Match the description with the correct emergency response plan's critical element.

1. _____ Includes the reasons for evacuation, the methods for accounting for patients, meeting locations, and maps.
2. _____ How to alert employees, law enforcement, and the fire department of the emergency.
3. _____ Includes the names of specific employees who must turn off the water, gas, electricity, and oxygen.
4. _____ Includes the names of workers who need to perform rescue and medical duties.
5. _____ Includes the floor plan, workplace map, safe areas, and procedures.

a. methods to report a fire and other emergencies
b. evacuation policy and procedure
c. critical shutdown procedures
d. emergency escape/exit routes and procedures
e. rescue and medical duties

Fill in the blank.

6. Floor maps with ________________________ and ________________________ should be posted throughout the facility.

7. ________________________ must be clearly marked and well-lit.

8. Exit routes should be clear of ________________________ and ________________________ at all times.

Match the evacuation priority by location.

9. _____ First priority
10. _____ Second priority
11. _____ Third priority
12. _____ Fourth priority

a. people on the rest of the floor
b. people in immediate danger
c. people on the floors immediately above and below the floor with the situation
d. people located on the floor where the emergency is occurring

Fill in the blank.

13. Evacuation priority by people means the people ______________________ leave first, followed by the ambulatory people, and last the ______________________ people.

Match the description with the correct type of evacuation.

14. _____ Involves evacuating people who are located on the floors above and below the situation
15. _____ Involves evacuating everyone from the building to a safe location outside the building
16. _____ Involves moving one or more people out of immediate danger
17. _____ Evacuation to an interior room with no windows
18. _____ Involves evacuating people off the same floor as the emergency situation

a. shelter-in-place evacuation
b. local evacuation
c. horizontal evacuation
d. vertical evacuation
e. building evacuation

Select the correct answer.

19. Which step is *not* part of the acronym RACE?
    a. Rescue individuals threatened by the fire.
    b. Activate the alarm if you discover the fire or respond if you hear the alarm.
    c. Confirm the location of the fire.
    d. Extinguish only small fires; otherwise evacuate individuals from the area.

20. Which step is *not* part of the PASS procedure for fire extinguishers?
    a. Pull the fire alarm.
    b. Aim the nozzle or hose at the base of the fire.
    c. Squeeze the handle to release the extinguishing agent.
    d. Sweep the nozzle or hose from side to side at the base of the fire until the fire is out.

Match the use with the correct class of fire extinguishers.

21. _____ Used on flammable liquids
22. _____ For fires involving combustible metals
23. _____ Used on ordinary combustibles
24. _____ Used on electrical equipment
25. _____ Used on ordinary combustibles, flammable liquids, or electrical equipment

a. Class C
b. Class A
c. Class B
d. Class ABC
e. Class D

L. Effects of Stress

Select the correct answer or fill in the blank.

1. ________________________ is a person's total response to environmental demands or pressures.
2. A(n) ________________________ is a stimulus that provokes a stress response.
3. Which are physical manifestations and emotional behaviors caused by the stress of being involved in an emergency?
   a. Shock, disbelief, irritability, crying, and anger
   b. Feelings of fear, anxiety, numbness, sadness, worry, powerlessness, or frustration
   c. Difficulty making decisions and trouble concentrating
   d. High blood pressure, high blood glucose levels
   e. All of the above

Match the description with the correct stage of the general adaptation syndrome.

4. _____ The body's resistance has been diminished by the continued stress.
5. _____ This is the immediate reaction to the stressor.
6. _____ If the stressor continues, the individual's body adapts to the stressor.

a. adaptation stage
b. alarm stage
c. exhaustion stage

Match the following strategies to indicate if they are either healthy or unhealthy. Answers can be used more than once.

7. _____ Lack of exercise and watching TV continuously
8. _____ Getting adequate sleep
9. _____ Eating healthy, well-balanced meals
10. _____ Using excessive amounts of alcohol and tobacco

a. healthy coping strategies
b. unhealthy coping strategies

CERTIFICATION PREPARATION

Circle the correct answer.

1. What is an opening task for the administrative medical assistant?
   a. Unlock supply cabinets.
   b. Perform quality-control tests on laboratory equipment.
   c. Update the voice mail message.
   d. Follow up on outstanding patient issues from the prior day.

2. What should be disinfected in the healthcare facility?
   a. Exam table
   b. Writing table
   c. Computer keyboard
   d. All of the above

3. How often do crash carts and other emergency supplies need to be inventoried?
   a. Every week
   b. Every other week
   c. Every month
   d. Every 6 months

4. What is *not* found on a routine maintenance log?
   a. Equipment name, serial number, and location of the machine
   b. Manufacturer's name and date of purchase
   c. Store name where the machine was purchased
   d. Warranty information and service provider information

5. What is the purpose of routine maintenance of administrative and clinical equipment?
   a. Prevent injury to the patients
   b. Prevent costly damage to the equipment
   c. Prevent injury to staff members
   d. All of the above

6. What is *not* a principle of proper body mechanics?
   a. When lifting an object, maintain a wide, stable base with your feet.
   b. Get help if the item is too heavy to lift by yourself.
   c. Keep your movements smooth.
   d. When reaching for an object, stand on tiptoes.

7. What is the correct way to operate most fire extinguishers?
   a. Pull the pin, squeeze the handle, aim the nozzle, and sweep the nozzle from side to side.
   b. Pull the pin, aim the nozzle, sweep the nozzle from side to side, and squeeze the handle.
   c. Pull the pin, sweep the nozzle from side to side, squeeze the handle, and aim the nozzle.
   d. Pull the pin, aim the nozzle, squeeze the handle, and sweep the nozzle from side to side.

8. What is a critical element of an emergency response plan?
   a. Evacuation policy and procedure
   b. Methods to report emergencies
   c. Critical shutdown procedures
   d. All of the above

9. Which is a dry chemical fire extinguisher that is used on fires related to electrical sources?
   a. Class A
   b. Class B
   c. Class C
   d. Class D

10. Which is *not* a symptom of stress?
   a. Anger
   b. Low blood pressure
   c. Anxiety
   d. Fear

WORKPLACE APPLICATION

1. Catherine is working at the reception desk and the procedure has been to place the cashbox on the receptionist's desk. Patients arrive, make payments, and the cashbox remains on the desk visible to all and in easy access to the public. How might Catherine safeguard the money in the cashbox?

____

____

2. Maria is lifting heavy boxes. Describe how she should lift and carry heavy boxes. ____________

____

____

____

____

3. Maria sometimes needs to room patients who make her uncomfortable. Describe four ways she could keep safe in these situations.

____

____

____

INTERNET ACTIVITIES

1. Obtain a vaccine name from the instructor and research the storage directions for that medication.
2. Research guidelines for storing vaccines in the refrigerator. Create a poster that provides the key guidelines that must be followed for safe storage.
3. Using the OSHA website (https://www.osha.gov/), research emergency action plans. Create a poster, PowerPoint, or paper summarizing your research. Focus on these areas:
   - The minimum requirements for the emergency action plan
   - Evacuation elements
   - Shelter-in-place requirements and procedures

Procedure 13.1 Perform an Equipment Inventory with Documentation

Name ______________________ **Date** __________ **Score** __________

Tasks: Perform an equipment inventory. Document the inventory on the equipment inventory form.

Equipment and Supplies:
- Equipment inventory form (Work Product 13.1)
- Pens
- Administrative or clinical equipment
- Purchase information (e.g., date, cost, and supplier) and warranty information (e.g., start and end date, warranty coverage)

Standard: Complete the procedure and all critical steps with a minimum score of 85% within two attempts (*or as indicated by the instructor*).

Scoring: Divide the points earned by the total possible points. Failure to perform a critical step, indicated by an asterisk (*), results in grade no higher than an 84% (*or as indicated by the instructor*).

Steps:	Point Value	Attempt 1	Attempt 2
1. For each piece of equipment to be inventoried, gather the following information: a. Name of equipment, manufacturer, and serial number b. Location and facility number (if applicable) c. Purchase date, cost, supplier, and warranty information	20		
2. Complete an equipment inventory form (Work Product 13.1) by adding the gathered information for each item inventoried.	60		
3. Review the document created. Make any necessary revisions.	20		
Total Points	**100**		

Comments

ABHES Competencies	Step(s)
7. Administrative Procedures f. Maintain inventory of equipment and supplies	Entire procedure

Work Product 13.1 Equipment Inventory Form

Name ______________________________ Date ____________ Score __________

To be used with Procedure 13.1.

Equipment Name	Manufacturer/ Serial Number	Location/Facility Number	Purchase Date/ Supplier	Cost	Warranty Information

Procedure 13.2 Perform Routine Maintenance of Equipment

Name ______________________ **Date** __________ **Score** __________

Tasks: Perform routine maintenance of administrative or clinical equipment. Document the maintenance on the log.

Equipment and Supplies:
- Maintenance log(s) (Work Product 13.2)
- Pens
- Information regarding the equipment (i.e., name, serial number, location, facility number, manufacturer, purchase date, warranty information, frequency of inspections, and service provider)
- Administrative or clinical equipment (e.g., oral thermometers)
- Supplies for routine maintenance (e.g., battery)
- User's guide or owner's manual, if needed

Standard: Complete the procedure and all critical steps with a minimum score of 85% within two attempts (*or as indicated by the instructor*).

Scoring: Divide the points earned by the total possible points. Failure to perform a critical step, indicated by an asterisk (*), results in grade no higher than an 84% (*or as indicated by the instructor*).

Steps:	Point Value	Attempt 1	Attempt 2
1. Gather information on the piece of equipment identified for routine maintenance including name, serial number, location, facility number, manufacturer, purchase date, warranty information, frequency of inspections, and service provider.	20		
2. Fill in the equipment details on the log (Work Product 13.2).	20*		
3. To perform the maintenance activities, gather the required supplies. If you are not familiar with the procedure or the required supplies, refer to the user's guide.	10		
4. Perform the maintenance activities as directed in the user's guide. Take any required safety precautions necessary to protect yourself and others.	20*		
5. Clean up the work area.	10		
6. Using a pen, document the date, time, the maintenance activity performed, and include your signature on the log.	20		
Total Points	**100**		

Comments

Work Product 13.2 Maintenance Logs

Name ______________________ **Date** __________ **Score** __________

To be used with Procedure 13.2.

Maintenance Log

Equipment: ____________ Serial #: ____________ Location: ____________

Facility #: ____________ Manufacturer: ____________ Purchased: ____________

Warranty Information: ____________

Frequency of Inspections: ____________

Service Provider: ____________

Date	Time	Maintenance Activities	Signature

Maintenance Log

Equipment: ____________ Serial #: ____________ Location: ____________

Facility #: ____________ Manufacturer: ____________ Purchased: ____________

Warranty Information: ____________

Frequency of Inspections: ____________

Service Provider: ____________

Date	Time	Maintenance Activities	Signature

Maintenance Log

Equipment: ____________ Serial #: ____________ Location: ____________

Facility #: ____________ Manufacturer: ____________ Purchased: ____________

Warranty Information: ____________

Frequency of Inspections: ____________

Service Provider: ____________

Date	Time	Maintenance Activities	Signature

Maintenance Log

Equipment: ____________ Serial #: ____________ Location: ____________

Facility #: ____________ Manufacturer: ____________ Purchased: ____________

Warranty Information: ____________

Frequency of Inspections: ____________

Service Provider: ____________

Date	Time	Maintenance Activities	Signature

Procedure 13.3 Perform a Supply Inventory with Documentation While Using Proper Body Mechanics

Name ______________________________ **Date** ____________ **Score** __________

Tasks: Perform a supply inventory using correct body mechanics. Document the inventory on the supply inventory form.

Equipment and Supplies:
- Supply inventory form (Work Product 13.3)
- Pens
- Administrative or clinical supplies to be inventoried
- Purchase information (e.g., item number, cost, and supplier) for supplies in inventory
- Reorder point and quantity to reorder for each item in inventory

Standard: Complete the procedure and all critical steps with a minimum score of 85% within two attempts (*or as indicated by the instructor*).

Scoring: Divide the points earned by the total possible points. Failure to perform a critical step, indicated by an asterisk (*), results in grade no higher than an 84% (*or as indicated by the instructor*).

Steps:	Point Value	Attempt 1	Attempt 2
1. For the supplies in inventory, gather the following information for each item: • Name, size, quantity (e.g., purchased individually, 100 per box) • Item number, supplier's name, cost • Reorder point and quantity to reorder	5		
2. For each supply item, enter information on the inventory form (Work Product 13.3). Make sure the appropriate entry is in the right location. Note: The "Stock Available" column will be empty for now.	15*		
3. Review the document. Make any necessary revisions.	10		
4. Using the supply inventory list, inventory the supplies in the department. Identify how the supply should be counted (e.g., individually, by the box) and count the number of items in stock.	15		
5. Add the number in the appropriate row under the "Stock Available" header.	10		
6. Compare the reorder point number to the stock available number. If the stock available number is at or below the reorder point, indicate that the item needs to be reordered by checking the appropriate column.	10*		
7. Make sure the supplies are neatly arranged. The older stock should be in front of the newer stock.	5		
8. Repeat steps 5 through 7 until all supplies are inventoried.	10		
9. Use proper body mechanics when lifting and moving supplies by maintaining a wide, stable base with your feet. Your feet should be shoulder-width apart, and you should have good footing. Bend at the knees, keeping your back straight. Lift smoothly with the major muscles in your arms and legs. Use the same technique when putting the item down.	10*		

10. Use proper body mechanics when reaching for an object. Clear away barriers and use a step-stool if needed. Your feet should face the object. Avoid twisting or turning with a heavy load.	**10***		
Total Points	**100**		

Comments

CAAHEP Competencies	Step(s)
VI.P.4. Perform an inventory of supplies	1-8
XII.P.3. Use proper body mechanics	9, 10
ABHES Competencies	**Step(s)**
7. Administrative Procedures f. Maintain inventory of equipment and supplies	1-8

Work Product 13.3 Supply Inventory Form

Name ______________________________ **Date** ____________ **Score** __________

To be used with Procedure 13.3.

Item Name	Size	Quantity	Item Number	Supplier's Name	Reorder Point	Quantity to Reorder	Cost	Stock Available	Order (✓)

Procedure 13.4 Evaluate the Work Environment

Name ______________________________ **Date** ______________ **Score** ___________

Tasks: Evaluate the work environment and identify unsafe working conditions.

Equipment and Supplies:
- Work environment evaluation form (Work Product 13.4)
- Pen

Standard: Complete the procedure and all critical steps with a minimum score of 85% within two attempts (*or as indicated by the instructor*).

Scoring: Divide the points earned by the total possible points. Failure to perform a critical step, indicated by an asterisk (*), results in grade no higher than an 84% (*or as indicated by the instructor*).

Steps:	**Point Value**	**Attempt 1**	**Attempt 2**
1. Observe the environment for slipping, tripping, or fall risks. Document your findings on the work environment evaluation form (Work Product 13.4).	**20**		
2. Observe the environment for safety and security issues. Document your findings.	**20**		
3. Observe the environment for fire risks and electrical issues. Document your findings.	**20**		
4. Observe the environment for fire containment and evacuation strategies. Document your findings.	**20**		
5. Based on your observations, summarize your findings. If risks are present, create a list of issues that need to be addressed. Describe what needs to be done for each risk.	**20***		
Total Points	**100**		

Comments

CAAHEP Competencies	**Step(s)**
XII.P.4. Evaluate an environment to identify unsafe conditions	Entire procedure

Work Product 13.4 Work Environment Evaluation Form

Name ______________________________ **Date** ____________ **Score** __________

To be used with Procedure 13.4.

Directions: *Check either in the "Yes" or "No" column for each question. Check "NA" if it is not applicable. Include any issues in the comment column. Summarize your findings for each area, using the space indicated.*

Slipping, tripping, or fall risks	Yes	No	NA	Comments
• Is the lighting appropriate?				
• Are any lights burned out? Are any areas dim?				
• Is the flooring and carpeting ripped or pulled up?				
• If rugs/mats are present, are they folded?				
• Is water on the floor?				
• Is signage present warning of the water?				
• Are items cluttering the hallway, making walking difficult?				
• Are cords, cables, and other items in the walkway?				
• Is trash on the floor?				
• Are heavy items on high shelves?				
• Is a sturdy step stool available?				
Safety and security issues	**Yes**	**No**	**NA**	**Comments**
• Are rooms available that can be locked and used during workplace violence?				
• Is there limited visibility from the hallway into the room?				
• Are there areas in the building with limited visibility?				
• If the building is accessible to the public, are there any safe zones or areas for staff?				
• Are the emergency call lights in the exam rooms and bathrooms functioning?				
• Are the oxygen tanks (if available) checked per the facility's policy?				
Fire risks and electrical issues	**Yes**	**No**	**NA**	**Comments**
• Are electrical cords and plugs free from cracks, fraying, or other damage?				
• Are power strips overloaded?				
• Is electricity being used near a water source?				
• Are flammable chemicals and supplies stored according to manufacturers' guidelines?				
• Are combustibles (e.g., paper, cardboard, cloth, flammable chemicals) away from heat sources?				

Fire containment and evacuation strategies	Yes	No	NA	Comments
• Are building diagrams posted on walls indicating exit routes (two or more), fire alarms, and fire extinguishers?				
• Are exit routes uncluttered?				
• Are exit signs visible and lit?				
• Are fire doors unblocked and able to be closed in an emergency?				
• Are interior rooms available for severe storms?				
• Are smoke detectors located throughout the building?				
• Are fire alarms available?				
• Are fire extinguishers available and checked routinely (per the facility's policy)?				
• Are flammable products (e.g., oxygen tanks, chemicals) stored along the exit routes?				

Based on your observations, summarize your findings.

If risks are present, create a list of issues that need to be addressed. Describe what needs to be done for each risk.

Procedure 13.5 Participate in a Mock Exposure Event

Name ______________________________ **Date** ______________ **Score** ____________

Tasks: Demonstrate self-awareness in an emergency situation. Participate in a mock exposure event and document specific steps taken. Recognize the physical and emotional effects on individuals involved in an emergency situation.

Scenario: You and Beth are in the autoclave room and two chemicals spill, creating toxic fumes. Beth is having trouble breathing. The following staff, patients, and visitors are present:

Rooms	Staff and Reception Areas
1—Teen and his mother	Reception Area A—Four people waiting
2—Older woman in a wheelchair	Reception Area B—Five people waiting
3—Mother with three little children	
4—Adult female	**Staff**
5—Empty	Tim—In MA station 3
6—An older couple	Rose—At the insurance desk
7—Adult male	Dave and Patty—At the reception desk
8—Empty	Julie Walden, MD—In provider office 1
Procedure room—Empty	Angela Perez, MD—In room 3
	Jean Burke, NP—In room 7

Directions: Using word processing software, write a paper and address the procedure steps. Use reliable Internet resources to research the physical manifestations and emotional behaviors of persons involved in an emergency. Include your findings in the paper as indicated in the procedure steps. Use 1-inch margins, double spacing, and 12-point font. Length should be at least two pages.

Equipment and Supplies:
- Paper
- Pen
- Floor map (see Figure 13.11 in the textbook)
- Computer with internet access

Standard: Complete the procedure and all critical steps with a minimum score of 85% within two attempts (*or as indicated by the instructor*).

Scoring: Divide the points earned by the total possible points. Failure to perform a critical step, indicated by an asterisk (*), results in grade no higher than an 84% (*or as indicated by the instructor*).

Steps:	Point Value	Attempt 1	Attempt 2
1. Using the scenario, describe how you would handle the emergency exposure situation with Beth. • Identify four steps a medical assistant could take to demonstrate self-awareness while responding to this emergency situation. • Describe exposure control mechanisms or how you might limit the exposure to other people once you remove Beth from the room.	15*		

Scenario continues: Dr. Walden informed the staff to evacuate from the building. The outdoor safe meeting location is at the back of the parking lot. 2. Document the steps to handle the exposure event and evacuation from the building. • Describe what each staff member and provider should do to help with the evacuation procedure and notify 911. • Describe the steps (evacuations) in the order that they should occur. • Describe how the staff may ensure all individuals are out of the building.	**15***		
3. Dr. Walden is in charge during the emergency. Describe what her responsibilities include.	**5**		
4. Dave took the patient registry. Describe why the patient registry is important.	**5**		
Scenario continues: Two weeks after the event, Beth confides to you that she is not doing well. She recovered from the exposure, but since the event she has had difficulty sleeping. She is anxious when she goes into the autoclave room. She is having trouble concentrating on her job. She mentioned she has had two nightmares of emergencies occurring in the department in which she gets injured. 5. *Do the following:* • Describe what might be occurring with Beth and the symptoms that relate to it. • Discuss what you might encourage her to do about the situation.	**15***		
6. Research the physical manifestations and emotional behaviors of persons involved in an emergency. Identify four physical signs and four emotional behaviors of stress in persons involved in an emergency situation. Cite your resources.	**15***		
7. Describe how the physical and emotional effects of stress would be different for Beth, you, the providers, and the other employees present.	**15**		
8. Describe how a medical assistant could limit the physical and emotional effects of stress on each person/group: Beth, the providers, the other employees present in the facility, and yourself.	**15**		
Total Points	**100**		

Comments

CAAHEP Competencies	Step(s)
A.8. Demonstrate self-awareness	1

Procedure 13.6 Use a Fire Extinguisher

Name ______________________________ **Date** __________ **Score** ________

Tasks: Select the correct fire extinguisher and demonstrate its use.

Equipment and Supplies:
- Fire extinguisher

Scenarios:
a. You are working in the medical laboratory, and an electrical fire starts.
b. You are working in the clinic, and a fire starts in a wastebasket.
c. You are working in the medical laboratory, and a chemical fire starts (combustible metal fire).

Standard: Complete the procedure and all critical steps with a minimum score of 85% within two attempts (*or as indicated by the instructor*).

Scoring: Divide the points earned by the total possible points. Failure to perform a critical step, indicated by an asterisk (*), results in grade no higher than an 84% (*or as indicated by the instructor*).

Steps:	**Point Value**	**Attempt 1**	**Attempt 2**
1. Using the scenario, identify the type of fire extinguisher required to put out the fire.	**20**		
2. Hold the extinguisher by the handle with the hose or nozzle pointing away from you. Pull out the pin that is located below the trigger.	**20**		
3. Stand about 10 feet from the fire. Aim the extinguisher hose or nozzle at the base of the fire. Keep the extinguisher in an upright position as you work.	**20**		
4. Squeeze the trigger slowly and evenly.	**20**		
5. Sweep from side to side until the fire is out.	**20**		
Total Points	**100**		

Comments

CAAHEP Competencies	**Step(s)**
XII.P.2.b. Demonstrate proper use of: fire extinguishers	Entire procedure

Student Name____________________ Date____________

Principles of Pharmacology

chapter **14**

CAAHEP Competencies	Assessment
I.C.10.a. Identify the classifications of medications including: indications for use	Certification Preparation – 9; Workplace Applications – 1; Internet Activities – 3
I.C.10.b. Identify the classifications of medications including: desired effects	Vocabulary Review – A. 1, 3, 4, 6, 8; Certification Preparation – 10; Workplace Applications – 1; Internet Activities – 3
I.C.10.c. Identify the classifications of medications including: side effects	Workplace Applications – 2; Internet Activities – 3
I.C.10.d. Identify the classifications of medications including: adverse reactions	Workplace Applications – 2; Internet Activities – 3

ABHES Competencies	Assessment
1. General Orientation d. List the general responsibilities and skills of the medical assistant	Skills and Concepts – E. 2
1.f. Comply with federal, state, and local health laws and regulations as they relate to healthcare settings	Skills and Concepts – F. 2-5
6. Pharmacology a. Identify drug classification, usual dose, side effects and contraindications of the top most commonly used medications.	Workplace Applications – 1-2; Internet Activities – 3
6.c. 1) Identify parts of prescriptions	Skills and Concepts – K. 2-5
6.c. 2) Identify appropriate abbreviations that are accepted in prescription writing	Abbreviations – 5-9, 16, 18-24, 26-48; Procedure 14.1
6.c. 3) Comply with legal aspects of creating prescriptions, including federal and state laws	Procedure 14.1
6.d. Properly utilize the *Physician's Desk Reference (PDR),* drug handbooks, and other drug references to identify a drug's classification, usual dosage, usual side effects, and contraindications	Internet Activities – 3

VOCABULARY REVIEW

Using the word pool on the right, find the correct word to match the definition. Write the word on the line after the definition.

Group A

1. A medication that prevents or reduces inflammation ____________________
2. A medication that slows down the cell's activity ____________________
3. A drug that reduces or eliminates pain ____________________
4. A drug that destroys or inhibits the growth of bacteria ____________________
5. By-products of drug metabolism ____________________
6. A drug that prevents or alleviates heart arrhythmias ____________________
7. A medication that increases the cell's activity ____________________
8. A substance (i.e., medication or chemical) that prevent the clotting of blood ____________________
9. A substance that inhibits the growth of microorganisms on living tissue ____________________
10. A medication that kills cells or disrupts parts of cells ____________________

Word Pool
- antiarrhythmic
- anticoagulant
- antiinflammatory
- antiseptic
- antibiotic
- analgesic
- depressing
- destroying
- metabolites
- stimulating

Group B

1. Information that appears on the drug label and addresses serious or life-threatening risks ____________________
2. Comparing a document with another document to ensure that they are consistent ____________________
3. A disease that occurs when a person cannot stop or limit the use of a drug, even after negative consequences have been experienced ____________________
4. Medical doctors who have been specially trained to diagnose and treat patients with mental, emotional, and behavioral conditions ____________________
5. Directions given by a provider for a specific medication to be administered to a patient ____________________
6. An identifier assigned by the Centers for Medicare and Medicaid Services (CMS) that classifies the healthcare provider by license and medical specialties ____________________
7. Indicates the greatest amount of medication a person should have within a 24-hour period ____________________
8. Physical characteristics of a medication (e.g., tablet and suspension) ____________________

Word Pool
- addiction
- boxed warning
- form
- maximum dosage
- medication order
- National Provider Identifier
- psychiatrists
- reconciling

ABBREVIATIONS

Write out what each of the following abbreviations stands for.

1. IV ____________
2. ID ____________
3. NAS ____________
4. SUBQ ____________
5. PO ____________
6. ung ____________
7. soln, sol. ____________
8. cap ____________
9. tinct ____________
10. IM ____________
11. C ____________
12. F ____________
13. m ____________
14. cm ____________
15. mm ____________
16. tab(s) ____________
17. kg ____________
18. g ____________
19. mg ____________
20. mcg ____________
21. gr ____________
22. gtt(s) ____________
23. L ____________
24. mL ____________
25. lb ____________
26. fl oz ____________
27. qt ____________
28. pt ____________
29. Tbs, tbsp ____________

30. tsp ________________
31. AM, a.m. ________________
32. PM, p.m. ________________
33. pc ________________
34. ac ________________
35. ad lib ________________
36. d ________________
37. noc, noct ________________
38. hr, h ________________
39. $\bar{p}$ ________________
40. min ________________
41. qh ________________
42. prn ________________
43. q4h ________________
44. q6h ________________
45. qam ________________
46. tid ________________
47. bid ________________
48. qid ________________
49. STAT ________________
50. ASA ________________
51. K ________________
52. Fe ________________
53. NS ________________
54. MOM ________________
55. NSAID ________________
56. PPD ________________
57. OTC ________________
58. aq ________________
59. med ________________
60. NKA ________________

61. NKDA ______________________________

62. NPO ______________________________

63. $\overline{aa}$ ______________________________

64. $\bar{c}$ ______________________________

65. $\bar{s}$ ______________________________

66. x ______________________________

67. qs ______________________________

68. Rx ______________________________

69. Sig ______________________________

70. VO ______________________________

SKILLS AND CONCEPTS

Answer the following questions.

A. Introduction

Fill in the blank.

1. ______________________ is the study of the properties, actions, and uses of drugs.
2. A(n) ______________________ is a chemical substance used to cure, treat, prevent, or diagnose disease.
3. Unpleasant effects of a drug in addition to the desired or therapeutic effect are called ______________________.

B. Pharmacology Basics

Match the medication with the correct sources of drug.

1. _____ Synthetic insulin
2. _____ Iron, iodine, and zinc
3. _____ *Penicillium chrysogenum*
4. _____ Heparin and lanolin
5. _____ Digitalis and quinidine

a. natural – animals
b. natural – plants
c. natural – minerals
d. natural – microbiologic substances
e. synthetic

Match the descriptions with the correct uses of drugs.

6. _____ Drugs that do not cure or treat the disease but improve the quality of life
7. _____ Drugs used to diagnose or monitor a condition
8. _____ Drugs that relieve the symptoms while the body fights off the disease
9. _____ Drugs used to prevent pregnancy
10. _____ Drugs used to increase the blood levels of naturally occurring substances in the body
11. _____ Drugs used to prevent diseases
12. _____ Drugs that eliminate the disease
13. _____ Medications used to maintain or enhance health

a. prevention
b. treatment
c. diagnosis
d. cure
e. contraceptive
f. health maintenance
g. palliation
h. replacement

C. Pharmacokinetics

Match the description with the correct term.

1. _____ Placed under the tongue to dissolve
2. _____ Injected into the muscle
3. _____ The study of drug absorption, distribution, metabolism, and excretion in the body
4. _____ Placed between the cheek and the gums to dissolve and absorb quickly
5. _____ The harmful and deadly effect of a medication that can develop due to the buildup of medication or by-products in the body
6. _____ The means by which a drug enters the body
7. _____ Injected just below the skin; moves into the capillaries or the lymphatic vessels and is brought to the bloodstream
8. _____ Where a drug enters the body
9. _____ Injected directly into the bloodstream
10. _____ The movement of drug from the site of administration to the bloodstream

a. pharmacokinetics
b. route
c. site of administration
d. absorption
e. toxicity
f. sublingual
g. buccal
h. intramuscular
i. subcutaneous
j. intravenous

Match the description with the correct term.

11. _____ A series of chemical processes whereby enzymes change drugs in the body
12. _____ Medications that are administered in an inactive form
13. _____ Tissues where drugs accumulate, and the drugs are slowly released into the bloodstream
14. _____ The movement of metabolites out of the body
15. _____ The movement of absorbed drug from the blood to the body tissues

a. distribution
b. reservoirs
c. metabolism
d. prodrugs
e. excretion

Fill in the blank.

16. Most metabolites are excreted through the ______________________ and ______________________.

17. Medications are limited when a female is breastfeeding her baby, because drugs can be ______________________ in the breast milk.

18. Drugs are ______________________ by the body through stool, urine, breast milk, sweat, exhaled air, and saliva.

19. Young children, older adults, and those with kidney disease are at risk for the______________________ of metabolic drug by-products in the body.

D. Drug Action

Fill in the blank or select the correct answer.

1. Which statement is correct regarding drug action?
   a. Infants and older adults have problems metabolizing and excreting medications.
   b. Thinner people require less medication than heavier people.
   c. Women can react differently to some medications compared to men.
   d. Certain foods affect a drug's action.
   e. All of the above.

2. Pharmacogenomics or ______________________ is the study of how genetic factors influence a person's metabolic response to a specific medication.

3. Medication effects that are seen at the site of administration are ______________________ effects and medication effects that are seen throughout the body are ______________________ effects.

4. ______________________ are also called *desired effects*.

5. The provider may prescribe a higher initial dose, called a(n) ______________________, which helps to quickly increase the medication level in the blood.

6. The blood concentrations of a medication that are high enough to produce the drug's therapeutic effect is called the ______________________.

7. A(n) ______________________ is the amount of medication needed to keep the blood levels within the therapeutic range.

8. An unexpected or life-threatening reaction to a medication is called a(n) ______________________.

9. ______________________ is an extreme hypersensitivity to a specific drug that can cause life-threatening symptoms, including swelling of the mouth and airway, dyspnea, wheezing, loss of consciousness, and death.

10. ______________________ is a peculiar response to a certain drug.

11. ______________________ is the need for a larger dose to get the same therapeutic or desired effect.

12. ______________________ is the strong psychological or physical need to take a certain drug.

E. Drug Legislation and the Ambulatory Care Setting

Fill in the blank.

1. ______________________ means to order a medication as a treatment for a condition, which is done by doctors and advanced-practice professionals.

2. ______________________ means to give a prescribed dose of medication to a patient, which is done by medical assistants, nurses, and providers.

3. ______________________ means to give a supply of medication that the patient will take later, which is the role of the pharmacist.

4. The ______________________ enforces the Food, Drug, and Cosmetic Act and is responsible for the safety, effectiveness, security, and quality of drugs and cosmetics.

5. The ______________________ enforces the Controlled Substances Act and oversees the manufacturing, importation, possession, use, and distribution of legal controlled substances.

F. Compliance with the Controlled Substance Act

Fill in the blank or select the correct answer.

1. Providers prescribing controlled substances need a DEA registration number, which is good for _____ years.

2. Which is correct regarding the storage of controlled substances?
   a. They need to be kept in a locked cabinet or safe of substantial construction.
   b. Keys should be placed in a locked area accessible only to authorized persons.
   c. They should be stored in a different location than non-narcotic medications.
   d. All of the above

3. Periodic ______________________ of the log with the actual inventory count is important to identify missing medications.

4. An inventory of all controlled substances must be done at least ______________________, unless required more often by law.

5. The controlled substance inventory and log records need to be kept for _____ years.

6. ______________________ of controlled substances means using the medication for personal reasons.

G. Brand and Generic Drugs

1. The ______________________ name or ______________________ name is assigned by the manufacturer and no other company can use that name.

2. The ______________________ name is assigned by the U.S. Adopted Name Council.

3. The ______________________ name represents the exact formula of the medication.

4. The ______________________ name is used to list the medication in the U.S. Pharmacopeia and in the National Formulary (USP-NP).

H. Drug Reference Information

Match the description with the correct term.

1. _____ Indicates recommended changes in dosages for special populations
2. _____ Indicates necessary actions or special care that needs to be taken when the patient is on the medication
3. _____ Conditions or diseases for which the drug is used
4. _____ The time during which the drug is present in the blood at great enough levels to produce a response
5. _____ Provides information on how the medication should be given
6. _____ The time it takes for the drug to produce a response
7. _____ How the drug provides therapeutic results in the body, or the use of the drug
8. _____ This section describes known undesirable experiences associated with the medication
9. _____ The time it takes for the drug to reach its greatest effective concentration in the blood
10. _____ Includes medications, foods, and beverages that may either increase or reduce the medication level in the blood
11. _____ Reasons or conditions that make administration of the drug improper or undesirable
12. _____ The time it takes half of the drug to be metabolized or eliminated by normal biologic processes

a. indications
b. dosage considerations
c. administration
d. action
e. adverse reactions
f. duration
g. interactions
h. contraindications
i. precautions
j. biologic half-life
k. onset
l. peak

I. Forms of Medications

Match the description with the correct form of medication.

1. _____ Designed to break down over time
2. _____ Clear sweetened liquid preparation that contains alcohol
3. _____ A sugar and water solution that contains flavoring and medicinal substance
4. _____ Medication in a hard or soft gelatin shell
5. _____ A suspension of medication in a gas, usually used for respiratory or sinus conditions
6. _____ A solid medication containing the active medication and an antacid
7. _____ Semisolid, greasy drug preparations that are applied to the skin, rectum, or nasal mucosa
8. _____ Solid formed by compressed powdered medication; may be coated
9. _____ Coated to pass through the acidic environment of the stomach and break down in the base environment of the intestines
10. _____ A notched tablet, which can be split into half with a pill cutter or splitter

a. tablet
b. capsule
c. scored tablet
d. buffered
e. enteric-coated tablet or capsule
f. extended-release tablet or capsule
g. ointment and paste
h. elixir
i. syrup
j. aerosol

J. Types of Medication Orders

Fill in the blank.

1. A(n) ______________________ order is given over the phone or in person, whereas a(n) ______________________ order is given in writing, such as an electronic message.

Match the description with the correct type of order.

2. _____ Medication that is given on an "as needed" basis for specific signs and symptoms.
3. _____ Medication taken at a regular interval until it is canceled or expired.
4. _____ Medication is administered one time right now.
5. _____ Order applies to all patients who meet specific criteria.
6. _____ Medication is administered one time.

a. routine order
b. standing order
c. PRN order
d. single or one-time order
e. stat order

K. Prescriptions

Fill in the blank.

1. A(n) ______________________ is a written order by a provider to the pharmacist.

Match the description with the correct part of a prescription.

2. _____ Medication name and strength
3. _____ Directions to the pharmacist, how much to dispense, refills, and if generics are permitted
4. _____ The Rx symbol; means take
5. _____ Directions to the patient regarding the dose and timing of the medication

a. superscription
b. inscription
c. signature
d. subscription

CERTIFICATION PREPARATION

Circle the correct answer.

1. The rate of medication absorption is influenced by the
   a. blood flow to the absorption area.
   b. route.
   c. conditions at the site of the absorption.
   d. all of the above.

2. Which statement is true regarding metabolism?
   a. Most drug metabolism occurs in the liver.
   b. Young children, older adults, and those with kidney disease have issues metabolizing medications.
   c. Prodrugs change to inactive forms of drugs during metabolism.
   d. a and c

3. ______ means one drug reduces or blocks the effect of another drug.
   a. Toxicity
   b. Synergism
   c. Antagonism
   d. Potentiation

4. ______ means one drug increases the effect of the second drug.
   a. Toxicity
   b. Synergism
   c. Antagonism
   d. Potentiation

5. ______ means to give a prescribed dose of medication to a patient.
   a. Dispense
   b. Administer
   c. Prescribe
   d. Treatment

6. What is the classification of amoxicillin?
   a. Analgesic
   b. Antianxiety
   c. Antibiotic
   d. Antidepressant

7. What is the classification of atenolol?
   a. Antianxiety
   b. Anticonvulsant
   c. Antidepressant
   d. Antihypertensive

8. What is the classification of albuterol?
   a. Cholesterol-lowering agent
   b. Bronchodilator
   c. Corticosteroid
   d. Antihypertensive

9. Which classification of medication increases urinary output and lowers blood pressure?
   a. Laxative
   b. Corticosteroid
   c. Antihypertensive
   d. Diuretic

10. What is the action of an antiemetic?
    a. Treats depression
    b. Reduces nausea and vomiting
    c. Treats bacterial infections
    d. Reduces blood glucose level

WORKPLACE APPLICATIONS

1. Using Table 14.4, Information on Commonly Prescribed Medications, complete the table. Identify the indications for use and the desired effects for the medication classifications listed.

Medication Classification	Indications for Use	Desired Effects
Analgesics (narcotic)		
Antianxiety		
Antibiotics		
Anticoagulants		
Anticonvulsants		
Antidepressants (SSRIs)		
Antigout		
Antihyperglycemics		
Antihypertensives		
Antiinflammatories		
Antiplatelets		

Medication Classification	Indications for Use	Desired Effects
Bronchodilators		
Cholesterol-lowering agents		
Contraceptive (oral)		
Corticosteroids (oral)		
Diuretics		
Hormone replacement (insulin)		
Muscle relaxants		
Stimulants		

2. Using Table 14.4, Information on Commonly Prescribed Medications, complete the table. Identify the two side effects and two adverse reactions for the following medication classifications.

Class	Generic Name	Side Effects	Adverse Reaction
Analgesics (narcotic)	hydrocodone/ acetaminophen		
Antianxiety (benzodiazepines)	alprazolam		
Antibiotics (penicillin)	amoxicillin		
Anticoagulants	warfarin		
Anticonvulsants	gabapentin		
Antidepressant	escitalopram		
Antihyperglycemics	metformin		
Antihypertensive	propranolol		

Class	Generic Name	Side Effects	Adverse Reaction
Bronchodilators	albuterol		
Cholesterol-lowering agents	atorvastatin		
Diuretics	furosemide		
Proton-pump inhibitors	omeprazole		

INTERNET ACTIVITIES

1. Using online resources, identify four reliable websites that can be used for medication information. Cite the websites.

2. Using the internet, research the Prescribers' Digital Reference website (https://www.pdr.net/) or the MedlinePlus website (https://medlineplus.gov/). Summarize the following points in a paper, PowerPoint Presentation, or in a poster.
   a. What types of drug information are available?
   b. How can a medical assistant use this website?
   c. What resources are available on this website?

3. Using appropriate online drug reference resources, research one medication from 12 different classifications listed in Table 14.3. The medications should not be listed on Table 14.4. Cite your references. In a paper, PowerPoint presentation, or poster, address the following points for each of the 12 medications:
   a. Generic name
   b. Trade names (in the U.S. only)
   c. Usual adult dose
   d. Classification
   e. Indication for use
   f. Desired effects
   g. Contraindications (list two or more)
   h. Side effects (list five or more)
   i. Adverse reactions (list three or more)

Procedure 14.1 Prepare a Prescription

Name ______________________________ **Date** ____________ **Score** __________

Tasks: Prepare prescriptions using a prescription refill protocol. Use approved abbreviations.

Scenario: You receive a call from Noemi Rodriguez (DOB 11/04/19XX). She is requesting refills on three of her prescriptions from Jean Burke, NP. She saw Jean Burke 10 months ago. Noemi has no known allergies (NKA). She is doing well with the prescriptions and has no concerns. You determine it is time for refills. Her prescriptions include Coumadin 5 mg, 1 tablet orally daily; Tenormin 50 mg, 1 tablet orally daily; and Plendil 5 mg, 1 tablet orally daily.

Prescription Refill Protocol
Walden-Martin Family Medicine Clinic

Description: A Certified Medical Assistant (CMA) can refill current hypertensive medications that fall within the guidelines of this protocol.

Step 1	Step 2	
For medications to be refilled, the following points need to be addressed.	**Qualifying Medications**	**Prescription Refill**
• Has the person seen the provider within the last year? • Is the prescription for a hypertensive, hyperlipidemia, or hyperthyroidism medication, a current prescription? • Is the person free of concerns or complications due to the medication? • Is it time for a refill? (The medical assistant must verify that it is time for a refill.) If the answers to the above questions are all YES, then proceed to Step 2. If any of the answers to the above questions are NO, then schedule the person for an appointment with the provider.	amlodipine amlodipine/benazepril atenolol atenolol/chlorthalidone benazepril captopril diltiazem enalapril felodipine fosinopril irbesartan isradipine lisinopril losartan nifedipine quinapril ramipril	Extend the current prescription for 6 months. Instruct patient that in 6 months: • A visit to the provider will be required • Blood pressure reading will be required • Lab work may be required

Equipment and Supplies:
- SimChart for the Medical Office (SCMO) or paper prescriptions (Work Product 14.1) and pen
- Prescription refill protocol
- Drug reference book or online resource

Standard: Complete the procedure and all critical steps in _______ minutes with a minimum score of 85% within two attempts (or as indicated by the instructor).

Scoring: Divide the points earned by the total possible points. Failure to perform a critical step, indicated by an asterisk (*), results in grade no higher than an 84% (or as indicated by the instructor).

Time: Began_________ Ended_________ Total minutes: _________

Steps:	**Point Value**	**Attempt 1**	**Attempt 2**
1. Using the scenario, look up the generic medication names using the drug reference book or online resource.	**10**		
2. Read the prescription refill protocol. Compare the generic names to the list of medications given. Identify medication(s) that meet the protocol.	**10**		
3. Prepare prescription(s) for refill according to the protocol using SCMO or paper prescriptions. • Using SCMO: Search for the patient. Verify the date of birth before selecting the patient. On the INFO PANEL, select Phone Encounter. Complete the fields on the Create New Encounter window and save. Check the box beside the No known allergy statement on the allergy screen and save. Select Order Entry from the Record dropdown list and select Add in the Out-of-office section. • Using paper prescriptions: Add in the patient's complete name, date of birth, and address.	**20**		
4. Using the information in the scenario, complete the prescription information on either the paper prescription or in the SCMO fields. Use only approved abbreviations.	**20**		
5. Complete any additional prescription(s) as needed by the prescription refill protocol.	**30**		
6. Review the prescriptions for any errors. Void the prescription and redo if needed. Note: After the provider signs the prescriptions and depending on the facility's policy, the medical assistant may need to document the refill in the health record. This cannot be done until the provider approves the prescriptions.	**10**		
Total Points	**100**		

Comments

ABHES Competencies	**Step(s)**
6. Pharmacology c.2) Identify appropriate abbreviations that are accepted in prescription writing	4
6.c.3) Comply with legal aspects of creating prescriptions, including federal and state laws	Entire procedure

Work Product 14.1 Prescriptions

To be used with Procedure 14.1.

Walden-Martin Family Medical Clinic
1234 AnyStreet, AnyTown, AnyState, 12345
Phone: 123-123-1234 Fax: 123-123-5678

Jean Burke NP, Family Nurse Practitioner

Patient: ______________________ DOB: ______________________

Address: ______________________ Date: ______________________

℞

Route:

Sig:

Disp:

Refills:

❑ Generics permitted

____

Jean Burke, NP
NPI#:1234567891

Walden-Martin Family Medical Clinic
1234 AnyStreet, AnyTown, AnyState, 12345
Phone: 123-123-1234 Fax: 123-123-5678

Jean Burke NP, Family Nurse Practitioner

Patient: ______________________ DOB: ______________________

Address: ______________________ Date: ______________________

℞

Route:

Sig:

Disp:

Refills:

❑ Generics permitted

____

Jean Burke, NP
NPI#:1234567891

Walden-Martin Family Medical Clinic
1234 AnyStreet, AnyTown, AnyState, 12345
Phone: 123-123-1234 Fax: 123-123-5678

Jean Burke NP, Family Nurse Practitioner

Patient: ______________________ DOB: ______________

Address: ______________________ Date: ______________

℞

Route:

Sig:

Disp:

Refills:

❑ Generics permitted

____
Jean Burke, NP
NPI#:1234567891

Student Name______________________ Date______________

chapter 15 Health Insurance Essentials

CAAHEP Competencies	Assessment
VIII.C.1.a. Identify: types of third party plans	Skills and Concepts – B. 1
VIII.C.2. Identify managed care requirements for patient referral	Skills and Concepts – C. 4
VIII.C.3.a. Identify processes for: verification of eligibility for services	Skills and Concepts – D. 2
VIII.C.3.b. Identify processes for: precertification/ preauthorization	Skills and Concepts – D. 3, 4
VIII.P.1. Interpret information on an insurance card	Procedure 15.1

ABHES Competencies	Assessment
5. Human Relations c. Assist the patient in navigating issues and concerns that may arise (i.e., insurance policy information, medical bills, and physician/ provider orders)	Case Scenario – 2
7. Administrative Procedures a. Gather and process documents	Procedure 15.1
7. Administrative Procedures c. Perform billing and collection procedures	Procedure 15.1

VOCABULARY REVIEW

Using the word pool on the right, find the correct word to match the definition. Write the word on the line after the definition.

Group A

1. A set dollar amount that the policyholder must pay before the insurance company starts to pay for services ______________________
2. Poor, needy, impoverished ______________________
3. The amount paid or to be paid by the policyholder for coverage under the contract, usually in periodic installments ______________________
4. Services provided to help prevent certain illnesses or that lead to an early diagnosis ______________________
5. When the policyholder pays a certain percentage of the bill and the insurance company pays the rest ______________________
6. A formal request for payment from an insurance company for services provided ______________________
7. A written agreement between two parties, in which one party (the insurance company) agrees to pay another party (the patient) if certain specified circumstances occur ______________________
8. Services that are proper and needed for the diagnosis or treatment of the medical condition ______________________
9. A set dollar amount that the policyholder must pay for each office visit ______________________
10. The person responsible for the payment of the premium ______________________

Word Pool
- policy
- premium
- subscriber
- deductible
- coinsurance
- copayment
- claim
- medically necessary
- preventive care
- indigent

Group B

1. Government insurance plan for dependents of military personnel ______________________
2. Those covered by Medicare; a designated person who receives funds from an insurance policy ______________________
3. Insurance plan funded by a large company or organization for its own employees ______________________
4. Low-income Medicare patients who qualify for Medicaid for their secondary insurance ______________________
5. Government insurance plan for those age 65 or older ______________________
6. A list of fixed prices for services ______________________
7. Government insurance plan for surviving spouses and dependent children of veterans who died in the line of duty ______________________

Word Pool
- Medicare
- Medicaid
- TRICARE
- Civilian Health and Medical Program of the Veterans Administration
- beneficiary
- resource-based relative value scale
- explanation of benefits
- fee schedule
- Qualified Medicare Beneficiaries
- self-funded plan

8. A document sent by the insurance company to the provider and the patient explaining the allowed charge amount, the amount reimbursed for services, and the patient's financial responsibilities ____________________
9. Government insurance plan for those with low income ____________________
10. A system used to determine how much providers should be paid for services provided; used by Medicare and many other health insurance companies ____________________

Group C

1. In charge of coordinating the patient's care ____________________
2. When the patient has authorized the insurance company to make the payment directly to the provider ____________________
3. An organization that processes claims and provides administrative services for another organization ____________________
4. A process required by some insurance carriers in which the provider obtains permission to perform certain procedures or services ____________________
5. An online marketplace where you can compare and buy individual health insurance plans ____________________
6. The primary care provider who is in charge of a patient's treatment ____________________
7. The amount paid for a medical service in a geographic area based on what providers in the area usually charge for the same or similar service ____________________
8. Providers are contracted with the insurance plan and have agreed to accept the contracted fee schedule as payment in full ____________________
9. The maximum that the insurance plan will pay for a procedure or service ____________________
10. An order from a primary care provider for the patient to see a specialist or get certain medical services ____________________

Word Pool

- third-party administrator
- health insurance exchange
- participating provider
- allowable charge
- assignment of benefits
- usual, customary, and reasonable
- primary care provider
- referral
- preauthorization
- gatekeeper

Group D

1. Reviews individual cases to ensure that services are medically necessary ____________________
2. The provider is paid a set amount for each enrolled person assigned to him or her, per period of time, whether or not that person has received services ____________________
3. The length of time a patient waits for disability insurance to pay after the date of injury ____________________
4. Low- to middle-income Americans can compare plans and lower their costs for healthcare coverage ____________________
5. An approved list of physicians, hospitals, and other providers ____________________
6. A health problem that was present before new health insurance coverage started ____________________
7. A service provided by various insurance companies for providers to look up a patient's insurance benefits, eligibility, claims status, and explanation of benefits ____________________
8. A decision-making process used by managed care organizations to manage healthcare costs; involves case-by-case assessments of the appropriateness of care ____________________
9. Government insurance plan for employees who are injured or become ill due to work-related issues ____________________

Word Pool

- provider network
- capitation
- utilization management
- utilization review committee
- online insurance web portal
- workers' compensation
- waiting period
- preexisting condition
- health insurance marketplaces

ABBREVIATIONS

Write out what each of the following abbreviations stands for.

1. ACA ____________________
2. STI ____________________
3. CHAMPVA ____________________
4. ESRD ____________________
5. CMS ____________________
6. HHS ____________________
7. RBRVS ____________________
8. UCR ____________________
9. EOB ____________________
10. QMBs ____________________
11. CHIP ____________________
12. TPA ____________________
13. MCO ____________________
14. PCP ____________________

15. HMO ______________________________

16. PPO ______________________________

17. EPO ______________________________

18. IPA ______________________________

19. PAR ______________________________

SKILLS AND CONCEPTS

Answer the following questions. Write your answer on the line or in the space provided.

A. Health Insurance Basics

1. Which of the following is *not* considered cost-sharing?
   a. Deductible
   b. Coinsurance
   c. Premium
   d. Copayment
   e. All of the above

2. A(n) ______________________ is submitted to the insurance carrier so the provider can be paid for services rendered.

3. The federal government requires all health plans cover ______________________ essential health benefits.

B. Health Insurance Plans

1. Match the following terms and definitions:

_____ Medicaid

_____ Medicare

_____ Medigap

a. A federally funded health insurance program for those older than 65 years or disabled individuals younger than 65 years
b. A term sometimes applied to private insurance products that supplement Medicare insurance benefits
c. A health insurance program that is funded by both federal and state governments for the medically indigent

2. List two different populations that qualify for Medicare. ______________________________

____

3. The RBRVS includes the following three parts:

   a. ______________________________

   b. ______________________________

   c. ______________________________

4. The intermediary and administrator who coordinates patients and providers and processes claims for self-funded plans is called a(n) ______________________.

5. Prescription drugs are covered by Medicare ______________________.

6. List four different populations that qualify for Medicaid. ______________________

____

7. Active-duty military personnel, family members of active duty personnel, and military retirees and their eligible family members younger than age 65 are covered by ______________________.

8. The health benefits program run by the Department of Veterans Affairs (VA) that helps eligible beneficiaries pay the cost of specific healthcare services and supplies is the (give acronym) ______________________.

9. Private health insurance plans are obtained from which two sources? ______________________

____

10. A(n) ______________________ is a healthcare provider who enters into a contract with a specific insurance company or program and agrees to accept the contracted fee schedule.

11. The ______________________ is the maximum that third-party payers will pay for a procedure or service.

C. Health Insurance Models

1. Traditional health insurance plans are also referred to as ______________________ plans.

2. For each of the following managed care plans, describe the deductible, coinsurance, and copayment requirements:

   a. Health maintenance organization (HMO): ______________________

   ____

   ____

   ____

   ____

   ____

   b. Preferred provider organization (PPO): ______________________

   ____

   ____

   ____

   ____

   ____

c. Exclusive provider organization (EPO): ______________________________

____

____

____

____

____

3. A(n) ______________________________ is a review of individual cases by a committee to make sure services are medically necessary and to study how providers use medical care resources.

4. Describe the managed care requirements for a patient referral. ______________________________

____

____

____

____

D. The Medical Assistant's Role

1. One of the medical assistant's responsibilities is verifying eligibility. Describe the processes available for the verification of eligibility for services.

____

____

____

2. Describe how the patient's insurance eligibility is confirmed. ______________________________

____

____

____

3. What items should the medical assistant gather when using the paper method to obtain a precertification for a service or procedure?

____

____

____

4. Describe the processes for precertification using the paper method. What does the medical assistant need to do?

____

____

____

E. Other Types of Insurance

1. List the services covered by workers' compensation plans.______________________________

____

____

____

2. Match the types of insurance benefits with their description.

_____ Disability
_____ Liability insurance
_____ Life insurance
_____ Long-term care insurance

a. Provides payment of a specified amount upon the insured's death
b. Covers a continuum of broad-range maintenance and health services to chronically ill, disabled, or mentally disabled individuals
c. A form of insurance that provides income replacement if the patient has a non-work–related injury
d. Often includes benefits for medical expenses related to traumatic injuries and lost wages payable to individuals who are injured in the insured person's home or in an automobile accident

CERTIFICATION PREPARATION

Circle the correct answer.

1. A policy that covers a number of people under a single master contract issued to the employer or to an association with which they are affiliated and that is not self-funded is usually called a(n)
   a. group policy.
   b. individual policy.
   c. government plan.
   d. self-insured plan.

2. The maximum amount of money third-party payers will pay for a specific procedure or service is called the
   a. benefit.
   b. allowed amount.
   c. allowable service.
   d. incurred amount.

3. A provider who enters into a contract with an insurance company and agrees to certain rules and regulations is called a _____ provider.
   a. paying
   b. physician
   c. participating
   d. none of the above

4. A review of individual cases by a committee to make sure that services are medically necessary and to study how providers use medical care resources is called a(n)
   a. credentialing committee review.
   b. peer review committee evaluation.
   c. utilization review.
   d. audit committee review.

5. Which type of HMO model consists of physicians with separately owned practices who formally organize into a group but continue to practice in their own offices?
   a. Staff model
   b. Independent practice association
   c. Group model
   d. None of the above

6. Which individuals would *not* normally be eligible for Medicare?
   a. A 66-year-old retired woman
   b. A blind teenager
   c. A 23-year-old recipient of Temporary Assistance for Needy Families (TANF)
   d. A person on dialysis

7. Which expenses would be paid by Medicare Part B?
   a. Inpatient hospital charges
   b. Hospice services
   c. Home healthcare charges
   d. Physician's office visits

8. A type of insurance that protects workers from loss of wages after an industrial accident that happened on the job is called
   a. an individual policy.
   b. workers' compensation.
   c. unemployment insurance.
   d. disability insurance.

9. A payment method in which providers are paid for each individual enrolled in a plan, regardless of whether the person sees the provider that month, is called a _____ plan.
   a. capitation
   b. self-insured
   c. managed care
   d. fee-for-service

10. What should the medical assistant always verify prior to the patient's appointment?
    a. Eligibility
    b. Benefits and exclusions
    c. Effective date of insurance
    d. All of the above

WORKPLACE APPLICATIONS

1. After reading the following paragraph, fill the blanks in the statements.

   The medical assistant's tasks related to health insurance processing are initiated when the patient encounters the provider by appointment, as a walk-in, or in the emergency department or hospital. To complete insurance billing and coding properly, the medical assistant must perform the following tasks:

   a. Obtain information from the patient and/or the guarantor, including ______________________ and ______________________ data.

   b. Verify the patient's ______________________ for insurance payment with the insurance carrier or carriers, as well as insurance ______________________, exclusions, and whether ______________________ is required to refer patients to specialists or to perform certain services or procedures such as surgery or diagnostic tests.

   c. Obtain ______________________ for referral of the patient to a specialist or for special services or procedures that require advance permission.

2. Julia Berkley has just gotten a new insurance policy and is struggling with all of the terminology she is seeing in her policy. She would like you to explain just what *premium, deductible, coinsurance,* and *copayment* really mean.

____

____

____

____

INTERNET ACTIVITIES

1. Using online resources, research TRICARE and CHAMPVA. Create a poster presentation, a PowerPoint presentation, or write a paper summarizing your research. Include the following points in your project:
   a. Describe both TRICARE and CHAMPVA.
   b. List who is eligible for TRICARE and who is eligible for CHAMPVA.
   c. Explain what is involved when a provider participates in TRICARE.

2. Using online resources, research preferred provider organizations (PPO). Create a poster presentation, a PowerPoint presentation, or write a paper summarizing your research. Include the following points in your project:
   a. Describe what a PPO is.
   b. List the ranges for deductibles and coinsurance amounts found.
   c. Explain how a PPO is different from an HMO.
   d. Describe why a patient might want to have a PPO policy instead of traditional insurance.

Procedure 15.1 Interpret Information on an Insurance Card

Name ______________________________ **Date** __________ **Score** _________

Task: To identify essential information on the health insurance identification (ID) card to confirm copayment obligations and obtain accurate health insurance information for claims submission.

Equipment and Supplies:
- Patient's health insurance ID, both sides (Figure 15.1)

Standard: Complete the procedure and all critical steps in _______ minutes with a minimum score of 85% within two attempts (*or as indicated by the instructor*).

Scoring: Divide the points earned by the total possible points. Failure to perform a critical step, indicated by an asterisk (*), results in grade no higher than an 84% (*or as indicated by the instructor*).

Time: Began_________ Ended_________ Total minutes: _________

Steps:	**Point Value**	**Attempt 1**	**Attempt 2**
1. Review the patient's health insurance ID card and identify the insured on the health insurance ID card. If the patient is different than the insured, obtain the relationship with the insured and the insured's date of birth and gender.	**20***		
2. Identify the insurance plan.	**20**		
3. Identify the insured's identification number and group number.	**20**		
4. Identify the patient's copayment, which is due before the appointment. Collect the correct amount.	**20**		
5. On the back of the health insurance ID card, ensure that a customer service phone number and medical claims address is present.	**20**		
Total Points	**100**		

Comments

CAAHEP Competencies	**Step(s)**
VIII.P.1. Interpret information on an insurance card	Entire procedure
ABHES Competencies	**Step(s)**
7. Administrative Procedures c. Perform billing and collection procedures	Entire procedure

Figure 15.1 Patient's Health Insurance ID Card

Front

AETNA

INSURED: Tapia, Arnold

IDENTIFICATION #: CH1197845 **DEPENDENTS:** Tapia, Celia B

GROUP #: 33347H **EFFECTIVE DATE:** 06/26/2012

CO-PAY: $25
SPECIALIST CO-PAY: $35
EMERGENCY DEPT: $35

DRUG CO-PAY
GENERIC: $10
NAME BRAND: $50

Back

Submit claims to:

Aetna
1234 Insurance Way
Anytown, AK 12345

Member Services: 1-800-123-222

Insured: If a life threatening emergency exists, seek immediate attention.

Student Name______________________________ Date______________

Diagnostic Coding Essentials

chapter **16**

CAAHEP Competencies	Assessments
IX.C.1. Identify the current procedural and diagnostic coding systems, including Healthcare Common Procedure Coding Systems II (HCPCS Level II)	Skills and Concepts – B. 1
IX.C.3. Define medical necessity	Skills and Concepts – A. 1
IX.P.2. Perform diagnostic coding	Procedure 16.1
ABHES Competencies	**Assessments**
1. General Orientation d. List the general responsibilities and skills of the medical assistant	Procedure 16.1

VOCABULARY REVIEW

Using the word pool on the right, find the correct word to match the definition. Write the word on the line after the definition.

Group A

1. The relative frequency of deaths in a specific population ______________
2. Information about a patient's diagnosis or diagnoses that has been taken from the medical documentation ______________
3. Any meeting between a patient and a healthcare provider ______________
4. Radiology, pathology, and laboratory reports ______________
5. The study of the causes or origin of diseases ______________
6. The branch of medicine dealing with the incidence, distribution, and control of disease in a population ______________

Word Pool

- diagnosis
- reimbursement
- mortality
- epidemiology
- encounter
- encoder
- diagnostic statement
- ancillary diagnostic services
- medically necessary
- etiology

7. Determining the cause of a condition, illness, disease, injury, or congenital defect ______________________
8. Accepted healthcare services that are appropriate for the evaluation and treatment of a disease, condition, illness, or injury and are consistent with the applicable standard of care ______________________
9. Software that will apply diagnostic or procedure codes to medical conditions or procedures ______________________
10. To make repayment for an expense or a loss incurred ______________________

Group B

1. A mental disorder in which the individual experiences a progressive loss of memory, personality alterations, confusion, loss of touch with reality, and stupor ______________________
2. Patient's chief complaint or statements about why the patient is seeking medical care ______________________
3. Developing slowly and lasting for a long time, generally 3 or more months ______________________
4. Suggest that it should not be used ______________________
5. An abnormal condition resulting from a previous disease ______________________
6. A document used to capture the services/procedures and diagnoses for a patient visit ______________________
7. The quality or state of being specific ______________________
8. A statement in the patient's own words that describes the reason for the visit ______________________
9. Abbreviations, punctuation, symbols, instructional notations, and related entities ______________________
10. Collecting important information from the health record ______________________

Word Pool

- specificity
- chronic
- conventions
- sequela
- dementia
- abstract
- encounter form
- chief complaint
- contraindicate
- subjective findings

Group C

1. Progressive loss of transparency of the lens of the eye ______________________
2. The signs and symptoms of a disease ______________________
3. The period from the last month of pregnancy to 5 months postpartum ______________________
4. Imminently threatening ______________________
5. First 6 weeks after delivery ______________________
6. The study of body tissues ______________________

Word Pool

- objective findings
- manifestation
- cataract
- myxedema
- impending
- histologic
- antepartum
- postpartum
- peripartum

7. Any measurable indicators found during the physical examination ______________________
8. Pregnancy ______________________
9. Advanced hypothyroidism in adulthood ______________________

ABBREVIATIONS

Write out what each of the following abbreviations stands for.

1. ICD-10-CM______________________
2. CMS______________________
3. WHO______________________
4. EHR______________________
5. HPI ______________________
6. H&P ______________________
7. CC ______________________
8. HIV ______________________
9. AIDS ______________________
10. DM ______________________

SKILLS AND CONCEPTS

Answer the following questions. Write your answer on the line or in the space provided.

A. Understanding Diagnostic Coding

1. Define *medically necessary* and explain how it applies to diagnostic coding. Give an example. ______________________

____

____

____

____

B. Getting to Know the ICD-10-CM

1. Fill in the blanks in the following statements with terms from the word bank to describe how to use the most current diagnostic coding classification system.

   Word Bank:

code	coding guidelines	character
convention	diagnostic	diagnostic statements
essential modifier	exclusion	ICD-10-CM
main term	Tabular List	

   a. Abstract the correct diagnosis from the ____________________ found in the patient health record.

   b. Use the ____________________ to look up the diagnosis in the Alphabetic Index.

   c. Review the ____________________ under the main term.

   d. Choose the correct code based on the ____________________ statement.

   e. Look up the code from the Alphabetic Index in the ____________________.

   f. Check for any ____________________, ____________________, inclusion notes, ____________________ notes, or additional ____________________ symbol.

   g. Assign the final ____________________ diagnosis code.

2. ICD-10-CM codes can have up to ______ characters. A(n) ____________________ "x" is used to fill in for positions that don't have characters.

3. What are the seventh characters used for encounter types and what do they indicate? ________________

   ____

   ____

   ____

4. Four basic forms of punctuation are used in the Tabular Index. List them and what they are used for.

   ____

   ____

   ____

   ____

   ____

   ____

   ____

5. Match the following terms.

_____ Main terms
_____ Nonessential modifiers
_____ Subterms
_____ Essential modifiers

a. Indented under the main term; they change the description of the diagnosis in bold type
b. Appear in bold
c. Are found after the main term and are enclosed in parentheses
d. Indented under the essential modifier

6. Review the following diagnostic statements and determine the main term and essential modifier in the Alphabetic Index.

   a. Morgan Smith had an acute myocardial infarction, commonly referred to as a *heart attack*.

      Main Term: ______________________ Essential Modifier: ______________________

   b. Georgia Summers went into anaphylactic shock after drinking milk.

      Main Term: ______________________ Essential Modifier: ______________________

   c. Roger Costen has benign essential hypertension.

      Main Term: ______________________ Essential Modifier: ______________________

   d. Raul Castro has been diagnosed with iron-deficiency anemia.

      Main Term: ______________________ Essential Modifier: ______________________

   e. Stephanie Thompson has a urinary tract infection.

      Main Term: ______________________ Essential Modifier: ______________________

   f. Mabel Johnson has rheumatoid arthritis.

      Main Term: ______________________ Essential Modifier: ______________________

   g. Amanda Smith was diagnosed with multiple sclerosis.

      Main Term: ______________________ Essential Modifier: ______________________

   h. Hudson Madison suffered a ruptured abdominal aneurysm.

      Main Term: ______________________ Essential Modifier: ______________________

   i. Don Julius died last week from congestive heart failure.

      Main Term: ______________________ Essential Modifier: ______________________

   j. Betty White has allergic gastroenteritis.

      Main Term: ______________________ Essential Modifier: ______________________

C. Preparing for Diagnostic Coding

1. The SOAP notes system of documentation divides the information into what four areas?

   a. ______________________________

   b. ______________________________

   c. ______________________________

   d. ______________________________

2. To prepare for medical coding, the coder must analyze the patient's health record and ______________ the diagnostic statement.

3. Information pertinent to code selection can be abstracted from a variety of medical documents. List the documents where the diagnostic statement may be found.

   ____

   ____

   ____

   ____

   ____

4. The ______________ is the provider's health history evaluation and physical assessment of the patient.

5. The ______________ is a statement in the patient's own words that describes why the person is seeking medical attention.

6. The ______________ is used for extracting procedure and diagnostic information for patients who underwent surgery.

D. Steps in ICD-10-CM Coding

1. Code the following diagnoses to the highest level of specificity using either the ICD-10-CM coding manual or the TruCode encoder.

   a. Kayla Swift was diagnosed with infectious mononucleosis. ______________

   b. Gerald Weaver has osteoarthritis in his right shoulder region. ______________

   c. Jeffrey Rush has a personal history of alcoholism. ______________

   d. Barry White's alcoholism has caused cirrhosis of the liver without ascites. ______________

   e. Frank Emmett had atherosclerosis of the extremities with gangrene. ______________

   f. Ginger Chan experienced dermatitis from using facial cosmetics. ______________

   g. The Lewises' first child was born with Down syndrome. ______________

   h. Lee Anna has experienced painful menstruation during her last three cycles. ______________

i. Gary Stevens was diagnosed with cardiomegaly. _______________

j. Jerry Stein developed Kaposi's sarcoma in his lymph nodes during the final stages of AIDS. _______________

k. Terri Holden attempted suicide for the second time using a handful of lithium. _______________

l. Susan French was stung by a jellyfish while swimming off the coast of Mexico. _______________

m. Riley Brown has acute myocarditis. _______________

n. Ordell Thompson has acute esophagitis. _______________

o. Korney Ralphy was diagnosed with systemic lupus erythematosus. _______________

p. Marcia Radson had a skin condition known as *bullous pemphigoid,* in which blisters form in patches all over her skin. _______________

q. Osteomalacia caused by malnutrition made it impossible for Robbie Hernandez to walk. _______________

r. Henry Casper has oral leukoplakia, which may have been caused by smoking a pipe. _______________

s. Patricia Kielty has had uterine endometriosis for several years and may require a hysterectomy in the future. _______________

t. Robert Bauer dislocated his right shoulder while playing baseball; it was a closed anterior dislocation. _______________

E. Understanding Coding Guidelines

1. If the provider note states ___________________________, ___________________________, or ___________________________, the coder should code the documented signs and symptoms.
2. ___________________________ is the underlying cause of a disease. ___________________________ are the signs and symptoms of a disease. The ___________________________ code is always listed first.
3. Coding of sequelae usually requires two codes with the ___________________________ code sequenced second.
4. Place of occurrence codes come from category ___________________________.
5. Category Y93 are ___________________________ that define what the patient was doing at the time of injury or when the health condition developed.

F. Maximizing Third-Party Reimbursement

1. When using ICD-10-CM codes it is important to code to the highest level of ___________________________.
2. Correct diagnostic coding can impact ___________________________ for services provided, which in turn can impact the practice's ___________________________.

CERTIFICATION PREPARATION

Circle the correct answer.

1. Which term defines a malignant neoplasm as the absence of invasion of surrounding tissues?
   a. Primary
   b. Secondary
   c. In situ
   d. Benign

2. Which code will be used for a patient with a history of myocardial infarction with no symptoms but diagnosed by means of an electrocardiogram?
   a. I21
   b. I25.2
   c. I21.3
   d. None of the above

3. Which term applies to the period from the last month of pregnancy to 5 months after giving birth?
   a. Antepartum
   b. Childbirth
   c. Postpartum
   d. Peripartum

4. The abbreviation that is the equivalent of "unspecified" is _____.
   a. NEC
   b. NOS
   c. NOW
   d. NCL

5. If the provider has documented "rule out" in the diagnostic statement, the medical assistant must code what?
   a. Whatever phrase follows "rule out"
   b. Lab results
   c. Signs/symptoms
   d. None of the above

6. A diagnosis is
   a. a third party's opinion of a patient's illness.
   b. determining the cause of a patient's illness.
   c. the process of finding a patient's past medical history.
   d. both b and c.

7. Currently in the United States, the source used for coding diagnoses in providers' offices is the
   a. *Diagnostic Guide for Medicare and Medicaid Services.*
   b. *Diagnostic Codes for Third-Party Payers.*
   c. *International Classification of Disease, 10th Revision, Clinical Modifications.*
   d. *AMA Manual of Essential Diagnostic Codes, Volume 1.*

8. Morbidity is the presence of illness or disease, whereas mortality is
   a. the determination of the nature of a disease.
   b. the deaths that occur from a disease.
   c. classification of a disease.
   d. All of the above.

9. In ICD-10, codes longer than three characters always have a decimal point between the
   a. fourth and fifth characters.
   b. fifth and sixth characters.
   c. third and fourth characters.
   d. sixth and seventh characters.

10. In the ICD-10-CM coding system, a lowercase "x" is used
    a. as a placeholder character within a code.
    b. to denote an obsolete code.
    c. as a cross-reference guide.
    d. to indicate the external causes of morbidity.

WORKPLACE APPLICATIONS

1. Dr. Martin has diagnosed Maude Crawford in the past with congestive heart failure and diabetes mellitus type 2 (insulin-dependent, long-term). She comes to the clinic today complaining of chest pain and has a fever of 101.8° F. Code all of these conditions. In which order should these codes be sequenced?
   a. ______________
   b. ______________
   c. ______________
   d. ______________
   e. ______________

2. Dr. Perez has documented the following for Reuven Ahmad:

   CC: Shortness of breath, chest pain, nausea, and excessive sweating
   DX: 1. probable myocardial infarction, 2. rule out gastroesophageal reflux disease

   What are the correct diagnosis codes for this patient?

   Note to instructors: Remind students that codes may change with updated versions of ICD.

INTERNET ACTIVITIES

1. Using online resources, research diagnostic code encoders. Create a poster presentation, a PowerPoint presentation, or write a paper summarizing your research. Include the following points in your project:
   a. Describe the purpose of an encoder.
   b. List three reasons why a healthcare organization would want to use an encoder for diagnostic coding.
   c. Explain how using an encoder is different than using the ICD-10-CM coding manuals.

2. Using online resources, research the history and development of ICD. Create a poster presentation, a PowerPoint presentation, or write a paper summarizing your research. Include the following points in your project:
   a. Describe the ICD system.
   b. Explain how and why it was originally developed.
   c. List five reasons why ICD-10-CM was developed.

Procedure 16.1 Perform Coding Using the Current ICD-10-CM Manual or Encoder

Name ______________________________ **Date** ____________ **Score** __________

Task: To perform accurate diagnosis coding using the ICD-10-CM manual or encoder.

Scenario: The encounter form and progress notes both show that the diagnosis for this patient encounter is acute colitis. Locate the most accurate ICD-10-CM code for this diagnostic statement.

Equipment and Supplies:
- ICD-10-CM manual (current year) *or*
- Encoder software such as TruCode

Standard: Complete the procedure and all critical steps in _______ minutes with a minimum score of 85% within two attempts (*or as indicated by the instructor*).

Scoring: Divide the points earned by the total possible points. Failure to perform a critical step, indicated by an asterisk (*), results in grade no higher than an 84% (*or as indicated by the instructor*).

Time: Began_________ Ended_________ Total minutes: _________

Steps:	Point Value	Attempt 1	Attempt 2
Alphabetic Index			
1. Determine and locate the main terms from the diagnostic statement in the Alphabetic Index.	**10**		
2. Locate the essential modifiers listed under the main term in the Alphabetic Index.	**10**		
3. Review the conventions, punctuation, and notes in the Alphabetic Index.	**10**		
4. Choose a tentative code, codes, or code range from the Alphabetic Index that matches the diagnostic statement as closely as possible.	**15***		
Tabular List			
5. Look up the codes chosen from the Alphabetic Index in the Tabular List.	**10**		
6. Review notes, conventions, and the Official Coding Guidelines associated with the code and code description in the Tabular List. a. Review conventions and punctuation. b. Review instructional notations: • *Includes* and *excludes* notes • *Code first, code also,* and *code additional* notes • *And, or,* and *with* statements	**10**		
7. Verify the accuracy of the tentative code in the Tabular List. a. Make sure all elements of the diagnostic statement are included in the codes selected. b. Make sure the code description does not include anything not documented in the diagnostic statement.	**10**		
8. Extend the codes to their highest level of specificity (up to the 7th character, if required). If a 7th character is required, and no codes are present for the 4th, 5th, or 6th characters, it is appropriate to use the dummy placeholder "x" for these positions.	**10**		

9. Assign the code (or codes) selected from the Tabular List as the appropriate code for the patient's condition by documenting it in the patient's health record.	**15***		
Total Points	**100**		
Alternate - Using the TruCode Encoder Software			
1. Type in the main term from the diagnostic statement in the search box.	**20**		
2. The software will provide a list of main terms that could be related to the diagnosis typed in the search box. The coder chooses the main term that best represents the diagnostic statement.	**20**		
3. Based on the main term chosen, a list of essential modifiers is presented. The coder must review the diagnostic statement to ensure that all documented modifying terms are identified. If the provider does not document a modifying term, the coder should not assume that a modifying term was implied.	**20**		
4. To determine the most accurate code, follow these coding guidelines.	**20**		
5. Once all the menus of essential modifiers have been presented, choose the most accurate and specific code based on the diagnostic statement.	**20***		
Total Points	**100**		

CAAHEP Competencies	**Steps**
IX.P.2. Perform diagnostic coding	Entire procedure

Student Name____ Date______________________

chapter

17

Procedural Coding Essentials

CAAHEP Competencies	Assessments
IX.C.1. Identify the current procedural and diagnostic coding systems, including Healthcare Common Procedure Coding Systems II (HCPCS Level II)	Skills and Concepts – A. 15, K. 1
IX.C.2.a. Identify the effects of: upcoding	Skills and Concepts – A. 11
IX.C.2.b. Identify the effects of: downcoding	Skills and Concepts – A. 12
IX.C.3. Define medical necessity	Skills and Concepts – A. 13
IX.P.1. Perform procedural coding	Procedures 17.1, 17.2
A.7. Demonstrate tactfulness	Procedure 17.3

ABHES Competencies	Assessments
1. General Orientation d. List the general responsibilities and skills of the medical assistant	Skills and Concepts – A. 9

VOCABULARY REVIEW

Using the word pool on the right, find the correct word to match the definition. Write the word on the line after the definition.

Group A

1. An online journal, supported by the AMA, that addresses subjects such as appealing insurance denials, validating coding to auditors, training staff members, and answering day-to-day coding questions ______________________
2. The use of a lower-level procedure code than is justified ______________________
3. Pertaining to, involving, or affecting two or both sides ______________________
4. The regular collection of data to assess whether the correct processes are being performed and desired results are being achieved ______________________

Word Pool

- performance measurement
- eponym
- specificity
- CPT Assistant
- débridement
- special report
- upcoding
- downcoding
- modifiers
- bilaterally

5. Additional medical documentation required to confirm the need for the use of unlisted, unusual, or newly adopted medical procedures code ______________________
6. Two-digit numeric codes that report or indicate specific criteria, specific condition, or special circumstance ______________________
7. The quality or state of being specific ______________________
8. The use of a higher-level procedure code than is supported in the documentation or by medical necessity ______________________
9. In medical terms, a medical diagnosis or procedure named for the person who discovered it ______________________
10. The surgical removal of dead, damaged, or infected tissue to improve the function of healthy tissue ______________________

Group B

1. A list of questions related to each organ system designed to uncover potential disease processes ______________________
2. The process of collecting pertinent medical information needed to assign the correct code ______________________
3. A statement in the patient's own words that describes the reason for the visit ______________________
4. The relative incidence of disease ______________________
5. Special symbols used to provide additional information about specific codes ______________________
6. Relates to the number of deaths from a given disease ______________________
7. Determine the amount of drug present ______________________
8. Each step of the procedure is listed separately ______________________
9. Medical services and procedures performed for the patient before, during, and after a surgical procedure ______________________
10. Based on the type of drug found ______________________
11. Includes services related to prepping the patient for the procedure, performing the procedure, and suturing to complete the procedure ______________________
12. A nursing healthcare professional who is certified to administer anesthesia ______________________

Word Pool

- conventions
- abstract
- chief complaint
- review of systems
- morbidity
- mortality
- Certified Registered Nurse Anesthetist
- global services
- bundled code
- unbundled code
- qualitative
- quantitative

ABBREVIATIONS

Write out what each of the following abbreviations stands for.

1. CPT ____________________
2. HCPCS ____________________
3. AMA ____________________
4. EHR ____________________
5. H&P ____________________
6. E/M ____________________
7. POS ____________________
8. NP ____________________
9. EP ____________________
10. ROS ____________________
11. CRNA ____________________
12. NCCI ____________________
13. MRI ____________________
14. TURP ____________________
15. ASA ____________________
16. RVG ____________________

SKILLS AND CONCEPTS

Answer the following questions. Write your answer on the line or in the space provided.

A. Introduction to the CPT Manual

1. The CPT system was developed and is maintained by the ____________________.
2. The CPT manual is updated every year on ____________________.
3. The CPT code is a five-digit code also known as a(n) ____________________ code.
4. Category II codes are primarily used for ____________________ and are optional.
5. Category ____________________ codes are for new experimental procedures or emerging technology.
6. The CPT coding manual organizes codes into the Alphabetic Index and the ____________________.

7. The six sections of the CPT manual include:

   a. ______________________________

   b. ______________________________

   c. ______________________________

   d. ______________________________

   e. ______________________________

   f. ______________________________

8. When using an unlisted procedure code, a(n) ____________________ must be sent with the insurance claim.

9. ____________________ are found at the beginning of each of the six sections of the CPT coding manual, and the medical assistant refers to them often when coding procedures.

10. Code additions that explain circumstances that alter a provided service or provide additional clarification or detail are called ____________________.

11. Define *upcoding* and discuss the effects. ______________________________

    ____

12. Define *downcoding* and discuss the effects. ______________________________

    ____

    ____

13. Define *medical necessity* as it applies to procedural coding. ______________________________

    ____

    ____

B. Steps for Efficient CPT Procedural Coding

1. List the sources used for procedural coding. ______________________________

   ____

   ____

2. Describe how to use the most current procedural coding system. ______________________________

   ____

3. Describe the four primary classifications of main and modifying terms. ______________________________

   ____

4. Explain the difference between "see" and "see also." ______________________________

   ____

5. Provide the full description for CPT code 47563
   47562 Laparoscopy, surgical; cholecystectomy
   47363 Cholecystectomy with cholangiography

   ____

   ____

   ____

C. CPT Coding Guidelines: Evaluation and Management Section

1. ________________ codes provide information on the healthcare facility where services were rendered.

2. When determining an evaluation and management code, you first need to identify the ________________ and the ________________.

3. ________________ alone can be used to select the correct E/M code.

D. CPT Coding Guidelines: Anesthesia

1. CPT codes for anesthesia
   a. always start with a zero (0).
   b. identify the anatomic location of the surgery performed.
   c. are used for conscious and unconscious sedation.
   d. a and b.

2. Providing anesthesia services in an emergency situation is considered a(n) ________________.

3. Which of the following are part of the formula for determining the fee for anesthesia services?
   a. Basic unit value
   b. Modifying unit
   c. Time unit
   d. Conversion unit
   e. All of the above

E. CPT Coding Guidelines: Surgical Section

1. Patient prep, surgical care, and postsurgical are considered ________________ and the single code that is used is called a(n) ________________.

2. Codes in which the components of a procedure are separated and reported separately are called ________________ codes.

3. Code for the excision of benign lesions includes ________________ and ________________.

4. When coding fractures, a closed fracture is defined as the
   a. fracture is not surgically opened.
   b. fractured bone cuts through the skin layers and can be directly visualized.
   c. fractured bone does not protrude through the dermis or epidermis.
   d. none of the above.

5. Antepartum care includes which of the following?
   a. Monthly visits up to 28 weeks gestation.
   b. Management of uncomplicated labor.
   c. Hospital and office visits after vaginal or cesarean section delivery.
   d. All of the above

F. CPT Coding Guidelines: Radiology and Pathology and Laboratory Section

1. The radiology section of CPT includes codes for which of the following?
   a. Nuclear medicine procedures
   b. Radiation oncology
   c. MRIs
   d. X-ray studies
   e. All of the above

2. ______________________ codes are considered ______________________ codes and are billed under the single CPT code.

G. CPT Coding Guidelines: Medicine Section

1. Codes in the Medicine section of CPT include codes for which of the following?
   a. Therapeutic procedures
   b. Diagnostic testing
   c. Dialysis
   d. Acupuncture
   e. All of the above

2. When coding vaccinations, there should be one code for the ______________________ of the vaccine and one code for the actual ______________________.

H. HCPCS Code System

1. Describe how to use the most current HCPCS level II coding system. ______________________

____

____

____

____

____

____

____

CODING EXERCISES

Code the following procedures with modifiers if appropriate.

CPT Coding

1. Dr. Smith visits Eula Fairbanks, a patient with dementia, in the nursing home for less than 30 minutes and performs an expanded problem-focused examination with MDM of low complexity.

   ____

2. Jessica Lundy, a newborn, was admitted to the pediatric critical care unit after her birth, where Dr. Williams provided her initial care.

   ____

3. Dr. Partridge participated in a complex, lengthy telephone call lasting 30 minutes, regarding a patient who was scheduled for multiple surgeries.

   ____

4. When Terri Anderson was involved in a major car accident, the emergency department physician took a comprehensive history, performed a comprehensive examination, and then made highly complex decisions.

   ____

5. Tim Taylor is a new patient with a small cyst on his back. Dr. Young took a problem-focused history, performed a problem-focused examination, and then made straightforward medical decisions.

   ____

6. Jim Angelo, an established patient, saw the physician for a minor cut on the back of his hand. The physician spent approximately 10 minutes with Jim.

   ____

7. Because Lucille Westerman had multiple health problems, she was admitted for observation after a fainting spell. Dr. Adams took a comprehensive history and performed a comprehensive examination, then made medical decisions of high complexity regarding her care.

   ____

8. Dr. Wray saw Tammy Luttrell in the office as a new patient. He took a an appropriate history and examination, and then made medical decisions of low complexity. Total time spent with the patient was 30 minutes.

   ____

9. Dr. Tompkins visited a new patient at her home and spent about 20 minutes diagnosing and treating her for the flu. A problem-focused history and examination with straightforward MDM was performed.

   ____

10. Vera Carpenter was admitted to the hospital for diabetes mellitus, congestive heart failure, and an infection of unknown origin. Dr. Antonetti performed a consultation by doing a detailed history and examination, and MDM of low complexity that took about an hour, including the time spent writing orders in her medical record.

    ____

11. Sylvia Julius, an established patient, saw Dr. Bridges for her allergies. The physician took a medically appropriate history and examination and made straightforward decisions regarding her care. Total time spent with the patient was 15 minutes.

    ____

12. Anesthesia for vaginal delivery

    ____

13. Anesthesia was provided for a brain-dead patient whose organs were being harvested for donation.

    ____

14. Laparoscopic biopsy of the left ovary

    ____

15. Treatment of a clavicular fracture without manipulation

    ____

16. Removal of nasal polyp, right nostril

    ____

17. Tonsillectomy and adenoidectomy, younger than 12

    ____

18. Left ectopic pregnancy

    ____

19. Closed treatment of a coccygeal fracture

    ____

20. A radiologic examination of mastoids, two views

    ____

21. A chest x-ray examination, four views

    ____

22. Magnetic resonance imaging (MRI) of spinal canal

    ____

23. Computed tomography (CT) scan of abdomen with contrast medium

    ____

24. Outpatient kidney imaging with vascular flow

    ____

25. Creatine phosphokinase (CPK) total lab test

    ____

26. Electrolyte panel

____

27. Adrenocorticotropic hormone (ACTH) stimulation panel

____

28. Obstetric panel

____

29. Total protein urine test

____

30. Blood alcohol level

____

31. Acute hepatitis panel

____

32. Urine pregnancy test

____

33. Polio vaccine, intramuscular route

____

34. Human papillomavirus (HPV) vaccine, nine types, three-dose schedule, intramuscular route

____

35. Psychotherapy for crisis; first 60 minutes

____

HCPCS Coding

1. Standard wheelchair

____

2. Gradient compression stocking below-knee, 40-50 mm Hg each

____

3. Above-knee, short prosthesis, no knee joint (stubbies), with articulated ankle/foot, dynamically aligned, right leg

____

4. Disposable contact lens, per lens, one set

____

5. Ambulance waiting time, 1 hour

____

CERTIFICATION PREPARATION

Circle the correct answer.

1. The CPT coding manual is updated annually on
   a. January 1.
   b. December 1.
   c. October 1.
   d. June 1.

2. To find the most accurate code, coders use which progression?
   a. Categories, subcategories, sections, subsections
   b. Sections, subsections, categories, subcategories
   c. Sections, categories, subsections, subcategories
   d. Subsections, subcategories, sections, categories

3. The evaluation and management CPT codes are used for insurance reimbursement in the following healthcare settings *except*
   a. medical office.
   b. weight loss clinic.
   c. nursing home.
   d. hospital.

4. Which codes can be used to help measure performance?
   a. Category I codes
   b. Category II codes
   c. Category III codes
   d. Both a and b

5. Which section uses the code range between 70000 and 79999?
   a. Anesthesia section
   b. Surgery section
   c. Radiology section
   d. Medicine section

6. When searching the Alphabetic Index, "humerus" is an example of a(n)
   a. procedure or service.
   b. organ or anatomic site.
   c. condition, illness, or injury.
   d. eponym, synonym, abbreviation, or acronym.

7. Which level of history includes a review of the systems that relate to the chief complaint?
   a. Problem-focused history
   b. Expanded problem-focused history
   c. Detailed history
   d. Comprehensive history

8. Which HCPCS codes range from A4000 to A8999?
   a. Ambulance transport
   b. Medical supplies
   c. Surgical supplies
   d. Both b and c

9. Which modifier indicates a professional component and is used when a separate technician performs the service, but the provider reviews the report and makes a diagnosis?
   a. -50
   b. -62
   c. -26
   d. -RT, -LT

10. Which code is assigned to an urgent care facility as the place of service?
    a. 01
    b. 13
    c. 20
    d. 23

WORKPLACE APPLICATIONS

Identify all procedures that need to be coded for billing purposes in the following situations. Using the most current CPT manual or an encoder such as TruCode, determine the correct CPT codes.

1. Monique Jones is a new patient who saw Dr. Walden to report feeling tired all the time. She stated that she was exhausted even after a full 8 hours of sleep at night. Monique said that she did not have much of an appetite and that she had been eating mostly salads and chicken with a bowl of fruit as snacks. She is not overweight, and her blood pressure and other vital signs were normal. Dr. Walden decided to perform a complete blood count, an electrolyte panel, and a lipid panel. She also ordered a urinalysis, an iron-binding capacity, and a vitamin B_{12} test. The provider asked the patient if she had noticed any blood in her urine or stool, and she denied blood in the urine but did mention she had several episodes of diarrhea. Dr. Walden added an occult blood test and a stool culture to check for pathogens. The physician placed Monique on multivitamin therapy and told her to return in 1 week to discuss her laboratory test results. She spent approximately 30 minutes with Monique, taking a medically appropriate history and examination, making low-complexity medical decisions. Monique scheduled her appointment for the following week and left the clinic. Total time spent with the patient was 25 minutes.

   What are the appropriate CPT codes for Monique Jones' visit with Dr. Walden? ____________________

   ____

2. **Diagnosis:** Left cheek laceration

   Procedure: Repair left cheek laceration

   After the patient was prepped with local anesthetic to the left cheek area, the cheek was dressed and draped with Betadine. The 1.7-cm chin laceration of the skin was closed with three interrupted 6-0 silk sutures. Gentamicin ointment was applied to the lacerations and a dressing was placed on the left cheek. The patient tolerated the procedure well.

   What is the appropriate CPT code for this procedure? ____________________

   Can a modifier be used for this procedure? ____________________ If so, what would be the most appropriate? ____________________

   Because anesthesia was used, can an appropriate anesthesia CPT code be used?

   ____

3. **Diagnosis:** Abdominal pain

   Procedure: Esophagogastroduodenoscopy with biopsy

   The patient was premedicated and brought to the endoscopy suite where his throat was anesthetized with Cetacaine spray. He then was placed in the left lateral position and given 2 mg Versed, IV. An Olympus gastroscope was advanced into the esophagus, which was well visualized with no significant spasms. Subsequently the scope was advanced into the distal esophagus, which was essentially normal. Then the scope was advanced into the stomach, which showed evidence of erythema and gastritis. The pylorus was intubated, and the duodenal bulb visualized. The duodenal bulb showed severe erythema suggestive of duodenitis. Biopsies of both the duodenum and the stomach were obtained. The scope was withdrawn. The patient tolerated the procedure well.

   In the Alphabetic Index, which main term should be used to look up the correct CPT code?

   ____

   What is the appropriate CPT code for this procedure? ____________________

   CPT code 43236 is a similar code with submucosal injection. Can this be used if the physician usually performs it, but forgot to document? ____________________

INTERNET ACTIVITIES

1. Using online resources, research job postings on the Internet that relate to medical billing and coding. Review job qualifications and requirements to qualify for these positions. Create a poster presentation, a PowerPoint presentation, or write a paper summarizing your research. Include the following points in your project:
   a. List the qualifications and requirements for a position in the medical billing and coding field.
   b. Explain how a graduate from your program would meet the requirements.
   c. Explain what additional training would be beneficial for someone looking for a position in the medical billing and coding field.

2. Visit http://www.cms.gov/ and use the search words "CPT Coding" to explore the topics related to CPT and HCPCS coding. Create a poster presentation, a PowerPoint presentation, or write a paper summarizing your research. Include the following points in your project:
   a. Explain the differences between CPT coding and HCPCS coding.
   b. Explain when each would be used.
   c. Describe two things that you learned about CPT codes.
   d. Describe two things you learned about HCPCS codes.

Procedure 17.1 Perform Procedural Coding: Surgery

Name ______________________________ **Date** ____________ **Score** __________

Task: To use the steps for CPT procedural coding to find the most accurate and specific CPT surgery code.

Equipment and Supplies:
- CPT coding manual (current year) or TruCode encoder software
- Operative report (Figure 17.1)

Standard: Complete the procedure and all critical steps in _______ minutes with a minimum score of 85% within two attempts (*or as indicated by the instructor*).

Scoring: Divide the points earned by the total possible points. Failure to perform a critical step, indicated by an asterisk (*), results in grade no higher than an 84% (*or as indicated by the instructor*).

Time: Began_________ Ended_________ Total minutes: _________

Steps Using the CPT Coding Manual:	**Point Value**	**Attempt 1**	**Attempt 2**
1. Abstract the procedures and/or services from the procedural statement in the surgical report.	**10**		
2. Select the most appropriate main term to begin the search in the Alphabetic Index.	**10**		
3. Once the main term has been located in the Alphabetic Index, review and select the modifying term or terms if required. If the main term cannot be found in the Alphabetic Index, repeat steps 2 and 3 using a different main term, possibly based on the procedural statement.	**10**		
4. Once the CPT code or code range is identified in the Alphabetic Index, disregard any code or code range containing additional descriptions or modifying terms not found in the health record.	**10**		
5. Record the code or code ranges that best match the procedural statements in the surgical report.	**10**		
6. Turn to the Tabular List and find the first code or code range from your search of the Alphabetic Index. Compare the description of the code with the procedural statement in the surgical report. Verify that all or most of the health record documentation matches the code description and that there is no additional information in the code description that is not found in the documentation.	**10**		
7. Review the coding guidelines and notes for the section, subsection, and code to ensure that there are no contraindications to use of the code. Review the coding conventions and add-on codes, if any.	**10**		
8. Determine whether a modifier is needed.	**10**		
9. Determine whether a Special Report is required.	**10**		
10. Record the CPT code selected in the health record documentation next to the procedure or service performed and in the appropriate block of the insurance claim form.	**10***		
Total Points	**100**		

Alternate Method **Steps Using the TruCode Software:**			
1. Abstract the procedures and/or services from the procedural statement in the surgical report.	**20**		
2. Type the main term into the encoder search box and select the CPT. Then click on Show All Results.	**20**		
3. If the main term cannot be found through the search, repeat steps 2 and 3 using a different main term based on the procedural statement.	**20**		
4. Choose the procedure description that is closest to the procedural statement in the surgical report.	**20***		
5. Record the CPT code that best matches the procedural statements in the surgical report in the patient's health record.	**20**		
Total Points	**100**		

Comments

CAAHEP Competencies	Step(s)
IX.P.1. Perform procedural coding	Entire procedure

Figure 17.1 Operative Report

Name ______________________ Date ____________ Score __________

Operative Report

PATIENT NAME: Sonia Sample
ROOM NUMBER: 222 West
MR NUMBER: 12-34-56

DATE OF PROCEDURE: 04/22/00
PREOPERATIVE DIAGNOSIS: Acute cholecystitis
POSTOPERATIVE DIAGNOSIS: Acute cholecystitis
NAME OF PROCEDURE: 1. Laparoscopic cholecystectomy
2. Intraoperative cystic duct cholangiogram
SURGEON: Claude St. John, M.D.
ASSISTANT: Mark Weiss, D.O.
ANESTHESIOLOGIST: Angela Adams, M.D.
ANESTHESIA: General

DESCRIPTION OF THE OPERATION:

The patient was placed in the supine position under general anesthesia. The oral gastric tube was placed. The Foley catheter was placed. The patient received appropriate antibiotics. The abdomen was prepped with iodine and draped in the usual fashion. Using a midline subumbilical incision, we entered the subcutaneous fat to find the aponeurosis of the rectus abdominis. Two stay sutures were placed 0.5 cm from the midline bilaterally and we left on these sutures, creating an opening in the linea alba.

Under direct vision, the catheter was placed. The Hasson cannula was placed in the abdominal cavity and all was normal except an acute necrotizing and probably gangrenous gallbladder. There were multiple omental adhesions. Three other trocars were placed in the right subcostal plane in the midline, midclavicular line, and midaxillary line using a #10, #5, and #5 mm trocar, respectively. The gallbladder was punctured and emptied of clear white bile indicating a hydrops of the gallbladder. It was grasped at its fundus and at Hartmann's pouch retracted cephalad and to the right, respectively. We found the cystic duct and the cystic artery after circumferential dissection and isolated the cystic duct completely.

When we were sure that this structure was a deep cystic duct, the clip was placed at the most distal aspect to make an opening immediately proximally and we placed a Reddick cholangiocatheter into it via #14 gauge percutaneous catheter. The cholangiogram showed normal arborization of the liver radicals. Normal bifurcation of the common hepatic duct. Normal common hepatic duct. Long large cystic duct. The common bile duct had numerous stones within it. They could not be emptied from the common bile duct. There was good flow into the duodenum.

The impression was choledocholithiasis. This was corroborated by the radiologist. The decision was made to prepare the patient most probably for endoscopic retrograde cholangiopancreatography postoperatively, and no further intervention of the common bile duct was done in this setting.

The cholangiocatheter was removed. An attempt was made to milk the bile out, but no stones came out. Three clips were placed on the proximal aspect of the cystic duct and the duct was then cut distally. The artery was isolated and double clipped proximally and single clipped distally and cut in the intervening section. We then peeled the gallbladder off the gallbladder bed with some difficulty because of the intense edema and inflammation. It was then removed from the liver bed completely. Cautery, suctioning and irrigation were used copiously to create a bloodless field. A last check was made and there was no bleeding and no bile leaking. A #15 Jackson-Pratt type drain was placed into Morrison's pouch and brought out through the lateral most port. We then removed, with great difficulty, the gallbladder from the umbilicus. Because of its enormous size and a 3 cm stone within it that was very difficult to macerate, the opening of the umbilicus had to be enlarged.

As this was done, we removed the gallbladder completely and sent it for pathologic section. Two separate figure-of-eight 0 PDS were used to close the abdominal fascia. The Jackson-Pratt drain was then sutured in place with 2.0 nylon. The skin was closed throughout with subcuticular 3-0 PDS after copious irrigation of the subcutaneous plane. Mastisol and Steri-Strips were placed on the wound. The patient remained stable although she did have bigeminy during surgery and was on a Lidocaine drip. She will be going to the intensive care unit but as she left, she was extubated in the recovery room and was fully alert. She is moving all limbs.

I will discuss with the gastroenterologist postoperative endoscopic retrograde cholangiopancreatography.

SPECIMEN: Gallbladder.

____

Claude St. John, M.D.
CSJ/ld:
D: 04/22/00
T: 04/22/00 9:21 am
CC: Maria Acosta, M.D.

Procedure 17.2 Perform Procedural Coding: Office Visit and Immunizations

Name ______________________ **Date** ____________ **Score** __________

Task: To use the steps for CPT Evaluation and Management coding and HCPCS coding to find the most accurate and specific CPT E/M and HCPCS codes using the coding manuals or the TruCode encoder.

Equipment and Supplies:
- CPT coding manual (current year)
- HCPCS coding manual (current year) or TruCode encoder software
- Progress note

Progress Note for Erma Willis (DOB 12/09/19XX):
04/08/20XX Mrs. Willis was seen today for a follow-up visit for a recent case of bronchitis. The infection has completely cleared, and she would like to get the influenza vaccine. The office visit involved a medically appropriate history and examination, and medical decision-making of straightforward complexity.

Standard: Complete the procedure and all critical steps in _______ minutes with a minimum score of 85% within two attempts (*or as indicated by the instructor*).

Scoring: Divide the points earned by the total possible points. Failure to perform a critical step, indicated by an asterisk (*), results in grade no higher than an 84% (*or as indicated by the instructor*).

Time: Began_________ Ended_________ Total minutes: _________

Steps Part A: CPT E/M Coding	**Point Value**	**Attempt 1**	**Attempt 2**
1. Determine the place of service from the progress note.	**15**		
2. Determine the patient's status.	**15**		
3. Identify the subsection, category, or subcategory of service in the E/M section.	**10**		
4. Determine the level of service: • Determine the complexity of medical decision-making. If necessary, compare the medical documentation against examples in Appendix C, Clinical Examples, of the CPT manual.	**15**		
5. Select the appropriate level of E/M service code, and document it in the patient's health record.	**10**		
Part B: HCPCS Coding with TruCode Encoder Software			
6. Review the provider documentation.	**10**		
7. Type the main term into the search box of the encoder and choose the HCPCS Tabular code set for accurate coding. If no modifying term produces an appropriate code or code range, review the documentation again and choose another main term.	**10**		
8. Compare the description of the code with the medical documentation. Select the appropriate HCPCS immunization code, and document it in the patient's health record.	**15**		
Total Points	**100**		

Comments

CAAHEP Competencies	Step(s)
IX.P.1. Perform procedural coding	Entire procedure

Procedure 17.3 Working with Providers to Ensure Accurate Code Selection

Name ______________________________ **Date** ____________ **Score** __________

Task: Communicate respectfully and tactfully with medical providers to ensure accurate code selection.

Background: Using tactful communication skills means using good manners as you provide truthful sensitive information to another person, while considering the person's feelings. Tactful communication skills include verbal and nonverbal communication that shows respect, discretion, compassion, honesty, diplomacy, and courtesy. When you use tactful behaviors, you demonstrate professionalism and you preserve relationships by avoiding conflicts and finding common ground.

Many times, the medical coder is the expert on the accurate CPT and ICD code selections. The highest level of specificity must be used when coding so that appropriate reimbursement can occur. It is not uncommon for the medical coder to interact with providers and assist them in understanding the coding process. During these interactions, it is crucial that the medical coder provides the information in a professional, organized, and logical manner. Using tactful communication skills is critical to maintaining a healthy working relationship with the providers.

Scenario: You are a new medical coder for the medical practice. You have been on the job for 6 weeks and have been seeing a trend that charges are being downcoded. The required documentation is present in the health records, but the providers have been selecting less specific codes for the appointment types. Your goal today is to explain to the providers accurate code selection for the appointment types.

Directions: Using the scenario, role-play with two peers, who will play the providers. You need to discuss the importance of selecting the correct code for reimbursement. You need to demonstrate respect during the conversation and utilize tactful communication skills.

Standard: Complete the role-play in _______ minutes with a minimum score of 100% within two attempts (*or as indicated by the instructor*).

Scoring: Divide the points earned by the total possible points. Met competency: 100% (10 points). Not met competency: 0% (0 points).

Time: Began_________ Ended_________ Total minutes: _________

Affective Behavior	***Directions:*** *Check behaviors observed during the role-play.*					
Tactfulness	Improper and/or inappropriate			Proper and appropriate		
	Spoke and/or acted in a manner that was offensive to others; lacked compassion and/or courtesy			Spoke and acted without offending others; showed compassion and courtesy		
	Failed to be sensitive to others when explaining the situation			Explained the situation in a clear and diplomatic way		
	Failed to explain the downcoding issue and/or the importance of proper coding			Explained the issues with downcoding and the importance of accurate coding for reimbursement		
	Failed to offer a solution for the situation			Offered a solution for the situation		
	Failed to answer questions; or answers were inappropriate and/or inaccurate			Answered questions appropriately and accurately		
	Other:			Other:		

Grading		**Point Value**	**Attempt 1**	**Attempt 2**
Does not meet Expectation	• Response was disrespectful and/or not tactful. • Student demonstrated more than 2 negative, unprofessional behaviors during the interaction.	0		
Needs Improvement	• Response was disrespectful and/or not tactful. • Student demonstrated 1 or 2 negative, unprofessional behaviors during the interaction.	0		
Meets Expectation	• Response was respectful and tactful; no negative, unprofessional behaviors observed. • More practice is needed for behavior to appear natural and for student to appear comfortable and at ease.	10		
Occasionally Exceeds Expectation	• Response was respectful and tactful; no negative, unprofessional behaviors observed. • At times student appeared comfortable and at ease; but more practice is needed for behavior to become natural and consistent with a professional medical assistant.	10		
Always Exceeds Expectation	• Response was respectful and tactful; no negative, unprofessional behaviors observed. • Student's behaviors appeared natural and comfortable. Behaviors are consistent with a professional medical assistant.	10		

Comments

CAAHEP Competencies	**Step(s)**
A.7 Demonstrate tactfulness	Entire role-play

Student Name________________________ Date____________

chapter 18

Medical Billing and Reimbursement Essentials

CAAHEP Competencies	Assessment
VII.C.4. Identify patient financial obligations for services rendered	Skills and Concepts – E. 1- 4
VII.P.3. Inform a patient of financial obligations for services rendered	Procedures 18.6, 18.7
VIII.C.1.b. Identify: the steps for filing a third-party claim	Skills and Concepts – B. 7, 8
VIII.C.2 Identify managed care requirements for patient referral	Skills and Concepts – A. 7
VIII.C.3.a. Identify processes for: verification of eligibility for services	Skills and Concepts – A. 3
VIII.C.3.b. Identify processes for: precertification/preauthorization	Skills and Concepts – A. 5, 6
VIII.C.3.c. Identify processes for: tracking unpaid claims	Skills and Concepts – D. 1
VIII.C.3.d. Identify processes for: claim denials and appeals	Skills and Concepts - D. 9-12
VIII.C.4. Identify fraud and abuse as they relate to thrid-party reimbursement	Skills and Concepts – C. 1
VIII.C.5 b. Define the following: advanced beneficiary notice (ABN)	Skills and Concepts – E. 5
VIII.C.5.c. Define the following: allowed amount	Vocabulary Review – C. 5
VIII.C.5.d. Define the following: deductible	Vocabulary Review – D. 6
VIII.C.5.e. Define the following: co-insurance	Vocabulary Review – D. 3
VIII.C.5.f. Define the following: co-pay	Vocabulary Review – A. 8
VIII.C.6. Identify the purpose and components of the Explanation of Benefits (EOB) and Remittance Advice (RA) Statements	Skills and Concepts – D. 4-8
VIII.P.2. Verify eligibility for services	Procedures 18.1, 18.6
VIII.P.3. Obtain precertification or preauthorization with documentation	Procedure 18.1
VIII.P.4. Complete an insurance claim form	Procedures 18.2, 18.3
VIII.P.5. Assist a patient in understanding an Explanation of Benefits (EOB)	Procedure 18.5

CAAHEP Competencies	Assessment
IX.P.3. Utilize medical necessity guidelines	Procedure 18.4
A.1. Demonstrate critical thinking skills	Procedures 18.5, 18.6, 18.7
A.3. Demonstrate empathy for patient's concerns	Procedures 18.5, 18.6, 18.7
A.7. Demonstrate tactfulness	Procedures 18.5, 18.6, 18.7
ABHES Competencies	**Assessment**
7. Administrative Procedures c. Perform billing and collection procedures	Procedures 18.1-15.7
7. Administrative Procedures d. Process insurance claims	Procedures 18.2, 18.3

VOCABULARY REVIEW

Using the word pool on the right, find the correct word to match the definition. Write the word on the line after the definition.

Group A

1. The standard form used for all government and most commercial insurance companies ______________________
2. A document sent by the insurance company to the provider explaining the allowed charge amount, the amount reimbursed for services, and the patient's financial responsibilities ______________________
3. A document sent by the insurance company to the provider and the patient explaining the allowed charge amount, the amount reimbursed for services, and the patient's financial responsibilities ______________________
4. The process of determining if a procedure or service is covered by the insurance plan and what the reimbursement is for that procedure or service ______________________
5. Starts when a patient makes an appointment and is complete when payment for services has been received ______________
6. Meeting the stipulated requirements to participate in the healthcare plan ______________________
7. A secure online website that gives contracted providers a single point of access to insurance companies. ______________
8. A set dollar amount that the patient must pay for each office visit ______________________
9. A form completed by the patient that authorizes the medical office to release medical records to the insurance company for health insurance reimbursement ______________________
10. An organization that accepts the claim data from the provider, reformats the data to meet the specifications outlined by the insurance plan, and submits the claim ______________________

Word Pool

- provider web portals
- copayment
- explanation of benefits
- remittance advice
- medical billing process
- eligibility
- precertification
- CMS-1500 health insurance claim form
- claims clearinghouse
- release of information

Group B

1. Used when the provider believes that the patient must see a specialist to continue treatment. Usually takes 3 to 10 working days for review and approval _______________
2. A process completed before claims submission in which claims are examined for accuracy and completeness _______________________
3. Gives the provider approval to render the medical service _______________
4. Used in an emergency situation and can be approved online _______________
5. The electronic transfer of data between two or more entities _______________________
6. When the provider is paid a set amount for each enrolled person assigned to him or her, per period of time, whether or not that person has received services _______________________
7. Nonsurgical procedure that uses an endoscope to view inside the body _______________
8. The individual who is directly contracted with the insurance company _______________
9. Used when an urgent but not life-threatening situation occurs _______________
10. Used to determine primary and secondary insurance status _______________

Word Pool

- preauthorization
- endoscopy
- regular referral
- urgent referral
- STAT referral
- capitation
- electronic data interchange
- audit
- birthday rule
- insured

Group C

1. Done on purpose_______________________
2. Agrees to accept the terms of the agreement with the insurance company, as well as accept what the plan states as an allowed amount for the services provided _______________________
3. Claims without errors_______________________
4. Knowingly and willfully attempting to execute a scheme to take from any healthcare benefit program _______________________
5. The maximum amount that an insurance company will pay for covered health services _______________
6. To settle or determine judicially _______________________
7. Transfers the patient's legal right to collect benefits for medical expenses to the provider of those services, authorizing payment to be sent directly to the provider _______________
8. Unintended action that directly or indirectly results in an overpayment to the healthcare provider _______________________
9. Software that finds common billing errors before the claim is sent to the insurance company _______________________
10. A number assigned by the Centers for Medicare and Medicaid Services (CMS) that classifies the healthcare provider by license and medical specialties _______________________

Word Pool

- adjudicate
- assignment of benefits
- National Provider Identifier
- participating provider
- allowed amount
- fraud
- abuse
- intentional
- claims scrubber
- clean claim

Group D

1. Services or supplies that are used to treat the patient's diagnosis meet the accepted standard of medical practice ____________________
2. A document signed by the patient that authorizes a provider to bill the patient for services that Medicare may consider not medically necessary ______________
3. When the insured and the insurance company share the cost of covered medical services after the deductible has been met ____________________
4. Claims with incorrect, missing, or insufficient data ______________
5. The person legally responsible for the entire bill ____________________
6. A set dollar amount that the policyholder is responsible for each year before the insurance company begins to reimburse the healthcare provider ____________________
7. Where the insurance company indicates the conditions under which the claim was paid ______________

Word Pool

- dirty claim
- remark codes
- medical necessity
- deductible
- coinsurance
- guarantor
- advance beneficiary notice

ABBREVIATIONS

Write out what each of the following abbreviations stands for.

1. EOB ____
2. RA ____
3. H&P ____
4. CMS-1500 ____
5. HIPAA ____
6. MCOs ____
7. PCP ____
8. GI ____
9. NUCC ____
10. AMA ____
11. CMS ____
12. LMP ____
13. NPI ____
14. CPT ____
15. HCPCS ____
16. POS ____

17. EMG ____________________

18. EPSDT____________________

19. CHAMPVA ____________________

20. FECA____________________

21. SSN ____________________

22. EIN ____________________

23. PAR____________________

24. CMPs____________________

25. PPO ____________________

26. ABN ____________________

27. H&P ____________________

28. SSN ____________________

SKILLS AND CONCEPTS

Answer the following questions. Write your answer on the line or in the space provided.

A. Medical Billing Process

1. List four types of information collected when a patient calls to schedule an appointment.

   a. ____________________

   b. ____________________

   c. ____________________

   d. ____________________

2. At the time of the appointment, what two things are copied or scanned into the computer? ____________________

   ____

3. Describe how the patient's insurance eligibility is confirmed. ____________________

   ____

   ____

   ____

   ____

4. Referring to the information on the ID card, answer the following questions.

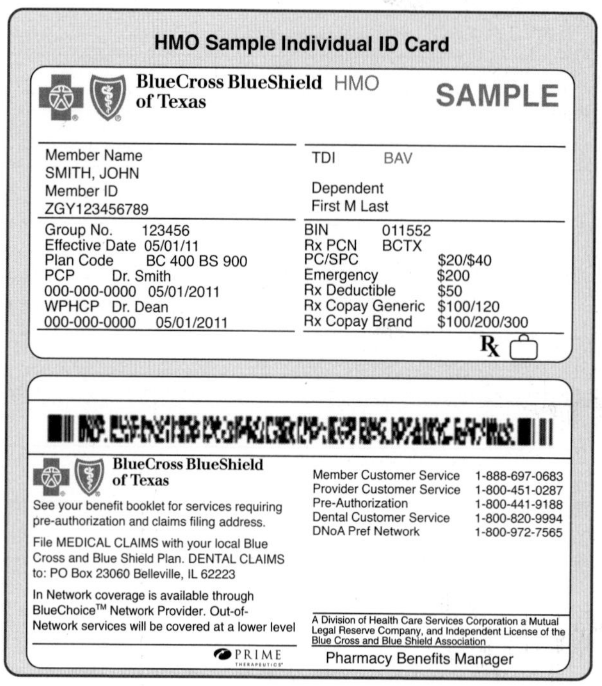

HMO Sample Individual ID Card

BlueCross BlueShield HMO
of Texas

SAMPLE

Member Name
SMITH, JOHN
Member ID
ZGY123456789

TDI BAV

Dependent
First M Last

Group No. 123456
Effective Date 05/01/11
Plan Code BC 400 BS 900
PCP Dr. Smith
000-000-0000 05/01/2011
WPHCP Dr. Dean
000-000-0000 05/01/2011

BIN 011552
Rx PCN BCTX
PC/SPC $20/$40
Emergency $200
Rx Deductible $50
Rx Copay Generic $100/120
Rx Copay Brand $100/200/300

BlueCross BlueShield
of Texas

See your benefit booklet for services requiring pre-authorization and claims filing address.

File MEDICAL CLAIMS with your local Blue Cross and Blue Shield Plan. DENTAL CLAIMS to: PO Box 23060 Belleville, IL 62223

In Network coverage is available through BlueChoice™ Network Provider. Out-of-Network services will be covered at a lower level

Member Customer Service	1-888-697-0683
Provider Customer Service	1-800-451-0287
Pre-Authorization	1-800-441-9188
Dental Customer Service	1-800-820-9994
DNoA Pref Network	1-800-972-7565

A Division of Health Care Services Corporation a Mutual Legal Reserve Company, and Independent License of the Blue Cross and Blue Shield Association

PRIME THERAPEUTICS

Pharmacy Benefits Manager

a. What is the member's name? ______________________________

b. What is the member's ID number? ______________________________

c. What is the group number? ______________________________

d. Who is the member's primary care provider (PCP)? ______________________________

e. What is the effective date of the plan? ______________________________

f. What is the deductible for prescriptions (Rx)? ______________________________

g. What is the copay for primary care (PC)? ______________________________

h. What number should the patient call if he has a concern? ______________________________

i. What number should you call if you need to get a preauthorization? ______________________________

j. What number should a healthcare professional working with Dr. Smith call if there is a question about the coverage?

____

5. The patient's billing record information is often found on the patient registration form. Using Figure 18.2 in the textbook, list the billing information found on the patient registration form.

____

____

____

____

____

6. What items should the medical assistant gather when using the paper method to obtain a precertification for a service or procedure?

____

____

____

____

____

7. Describe the processes for precertification using the paper method. What does the medical assistant need to do?

____

____

____

____

____

8. Describe the managed care requirements for a patient referral. _______________

____

____

____

____

____

B. Submitting Claims to Third-Party Payers

1. In your own words, identify the steps for filing a third-party claim. ______

2. Describe the electronic claim form. ______

3. Describe two ways electronic claims can be submitted. ______

4. Describe direct billing. ______

5. Explain the role of a claims clearinghouse.____

____

____

____

____

____

6. The medical assistant obtained precertification for a procedure. After the procedure was completed, what are six items needed to complete the CMS-1500 health insurance claim form?

   a. ____

   b. ____

   c. ____

   d. ____

   e. ____

   f. ____

7. Name the three sections of the claim form.

   a. ____

   b. ____

   c. ____

8. Identify information required to file a third-party claim.

   a. What information must be included in Section 1 of the claim form? ____________________

   ____

   b. Name 13 pieces of information required in Section 2.

      1. ____

      2. ____

      3. ____

      4. ____

      5. ____

      6. ____

      7. ____

      8. ____

      9. ____

      10. ____

11. ______
12. ______
13. ______

c. Name 19 pieces of information required in Section 3.

1. ______
2. ______
3. ______
4. ______
5. ______
6. ______
7. ______
8. ______
9. ______
10. ______
11. ______
12. ______
13. ______
14. ______
15. ______
16. ______
17. ______
18. ______
19. ______

C. Impact of Accurate Coding

1. Differentiate between fraud and abuse. ______

2. What are the possible consequences of coding fraud and abuse?____________________

3. What is the purpose of "claim scrubbers"?____________________

D. Claim Follow-up

1. Which of the following are included in claims tracking?
   a. Confirm that the claims submitted to the clearinghouse match the claims listed on the confirmation report.
   b. Inquire about the status of claims that have not been paid within 10-14 days of submittal.
   c. Resubmit the claim if not received by the insurance company.
   d. All of the above

2. Insurance companies will typically take ______ days to process insurance claims electronically.

3. What information is needed to verify the claim status with insurance company?____________________

Using the explanation below, answer the following questions:

01/20/20XX

XYZ Insurance Company Explanation of Benefits

Walden-Martin Family Medical Clinic
1234 Anystreet
Anytown, AK 12345-1234

Patient Name	Treatment Dates	CPT Code	Charge Amount	Reason Code	Covered Amount	Deductible Amount	Co-Pay Amount	Paid At	Payment Amount
Yan, Tai	01/06/20XX	99205	132.28	03	125.00	0.00	0.00	80%	100.00
	01/06/20XX	82947	15.00		15.00	0.00	0.00	80%	12.00
	01/06/20XX	86580	11.34		11.34	0.00	0.00	80%	9.07
	Totals		158.62		151.34				121.07
Gomez, Pedro	01/07/20XX	99212	28.55		28.55	0.00	0.00	80%	22.84
	Totals		28.55		28.55				22.84
Green, Jana	01/04/20XX	99203	70.92	03	69.23	0.00	0.00	80%	55.38
	01/04/20XX	71020	40.97	03	34.95	0.00	0.00	80%	27.96
	Totals		111.89		104.18				83.34

Reason Code: 03 Allowed amount per insurance contract

Check No: 56390 $227.25

4. For Tai Yan's office visit, 99205, there is a difference between the Charge Amount and Covered Amount. Based on the reason code supplied what will be done with the difference?

____

____

____

____

5. How much is Tai Yan responsible for? ____

____

6. How much will be written off for Jana Green? ____

____

7. How much is Jana Green responsible for? ____

____

8. What is the covered amount services provided to Pedro Gomez? ____

____

9. The process for claim denial starts with the review of ____________________ or ____________________.

10. When reviewing an EOB or RA, the ________________ can identify why a claim was denied.

11. If a claim was denied due to medical necessity the medical assistant should
    a. talk to the business supervisor to determine if the patient can billed for the services.
    b. contact the patient to make sure that they understand that the procedure was not covered.
    c. review the documentation to determine if the correct diagnosis and procedure codes were submitted.
    d. obtain the correct insurance plan information.

12. When a claim has been denied and the provider feels that it was coded correctly, an appeal letter should be sent including which of the following?
    a. Identity of the denied claim.
    b. A statement from the provider detailing the medical reasoning for performing the procedure.
    c. Additional medical reports.
    d. All of the above

E. The Patient's Financial Responsibility

Calculating Coinsurance and Deductible

Use the following information as you answer the following questions.

Patient: Zach Green Deductible: $750 Coinsurance: 80/20 Patient out-of-pocket expense maximum: $2000

1. During Zach's first visit of the year, he incurred a $500 bill. Who pays this bill?________________

    ____

    ____

2. During Zach's second visit of the year, he incurred a $450 bill. Describe how much is paid by Zach and the insurance carrier.

    ____

    ____

3. Zach had surgery, which was his third claim of the year. He had a bill of $5000. Considering the prior visits, what is Zach's portion of this bill and what is the responsibility of the insurance carrier?

    ____

    ____

    ____

4. How much is Zach responsible for so far this year considering his first three visits? ________________

    ____

    ____

    ____

5. When services that a provider suggests are not covered by Medicare, the patient can sign a(n) ________________ giving them the option to pay the provider's fee in full.

CERTIFICATION PREPARATION

Circle the correct answer.

1. To examine claims for accuracy and completeness before they are submitted is to _____ the claims.
   a. correct
   b. audit
   c. revise
   d. reject

2. Block 1 of the CMS-1500 form contains what information?
   a. Patient's name
   b. Insured's name
   c. Type of insurance coverage
   d. Carrier address

3. The patient's name is found in block
   a. 1.
   b. 2.
   c. 3.
   d. 4.

4. CPT codes are found in what block?
   a. 24a
   b. 24b
   c. 24d
   d. 24e

5. Claims with incorrect, missing, or insufficient data are called
   a. clean.
   b. dingy.
   c. incomplete.
   d. dirty.

6. Which is a common reason why insurance claims are rejected?
   a. When a procedure listed is not an insurance benefit
   b. Medical necessity
   c. Preauthorization not obtained
   d. All of the above

7. Which is a fixed amount per visit that is typically paid at the time of medical services?
   a. Copayment
   b. Deductible
   c. Coinsurance
   d. Both a and b

8. Patients sign a(n) _____ of benefits form so that the physician will receive payment for services directly.
   a. release
   b. assignment
   c. turning
   d. sending

9. Claims submitted to a _____ are forwarded to individual insurance carriers.
   a. direct biller
   b. third-party administrator
   c. clearinghouse
   d. post office

10. Electronic data interchange is
    a. transferring data back and forth between two or more entities.
    b. sending information to one insurance carrier.
    c. sending information to one clearinghouse for processing.
    d. None of the above

WORKPLACE APPLICATIONS

1. Sally is the only medical biller in her healthcare agency. One of the two providers orders and performs tests and procedures before getting the needed preauthorizations from the patients' insurance carriers. As a result, the insurance carriers are not covering the claims and the clinic has had to write off thousands of dollars. Discuss how Sally should deal with the situation.

   a. How might she display tactful behavior when communicating with the provider about the third-party requirements?

   ____

   ____

   ____

   b. How would you deal with this situation if you were Sally? ____________________

   ____

   ____

   ____

2. Christi Brown is meeting with you regarding the bill she received in the mail. When she called to make the appointment, she voiced her confusion about the bill, stating she thought her insurance covered everything. You check her record and see that she met her deductible and now needs to pay 20% of the billed amount. She owes $170. Explain what a deductible and coinsurance are.

   ____

   ____

   ____

INTERNET ACTIVITIES

1. Using online resources, research your insurance carrier or an insurance carrier popular in your area. Research the appeal process for denied claims. Create a poster presentation, a PowerPoint presentation, or write a paper summarizing your research. Include the following points in your project:
   a. Who can start the appeal process?
   b. What steps are involved in the appeal process?
   c. What is the time frame for getting a response to the appeal?

2. Visit http://www.nucc.org and research the resources available on this website. Create a poster presentation, a PowerPoint presentation, or write a paper summarizing your research. Include the following points in your project:
   a. What resources are available for a medical biller on this website?
   b. List three that you think would be most helpful to a medical assistant who does medical billing.
   c. What information is available about the CMS-1500 claim form?
   d. Describe two things you learned from this website.

3. Using online resources, research the most common errors that occur when submitting claims. Create a poster presentation, a PowerPoint presentation, or write a paper summarizing your research. Include the following points in your project:
   a. What are the most common errors?
   b. How can these errors be prevented?
   c. What can a medical assistant do to prevent those errors?

Procedure 18.1 Perform Precertification with Documentation

Name ______________________________ **Date** __________ **Score** __________

Task: To obtain precertification from a patient's insurance carrier for requested services or procedures.

Equipment and Supplies:
- Paper method: Patient's health record, prior authorization (precertification) request form, copy of patient's health insurance ID card, a pen
- Electronic method: Electronic health record system such as SimChart for the Medical Office (SCMO)

Scenario: You are working with Dr. Julie Walden at Walden-Martin Family Medical Clinic. Erma Willis (DOB 12/09/19XX) was seen for excessive snoring and Dr. Walden ordered a sleep study. You need to complete a prior authorization/certification form for the sleep study, which will be conducted by Dr. Jim Sandman. You checked and there is a signed release of information form.

Insurance Information Aetna 1234 Insurance Way Anytown, AL 112345-1234 Member ID Number: EW8884910 Group Number: 66574W	**Clinic and Provider Information** Walden-Martin Family Medical Clinic 1234 Anystreet Anytown, AL 12345 Provider: Julie Walden, MD Fax: 123-123-5678 Phone: 123-123-1234 Provider Contact Name: (your name)
Service Information Place: Walden-Martin Family Medicine Clinic Service Requested: Sleep study Starting Service Date: 1 week from today Ending Service Date: 1 week from today Service Frequency: once ICD-10-CM code: R06.83 CPT code: 95807 Not related to an injury or workers' compensation	

Standard: Complete the procedure and all critical steps in ______ minutes with a minimum score of 85% within two attempts (*or as indicated by the instructor*).

Scoring: Divide the points earned by the total possible points. Failure to perform a critical step, indicated by an asterisk (*), results in grade no higher than an 84% (*or as indicated by the instructor*).

Time: Began________ Ended________ Total minutes: ________

Steps:	**Point Value**	**Attempt 1**	**Attempt 2**
1. For the paper method, gather the health record, precertification/prior authorization request form, copy of the health insurance ID card, and a pen. For the electronic method, access the Simulation Playground in SCMO.	**20**		
2. Using the health record, determine the service or procedure that requires precertification/preauthorization.	**20***		

3. For the paper method, complete the Precertification/Prior Authorization Request form. For the electronic method, click on the Form Repository icon in SCMO. Select Prior Authorization Request from the left INFO PANEL. Use the Patient Search button at the bottom to find the patient. Complete the remaining fields of the form.	**20**		
4. Proofread the completed form and make any revisions needed.	**20**		
5. Paper method: File the document in the health record after it is faxed to the insurance carrier. Electronic method: Print and fax or electronically send the form to the insurance company and save the form to the patient's record.	**20**		
Total Points	**100**		

Comments

CAAHEP Competencies	**Step(s)**
VIII.P.2 Verify eligibility for services	Entire procedure
VIII.P.3. Obtain precertification or preauthorization with documentation	Entire procedure
ABHES Competencies	**Step(s)**
7. Administrative Procedures c. Perform billing and collection procedures	Entire procedure

Procedure 18.2 Generate an Insurance Claim

Name ______________________________ **Date** __________ **Score** ________

Task: To accurately generate an insurance claim using NUCC guidelines.

Equipment and Supplies:
- Patient's health record
- Copy of patient's insurance ID card or cards
- Patient registration / intake form
- Encounter form
- Insurance claims processing guidelines
- Electronic claims software such as SimChart for the Medical Office

Scenario: Mr. Walter Biller had an appointment with Dr. Walden on November 16, 20XX. He came in for an influenza vaccination, and while he was there, he wanted Dr. Walden to look at his ear because he was having problems hearing. His right ear canal was impacted with cerumen; the ear canal was irrigated, and the cerumen was removed during the visit.

Patient Demographics Walter B. Biller (patient and insured) 87 Willoughby Lane Anytown, AL 12345-1234 Phone: 123-237-3748 DOB: 01/04/1970 SSN: 285-77-7796 HIPAA form on file: Yes – March 19, 20XX Signature on file: Yes – March 19, 20XX	**Clinic and Provider Information** Walden-Martin Family Medical Clinic 1234 Anystreet Anytown, AL 12345 123-123-1234 POS – 11 Office Established patient of Julie Walden, MD Federal Tax ID# 651249831 NPI# 1467253823	
Insurance Information Account Number: 16611 Aetna Policy/ID Number: CH8327753 Group Number: 33347H		
Diagnosis:	**ICD-10-CM code**	
Impacted cerumen, right ear	H61.21	
Service	**CPT Code**	**Fee**
Est. minimal OV	99212	$24.00
Cerumen removal	69210	$46.00
Vaccine – Flu, 3 Y+	90658	$24.00
Preventive – Flu Administration	90471	$7.00

Standard: Complete the procedure and all critical steps in _______ minutes with a minimum score of 85% within two attempts (*or as indicated by the instructor*).

Scoring: Divide the points earned by the total possible points. Failure to perform a critical step, indicated by an asterisk (*), results in grade no higher than an 84% (*or as indicated by the instructor*).

Time: Began________ Ended________ Total minutes: ________

Steps:	Point Value	Attempt 1	Attempt 2
1. Gather the documents required to generate the claim.	**5**		
2. Perform a patient search to locate the correct patient. Verify name and date of birth.	**15***		
3. Ensure that all of the demographic information has been entered into the practice management software accurately.	**10**		
4. Select the correct encounter needed for claim.	**5**		
5. Review the autopopulated patient information and document any additional information needed. Save this information.	**10**		
6. Review the autopopulated provider information and document any additional information that is needed. Save this information.	**10**		
7. Review the autopopulated payer information and document any additional information that is needed. Save this information.	**10**		
8. Review the patient claim information, including diagnoses, if the condition is related to employment, auto accident, other accident, disability information, release of information, assignment of benefits, and referring physician. Document any additional information needed. Save this information.	**15***		
9. Verify or enter the date of service, CPT/HCPCS codes, POS codes, link the diagnoses to the correct charge, modifiers, fees, and units. Save this information.	**15***		
10. Submit the claim.	**5**		
Total Points	**100**		

Comments

CAAHEP Competencies	Step(s)
VIII.P.4. Complete an insurance claim form	Entire procedure
ABHES Competencies	**Step(s)**
7. Administrative Procedures c. Perform billing and collection procedures	Entire procedure

Procedure 18.3 Complete an Insurance Claim Form

Name ______________________________ **Date** __________ **Score** __________

Task: To accurately complete a CMS-1500 health insurance claim form using NUCC guidelines

Equipment and Supplies:
- Patient's health record
- Copy of patient's insurance ID card or cards
- Patient registration/intake form
- Encounter form
- Insurance claims processing guidelines (Table 18.2)
- Blank CMS-1500 health insurance claim form (Work Product 18.1)

Background: Almost all medical billing is done electronically through practice management billing software. The paper CMS-1500 health insurance claim form is provided only to help students practice and develop their medical billing skills.

Directions: Complete each block (as appropriate) of the CMS-1500 (see Table 18.2 for block descriptions).

Scenario: Kyle Reeves had an appointment with Dr. Walden on March 20, 20XX. He came in because he was experiencing extreme fatigue, fever, sore throat, head and body aches. On examination, Dr. Walden also discovered swollen lymph nodes in the neck and armpits along with a swollen liver and spleen. She ordered a CBC, mononucleosis test, and a urinalysis. The mononucleosis test came back positive.

<table>
<tr><td>Patient Demographics
Kyle T. Reeves (patient)
8448 Washington Ave
Anytown, AL 12345-1234
Phone: 123-255-6499
DOB: 01/01/2004
SSN: 933-35-3754
HIPAA form on file: Yes – March 19, 20XX
Signature on file: Yes – March 19, 20XX</td><td>Clinic and Provider Information
Walden-Martin Family Medical Clinic
1234 Anystreet
Anytown, AL 12345
123-123-1234
POS – 11 Office
Established patient of Julie Walden, MD
Federal Tax ID# 651249831
NPI# 1467253823</td><td rowspan="4"></td></tr>
<tr><td>Insurance Information
Account Number: 16611
Insured: Kim Reeves (mother)
Blue Cross Blue Shield
Policy/ID Number: K20568R
Group Number: 21548R</td><td></td></tr>
<tr><td>Diagnosis:</td><td>ICD-10-CM code</td></tr>
<tr><td>Infectious mononucleosis</td><td>O75</td></tr>
<tr><td>Service</td><td>CPT Code</td><td>Fee</td></tr>
<tr><td>Est. Expanded OV</td><td>99213</td><td>$43.00</td></tr>
<tr><td>CBC w/auto differential</td><td>85025</td><td>$35.00</td></tr>
<tr><td>Mononucleosis test</td><td>86663</td><td>$34.00</td></tr>
<tr><td>U/A, w/micro non-automated</td><td>81001</td><td>$27.00</td></tr>
</table>

Standard: Complete the procedure and all critical steps in _______ minutes with a minimum score of 85% within two attempts (*or as indicated by the instructor*).

Scoring: Divide the points earned by the total possible points. Failure to perform a critical step, indicated by an asterisk (*), results in grade no higher than an 84% (*or as indicated by the instructor*).

Time: Began_________ Ended_________ Total minutes: _________

Steps:	**Point Value**	**Attempt 1**	**Attempt 2**
1. Gather the documents required to complete the claim form.	**10**		
2. Complete the claim form using a pen. Use capital letters. Do not use punctuation (commas or dollar signs) unless indicated in the insurance manual or guidelines. Use a hyphen to hyphenate last names.	**10**		
3. Using the patient's health insurance ID card, determine the type of insurance, and the insurance ID number. Enter this information into block 1 and 1a.	**10**		
4. Using the ID card, the encounter form, and the registration/intake form, determine the patient's information and insured individual's information. Accurately complete blocks 2, 3, 5, 6, 9, and 10 a-c by entering in the patient's information. Complete 4, 7, and 11, a-d with the insured's information.	**10**		
5. Complete blocks 12 and 13 by entering "signature on file" and the date.	**10**		
6. Accurately enter the physician or supplier information by completing blocks 14 through 23. Use the eight (8)–digit format (MM/DD/YYYY) when needed.	**10**		
7. Using the encounter form, complete the appropriate blocks from 24A through 24H. **Note**: • Block 24A: Enter the dates of service, both From and To. For ambulatory services, enter the same date in the FROM and TO fields. Enter a date for each procedure, service, or supply in eight (8)–digit format (MM/DD/YYYY). • Block 24F: Enter the charge for the listed service or procedure. *Do not use commas when reporting dollar amounts.* The cents column is the small column to the right. • Block 24G: Enter the number of days or units. This block is usually used for multiple visits, units of supplies, anesthesia units or minutes, or oxygen volume. If only one service is performed, enter 1.0	**10**		
8. Complete blocks 24I through 27 by entering information on the provider's or healthcare facility where the service was provided and the patient's account number. Check the correct box to indicate acceptance of assignment of benefits.	**10**		
9. Complete blocks 28 through 29 by entering the total charges, total amount paid, and the total amount due. Complete blocks 31 through 33a by entering in the provider's and facility's information.	**10**		
10. Review the claim for accuracy and completeness before submitting. Correct any errors or missing information.	**10***		
Total Points	**100**		

Comments

CAAHEP Competencies	Step(s)
VIII.P.4. Complete an insurance claim form	Entire procedure
ABHES Competencies	**Step(s)**
7. Administrative Procedures d. Process insurance claims	Entire procedure

Work Product 18.1 CMS-1500 Health Insurance Claim Form

HEALTH INSURANCE CLAIM FORM

APPROVED BY NATIONAL UNIFORM CLAIM COMMITTEE (NUCC) 02/12

PICA | PICA

CARRIER

1. MEDICARE (Medicare#) MEDICAID (Medicaid#) TRICARE (ID#/DoD#) CHAMPVA (Member ID#) GROUP HEALTH PLAN (ID#) FECA BLK LUNG (ID#) OTHER (ID#)

1a. INSURED'S I.D. NUMBER (For Program in Item 1)

2. PATIENT'S NAME (Last Name, First Name, Middle Initial)

3. PATIENT'S BIRTH DATE MM DD YY SEX M F

4. INSURED'S NAME (Last Name, First Name, Middle Initial)

5. PATIENT'S ADDRESS (No., Street)

6. PATIENT RELATIONSHIP TO INSURED Self Spouse Child Other

7. INSURED'S ADDRESS (No., Street)

CITY STATE

8. RESERVED FOR NUCC USE

CITY STATE

ZIP CODE TELEPHONE (Include Area Code) ( )

ZIP CODE TELEPHONE (Include Area Code) ( )

9. OTHER INSURED'S NAME (Last Name, First Name, Middle Initial)

10. IS PATIENT'S CONDITION RELATED TO:

11. INSURED'S POLICY GROUP OR FECA NUMBER

a. OTHER INSURED'S POLICY OR GROUP NUMBER

a. EMPLOYMENT? (Current or Previous) YES NO

a. INSURED'S DATE OF BIRTH MM DD YY SEX M F

b. RESERVED FOR NUCC USE

b. AUTO ACCIDENT? YES NO PLACE (State)

b. OTHER CLAIM ID (Designated by NUCC)

c. RESERVED FOR NUCC USE

c. OTHER ACCIDENT? YES NO

c. INSURANCE PLAN NAME OR PROGRAM NAME

d. INSURANCE PLAN NAME OR PROGRAM NAME

10d. CLAIM CODES (Designated by NUCC)

d. IS THERE ANOTHER HEALTH BENEFIT PLAN? YES NO ***If yes**, complete items 9, 9a, and 9d.*

READ BACK OF FORM BEFORE COMPLETING & SIGNING THIS FORM.

12. PATIENT'S OR AUTHORIZED PERSON'S SIGNATURE I authorize the release of any medical or other information necessary to process this claim. I also request payment of government benefits either to myself or to the party who accepts assignment below.

SIGNED ______ DATE ______

13. INSURED'S OR AUTHORIZED PERSON'S SIGNATURE I authorize payment of medical benefits to the undersigned physician or supplier for services described below.

SIGNED ______

PATIENT AND INSURED INFORMATION

14. DATE OF CURRENT ILLNESS, INJURY, or PREGNANCY (LMP) MM DD YY QUAL.

15. OTHER DATE QUAL. MM DD YY

16. DATES PATIENT UNABLE TO WORK IN CURRENT OCCUPATION FROM MM DD YY TO MM DD YY

17. NAME OF REFERRING PROVIDER OR OTHER SOURCE 17a. 17b. NPI

18. HOSPITALIZATION DATES RELATED TO CURRENT SERVICES FROM MM DD YY TO MM DD YY

19. ADDITIONAL CLAIM INFORMATION (Designated by NUCC)

20. OUTSIDE LAB? YES NO $ CHARGES

21. DIAGNOSIS OR NATURE OF ILLNESS OR INJURY Relate A-L to service line below (24E) ICD Ind.

A. B. C. D.
E. F. G. H.
I. J. K. L.

22. RESUBMISSION CODE ORIGINAL REF. NO.

23. PRIOR AUTHORIZATION NUMBER

	24. A. DATE(S) OF SERVICE From MM DD YY	To MM DD YY	B. PLACE OF SERVICE	C. EMG	D. PROCEDURES, SERVICES, OR SUPPLIES (Explain Unusual Circumstances) CPT/HCPCS	MODIFIER	E. DIAGNOSIS POINTER	F. $ CHARGES	G. DAYS OR UNITS	H. EPSDT Family Plan	I. ID. QUAL.	J. RENDERING PROVIDER ID. #
1											NPI	
2											NPI	
3											NPI	
4											NPI	
5											NPI	
6											NPI	

PHYSICIAN OR SUPPLIER INFORMATION

25. FEDERAL TAX I.D. NUMBER SSN EIN

26. PATIENT'S ACCOUNT NO.

27. ACCEPT ASSIGNMENT? (For govt. claims, see back) YES NO

28. TOTAL CHARGE $

29. AMOUNT PAID $

30. Rsvd for NUCC Use

31. SIGNATURE OF PHYSICIAN OR SUPPLIER INCLUDING DEGREES OR CREDENTIALS (I certify that the statements on the reverse apply to this bill and are made a part thereof.)

SIGNED DATE

32. SERVICE FACILITY LOCATION INFORMATION

a. NPI b.

33. BILLING PROVIDER INFO & PH # ( )

a. NPI b.

NUCC Instruction Manual available at: www.nucc.org ***PLEASE PRINT OR TYPE*** APPROVED OMB-0938-1197 FORM 1500 (02-12)

Procedure 18.4 Use Medical Necessity Guidelines: Respond to a "Medical Necessity Denied" Claim

Name ______________________________ **Date** __________ **Score** __________

Task: To resolve the insurance company's denial of a claim for medical necessity by completing an accurate claim.

Equipment and Supplies:
- Paper method: Patient's health record, copy of patient's insurance ID card or cards, patient registration form, encounter form, blank CMS-1500 health insurance claim form (Work Product 15-2), and a pen
- Electronic method: SimChart for the Medical Office
- Insurance denial letter or scenario (see below)

Scenario: You are working at Walden-Martin Family Medical Clinic, 1234 Anystreet, Anytown, AL 12345 (phone: 123-123-1234). You receive a letter indicating that Medicare has denied the following claim for not being medically necessary:

Patient: Norma B. Washington   DOB: 08/07/19XX   Policy/ID Number: 847744144A

Date of Service: 06/13/20XX   ICD: G43.101 (Migraine)   CPT: J3420 (B-12 injection)

Provider: Julie Walden MD

You did some research and the information above was the only information sent to Medicare for that encounter. The following information was the correct information for the encounter:

Patient: Norma B. Washington   DOB: 08/01/19XX   Date of Service: 06/15/20XX

ICD: G43.101 (Migraine)   CPT: J1885 (Toradol 15 mg—$15.50) and 96372 (Injection, Ther/Proph/Diag—$25.00)

ICD: D51.0 (Vitamin B_{12} deficiency anemia)   CPT: J3420 (B_{12} injection—$24.00) and 96372 (Injection, Ther/Proph/Diag—$25.00)

To be billed to: Medicare, 1234 Insurance Road, Anytown, AL 12345-1234

Standard: Complete the procedure and all critical steps in ______ minutes with a minimum score of 85% within two attempts (*or as indicated by the instructor*).

Scoring: Divide the points earned by the total possible points. Failure to perform a critical step, indicated by an asterisk (*), results in grade no higher than an 84% (*or as indicated by the instructor*).

Time: Began________ Ended________ Total minutes: ________

Steps:	Point Value	Attempt 1	Attempt 2
1. Review the insurance denial letter (scenario) carefully. Compare the patient's information from the denial letter to the health record, claim, and encounter form. Look for errors in the patient's name and date of birth.	20*		
2. Compare the insurance denial letter (scenario) to the health record, claim, and encounter form. Look for errors in the date of service, the diagnosis, and the procedure codes. The procedure must be medically necessary for the diagnosis indicated.	20*		

3. Complete a claim (either CMS-1500 or an electronic claim using SimChart) by entering in the information about the carrier, patient, and insured.	**20**		
4. Enter the information regarding the physician, procedures, and diagnosis. Make sure to include all of the information from the encounter.	**20**		
5. Proofread the claim form for accuracy before submitting the claim.	**20**		
Total Points	**100**		

Comments

CAAHEP Competencies	**Step(s)**
IX.P.3. Utilize medical necessity guidelines	Entire procedure
ABHES Competencies	**Step(s)**
7. Administrative Procedures c. Perform billing and collection procedures	Entire procedure

Work Product 18.2 CMS-1500 Health Insurance Claim Form

HEALTH INSURANCE CLAIM FORM

APPROVED BY NATIONAL UNIFORM CLAIM COMMITTEE (NUCC) 02/12

PICA | PICA

CARRIER

1. MEDICARE (Medicare#) | MEDICAID (Medicaid#) | TRICARE (ID#/DoD#) | CHAMPVA (Member ID#) | GROUP HEALTH PLAN (ID#) | FECA BLK LUNG (ID#) | OTHER (ID#)

1a. INSURED'S I.D. NUMBER (For Program in Item 1)

2. PATIENT'S NAME (Last Name, First Name, Middle Initial)

3. PATIENT'S BIRTH DATE MM DD YY SEX M F

4. INSURED'S NAME (Last Name, First Name, Middle Initial)

5. PATIENT'S ADDRESS (No., Street)

6. PATIENT RELATIONSHIP TO INSURED Self Spouse Child Other

7. INSURED'S ADDRESS (No., Street)

CITY STATE

8. RESERVED FOR NUCC USE

CITY STATE

ZIP CODE TELEPHONE (Include Area Code) ( )

ZIP CODE TELEPHONE (Include Area Code) ( )

9. OTHER INSURED'S NAME (Last Name, First Name, Middle Initial)

10. IS PATIENT'S CONDITION RELATED TO:

11. INSURED'S POLICY GROUP OR FECA NUMBER

a. OTHER INSURED'S POLICY OR GROUP NUMBER

a. EMPLOYMENT? (Current or Previous) YES NO

a. INSURED'S DATE OF BIRTH MM DD YY SEX M F

b. RESERVED FOR NUCC USE

b. AUTO ACCIDENT? YES NO PLACE (State)

b. OTHER CLAIM ID (Designated by NUCC)

c. RESERVED FOR NUCC USE

c. OTHER ACCIDENT? YES NO

c. INSURANCE PLAN NAME OR PROGRAM NAME

d. INSURANCE PLAN NAME OR PROGRAM NAME

10d. CLAIM CODES (Designated by NUCC)

d. IS THERE ANOTHER HEALTH BENEFIT PLAN? YES NO ***If yes***, complete items 9, 9a, and 9d.

READ BACK OF FORM BEFORE COMPLETING & SIGNING THIS FORM.

12. PATIENT'S OR AUTHORIZED PERSON'S SIGNATURE I authorize the release of any medical or other information necessary to process this claim. I also request payment of government benefits either to myself or to the party who accepts assignment below.

SIGNED ____ DATE ____

13. INSURED'S OR AUTHORIZED PERSON'S SIGNATURE I authorize payment of medical benefits to the undersigned physician or supplier for services described below.

SIGNED ____

PATIENT AND INSURED INFORMATION

14. DATE OF CURRENT ILLNESS, INJURY, or PREGNANCY (LMP) MM DD YY QUAL.

15. OTHER DATE QUAL. MM DD YY

16. DATES PATIENT UNABLE TO WORK IN CURRENT OCCUPATION MM DD YY FROM TO MM DD YY

17. NAME OF REFERRING PROVIDER OR OTHER SOURCE

17a.

17b. NPI

18. HOSPITALIZATION DATES RELATED TO CURRENT SERVICES MM DD YY FROM TO MM DD YY

19. ADDITIONAL CLAIM INFORMATION (Designated by NUCC)

20. OUTSIDE LAB? YES NO $ CHARGES

21. DIAGNOSIS OR NATURE OF ILLNESS OR INJURY Relate A-L to service line below (24E) ICD Ind.

A. B. C. D.

E. F. G. H.

I. J. K. L.

22. RESUBMISSION CODE ORIGINAL REF. NO.

23. PRIOR AUTHORIZATION NUMBER

	24. A. DATE(S) OF SERVICE From MM DD YY	To MM DD YY	B. PLACE OF SERVICE	C. EMG	D. PROCEDURES, SERVICES, OR SUPPLIES (Explain Unusual Circumstances) CPT/HCPCS	MODIFIER	E. DIAGNOSIS POINTER	F. $ CHARGES	G. DAYS OR UNITS	H. EPSDT Family Plan	I. ID. QUAL.	J. RENDERING PROVIDER ID. #
1											NPI	
2											NPI	
3											NPI	
4											NPI	
5											NPI	
6											NPI	

25. FEDERAL TAX I.D. NUMBER SSN EIN

26. PATIENT'S ACCOUNT NO.

27. ACCEPT ASSIGNMENT? (For govt. claims, see back) YES NO

28. TOTAL CHARGE $

29. AMOUNT PAID $

30. Rsvd for NUCC Use

31. SIGNATURE OF PHYSICIAN OR SUPPLIER INCLUDING DEGREES OR CREDENTIALS (I certify that the statements on the reverse apply to this bill and are made a part thereof.)

SIGNED DATE

32. SERVICE FACILITY LOCATION INFORMATION

a. NPI b.

33. BILLING PROVIDER INFO & PH # ( )

a. NPI b.

PHYSICIAN OR SUPPLIER INFORMATION

NUCC Instruction Manual available at: www.nucc.org ***PLEASE PRINT OR TYPE*** APPROVED OMB-0938-1197 FORM 1500 (02-12)

Procedure 18.5 Assist a Patient in Understanding an Explanation of Benefits (EOB)

Name ______________________________ **Date** ____________ **Score** __________

Tasks: To explain an explanation of benefits (EOB) to a patient.

Equipment and Supplies:
- Explanation of benefits

Obtaining Payments – WMFM Clinic Policy

- For patients with copayments, all copayments must be collected before the patient leaves the clinic.
- For patients with balances overdue:
    - Patients must pay 20% of the balance before an appointment can be scheduled.
    - Or patients can establish a 6- or 12-month interest-free payment plan, making the first payment before the next visit can be scheduled.
- Payments can be made using VISA, MasterCard, personal check (no starter checks accepted), or cash. Payments can also be made online.

Scenario: Noemi Rodriguez has stopped in to WMFM Clinic with an explanation of benefits that she recently received from her insurance company (see next page). She states that her policy has a $1000 deductible and 80/20 coinsurance. She doesn't understand why the insurance company didn't pay the bill in full as she had services earlier in the year. She also is not clear on what she is financially responsible for.
WMFM Clinic is a participating provider with the Aetna Preferred Provider Plan that Ms. Rodriguez is part of.

Explanation of Benefits

Aetna 1234 Insurance Way Anytown, AL 12345-1234 800-333-444-5555 800-333-444-6666 (FAX)		Insured's Name:	Noemi Rodriguez
	Policy ID #	NR5006789	
		Date:	03/03/20XX
Patient Name:	Noemi Rodriguez 441 Hyacinth Way Anytown, AL 12345	Provider:	Walden-Martin Family Medical Clinic J.A. Martin NPI 1234567890 Claim No. 9885050333-XX Check No. 2034422

Date of Service	CPT Code	Charge Amount	Allowable Charges	Applied to Deductible	Co-Pay	Total Benefit	Reason Code(s)
01/14/20XX	99205	225.00	200.00	150.00	0.00	40.00	01/42
01/14/20XX	85025	35.00	30.00	0.00	0.00	24.00	42
01/14/20XX	82272	7.00	7.00	0.00	0.00	5.60	
01/14/20XX	80061	47.00	45.00	0.00	0.00	36.00	42
01/14/20XX	80076	39.00	32.50	0.00	0.00	26.00	42
01/14/20XX	80069	41.50	40.00	0.00	0.00	32.00	42
01/14/20XX	85652	16.00	16.00	0.00	0.00	12.80	
01/14/20XX	81001	27.00	25.00	0.00	0.00	20.00	42
Total		437.50	395.50	150.00	0.00	236.40	

Reason Code:
01 Deductible amount
42 Charges exceed our fee schedule or maximum allowed amount

Standard: Complete the procedure and all critical steps in _______ minutes with a minimum score of 85% within two attempts (*or as indicated by the instructor*).

Scoring: Divide the points earned by the total possible points. Failure to perform a critical step, indicated by an asterisk (*), results in grade no higher than an 84% (*or as indicated by the instructor*).

Time: Began_________ Ended_________ Total minutes: _________

Steps:	**Point Value**	**Attempt 1**	**Attempt 2**
1. Review the each of the columns found on the explanation of benefits. Have a clear understanding how the insurance company came up with the patient's responsibility.	**20**		
2. Determine if any amount has been applied to Ms. Rodriguez's deductible. Explain to Ms. Rodriguez how that impacts how much the insurance company will pay and her financial responsibility.	**20***		

3. Compare the charge amount for each service to the allowed amount. Explain to Ms. Rodriguez how the difference between those two is taken care of. Inform the patient of the clinic policy regarding copayments and how the payment can be made.	**20**		
4. Calculate what Ms. Rodriguez's financial responsibility is and explain to her how you came up with that amount.	**20***		
5. Ask if the patient has any further questions.	**20***		
Total Points	**100**		

Affective Behavior	***Directions:*** *Check behaviors observed during the role-play.*					
Tactfulness	**Negative, Unprofessional Behaviors**	**Attempt**		**Positive, Professional Behaviors**	**Attempt**	
		1	**2**		**1**	**2**
	Rude, unkind			Courteous, professional; assertive as required		
	Disrespectful, impolite			Polite, patient		
	Negative verbal communication (e.g., harsh words, disrespectful comments)			Professional verbal communication (e.g., respectful and understanding communication)		
	Brief, abrupt			Took time with person		
	Unconcerned with person's dignity			Maintained person's dignity		
	Negative nonverbal behaviors			Positive nonverbal behaviors		
	Other:			Other:		
Empathy	Distracted; not focused on the other person			Focused full attention on the other person		
	Judgmental attitude; not accepting attitude			Nonjudgmental, accepting attitude		
	Failed to clarify what the person verbally or nonverbally communicated			Used summarizing or paraphrasing to clarify what the person verbally or nonverbally communicated		
	Failed to acknowledge what the person communicated			Acknowledged what the person communicated		
	Rude, discourteous			Pleasant and courteous		
	Disregarded the person's dignity and rights			Maintained the person's dignity and rights		
	Other:			Other:		

Critical Thinking	Coached or told of an issue or problem			Independently identified the problem or issue		
	Failed to ask relevant questions related to the condition			Asked appropriate questions to obtain the information required		
	Failed to consider alternatives; failed to ask questions that demonstrated understanding of principles/concepts			Willing to consider other alternatives; asked appropriate questions that showed understanding of principles/concepts		
	Failed to make an educated, logical judgment/decision; actions or lack of actions demonstrated unsafe practices and/or did not follow the protocol			Made an educated, logical judgment/decision based on the protocol; actions reflected principles of safe practice		
	Other:			Other:		

Grading for Affective Behaviors		**Point Value**	**Attempt 1**	**Attempt 2**
Does not meet Expectation	• Response was insensitive and/or disrespectful. • Student demonstrated more than 2 negative, unprofessional behaviors during the interaction.	0		
Needs Improvement	• Response was insensitive and/or disrespectful. • Student demonstrated 1 or 2 negative, unprofessional behaviors during the interaction.	0		
Meets Expectation	• Response was sensitive and respectful; no negative, unprofessional behaviors observed. • More practice is needed for behavior to appear natural and for student to appear comfortable and at ease.	15		
Occasionally Exceeds Expectation	• Response was sensitive and respectful; no negative, unprofessional behaviors observed. • At times student appeared comfortable and at ease; but more practice is needed for behavior to become natural and consistent with a professional medical assistant.	15		
Always Exceeds Expectation	• Response was sensitive and respectful; no negative, unprofessional behaviors observed. • Student's behaviors appeared natural and comfortable. Behaviors are consistent with a professional medical assistant.	15		

Comments

CAAHEP Competencies	Step(s)
VIII.P.5. Assist a patient in understanding an Explanation of Benefits (EOB)	Entire procedure
A.1. Demonstrate critical thinking skills	Entire procedure
A.3. Demonstrate empathy for patients' concerns	5
A.7. Demonstrate tactfulness	Entire procedure
ABHES Competencies	**Step(s)**
7. Administrative Procedures c. Perform billing and collection procedures	Entire procedure

Procedure 18.6 Inform a Patient of Financial Obligations for Services Rendered

Name ______________________________ **Date** ____________ **Score** __________

Tasks: Inform patient of his/her financial obligation and to demonstrate professionalism and sensitivity when discussing the patient's billing record.

Equipment and Supplies:
- Facility's payment policy
- Copy of patient's insurance card (or see information in the scenario)
- Patient's account record (or see information in the scenario)

Obtaining Payments – WMFM Clinic Policy
- For patients with copayments, all copayments must be collected before the patient leaves the clinic.
- For patients with balances overdue:
  - Patients must pay 20% of the balance before an appointment can be scheduled.
  - Or patients can establish a 6- or 12-month interest-free payment plan, making the first payment before the next visit can be scheduled.
- Payments can be made using VISA, MasterCard, personal check (no starter checks accepted), or cash. Payments can also be made online.

Scenario #1: Mr. Walter Biller arrives for his appointment. You need to check his eligibility for services and also if he has a copayment for today's visit. His insurance information: account number: 16611; Aetna, Policy/ID Number: CH8327753; and Group Number: 33347H

Scenario #2: Christi Brown is meeting with you regarding the bill she received in the mail. She called to make the appointment and she voiced her confusion about the bill. She stated that she thought her insurance covered everything. You check her record and see that she met her deductible and now needs to pay 20% of the billed amount. She owes $170.

Directions: Role-play the scenarios with a peer. The peer will be the insurance representative in Scenario #1, and then the patient in Scenario #2. You will be the medical assistant. You need to be professional and sensitive when working with patients regarding payments. You also need to follow the clinic's policy.

Standard: Complete the procedure and all critical steps in _______ minutes with a minimum score of 85% within two attempts (*or as indicated by the instructor*).

Scoring: Divide the points earned by the total possible points. Failure to perform a critical step, indicated by an asterisk (*), results in grade no higher than an 84% (*or as indicated by the instructor*).

Time: Began_________ Ended_________ Total minutes: _________

Steps:	**Point Value**	**Attempt 1**	**Attempt 2**
Scenario #1: Role-play with a peer who will be the insurance representative.			
1. Contact the patient's insurance company and verify the patient's eligibility for services. Provide the representative with the patient's information. Find out if the patient has a copayment for today's visit. Document the information obtained.	20*		
Scenario #1 update: You need to provide the patient with the information that he owes a copayment for today's visit.			
2. Inform the patient of his financial obligation of the copayment.	10*		

Scenario update: He states he does not have the cash with him.			
3. Inform the patient of the clinic policy regarding copayments and how the payment can be made.	**10**		
4. Demonstrate sensitivity and professionalism when discussing the payment.	**15***		
Scenario #2: Role-play with a peer who will be the patient.			
5. Determine the amount the patient owes by reviewing the patient's account record. Inform the patient the amount owed for services rendered.	**15***		
Scenario update: Patient stated she does not have the money to pay the entire bill today.			
6. Inform the patient of the clinic policy regarding overdue accounts and scheduling appointments. Provide the patient with options for the overdue amount based on the clinic policy.	**15**		
7. Demonstrate sensitivity and professionalism when discussing the payment and the situation.	**15***		
Total Points	**100**		

Affective Behavior	***Directions:*** *Check behaviors observed during the role-play.*					
Tactfulness	**Negative, Unprofessional Behaviors**	**Attempt**		**Positive, Professional Behaviors**	**Attempt**	
		1	**2**		**1**	**2**
	Rude, unkind			Courteous, professional; assertive as required		
	Disrespectful, impolite			Polite, patient		
	Negative verbal communication (e.g., harsh words, disrespectful comments)			Professional verbal communication (e.g., respectful and understanding communication)		
	Brief, abrupt			Took time with person		
	Unconcerned with person's dignity			Maintained person's dignity		
	Negative nonverbal behaviors			Positive nonverbal behaviors		
	Other:			Other:		

Empathy	Distracted; not focused on the other person			Focused full attention on the other person		
	Judgmental attitude; not accepting attitude			Nonjudgmental, accepting attitude		
	Failed to clarify what the person verbally or nonverbally communicated			Used summarizing or paraphrasing to clarify what the person verbally or nonverbally communicated		
	Failed to acknowledge what the person communicated			Acknowledged what the person communicated		
	Rude, discourteous			Pleasant and courteous		
	Disregarded the person's dignity and rights			Maintained the person's dignity and rights		
	Other:			Other:		
Critical Thinking	Coached or told of an issue or problem			Independently identified the problem or issue		
	Failed to ask relevant questions related to the condition			Asked appropriate questions to obtain the information required		
	Failed to consider alternatives; failed to ask questions that demonstrated understanding of principles/concepts			Willing to consider other alternatives; asked appropriate questions that showed understanding of principles/concepts		
	Failed to make an educated, logical judgment/decision; actions or lack of actions demonstrated unsafe practices and/or did not follow the protocol			Made an educated, logical judgment/decision based on the protocol; actions reflected principles of safe practice		
	Other:			Other:		

Grading for Affective Behaviors		**Point Value**	**Attempt 1**	**Attempt 2**
Does not meet Expectation	• Response was insensitive and/or disrespectful. • Student demonstrated more than 2 negative, unprofessional behaviors during the interaction.	0		
Needs Improvement	• Response was insensitive and/or disrespectful. • Student demonstrated 1 or 2 negative, unprofessional behaviors during the interaction.	0		
Meets Expectation	• Response was sensitive and respectful; no negative, unprofessional behaviors observed. • More practice is needed for behavior to appear natural and for student to appear comfortable and at ease.	15		
Occasionally Exceeds Expectation	• Response was sensitive and respectful; no negative, unprofessional behaviors observed. • At times student appeared comfortable and at ease; but more practice is needed for behavior to become natural and consistent with a professional medical assistant.	15		
Always Exceeds Expectation	• Response was sensitive and respectful; no negative, unprofessional behaviors observed. • Student's behaviors appeared natural and comfortable. Behaviors are consistent with a professional medical assistant.	15		

Comments

CAAHEP Competencies	**Step(s)**
A.1. Demonstrate critical thinking skills	Entire procedure
A.3. Demonstrate empathy for patient's concerns.	4, 7
A.7. Demonstrate tactfulness	4, 7
VII.P.3. Inform a patient of financial obligations for services rendered	2, 5
VIII.P.2. Verify eligibility for services	1
ABHES Competencies	**Step(s)**
7. Administrative Procedures c. Perform billing and collection procedures	Entire procedure

Procedure 18.7 Show Sensitivity when Communicating with Patients Regarding Third-Party Requirements

Name ______________________________ **Date** __________ **Score** __________

Tasks: Communicate in an assertive, professional manner with a third-party representative. Demonstrate sensitivity through verbal and nonverbal communication when discussing third-party requirements with a patient. Display tactful behavior when communicating with a provider regarding third-party requirements.

Equipment and Supplies:
- Copy of patient's health insurance ID card
- Prescription for new medication

Scenario: Ken Thomas saw Jean Burke N.P. for his asthma today. He was prescribed a fluticasone inhaler 220 mcg and a refill on his albuterol inhaler. When Ken stops at the checkout desk to make a follow-up appointment, he looks concerned. You inquire how you can help him and he states that he is wondering if his new insurance will pick up the fluticasone inhaler. He further explains that he has used it in the past with great results, but he recently switched insurance plans and he is finding it doesn't have the same coverage as his old plan.

- *Role-play #1:* You call the insurance company and discuss the coverage with the insurance carrier's representative. The representative tells you that the fluticasone inhaler is not covered for his condition. The representative gave you names of two other inhalers that would be covered.
  When you ask if the drug would be covered through the exceptions process, the representative indicated that the provider must send a letter indicating the drug is appropriate for the patient's condition because all other drugs covered by the plan have not been effective, those drugs have side effects that may be harmful to the patient, or the patient is allergic to the other drugs.
- *Role-play #2:* You must explain to Ken, who is upset with his insurance coverage, that he would have to cover the $250 inhaler.
- *Role-play #3:* Ken explains he does not have $250 for the inhaler. He asks what else he should do. You mention the exception process and Ken requests the provider to send a letter. You need to role-play notifying the provider of the third-party requirements.

Directions: Role-play the scenarios with a peer. The peer will play the part of the insurance representative, the patient, and the provider. You need to be professional and assertive with the insurance representative. When working with the patient, you need to show sensitivity. When communicating with the provider, you need to be professional and tactful.

Standard: Complete the procedure and all critical steps in _______ minutes with a minimum score of 85% within two attempts (*or as indicated by the instructor*).

Scoring: Divide the points earned by the total possible points. Failure to perform a critical step, indicated by an asterisk (*), results in grade no higher than an 84% (*or as indicated by the instructor*).

Time: Began_________ Ended_________ Total minutes: _________

Steps:	Point Value	Attempt 1	Attempt 2
1. Obtain a copy of the patient's health insurance ID card and the prescription for the new medication.	**10**		
2. Review the insurance card for coverage information and the phone number for providers.	**20**		

3. *Scenario: Role-play #1 with a peer. The peer will be the insurance representative.* Contact the insurance company and clearly state the patient's information, the patient's question, and the new medication. Write down information provided by the representative.	**10***		
4. Demonstrate professionalism through verbal communication skills, by stating a respectful, assertive, clear, organized message while pronouncing medical terminology and medications correctly.	**10***		
5. *Scenario: Role-play #2 with a peer. The peer will be the patient.* Explain to the patient the message from the insurance representative using language that can be understood by the patient. *(Refer to the Checklist for Affective Behaviors - Respect and Sensitivity)*	**10***		
6. Demonstrate sensitivity to the patient by paying attention to and responding appropriately to the patient's nonverbal body language and verbal message.	**10***		
7. Demonstrate sensitivity to the patient by showing empathy and clarifying that you understand what the patient is stating. Give the patient your full attention during the conversation and reserve judgment.	**10***		
8. Demonstrate sensitivity to the patient by using a pleasant, courteous tone of voice. Use body language to communicate respect (e.g., eye contact if culturally appropriate, keep arms uncrossed and relaxed).	**10***		
9. *Scenario: Role-play #3 with a peer. The peer will be the provider.* Demonstrate tactful behavior when explaining the third-party requirements to the provider. *(Refer to the Checklist for Affective Behaviors - Tactful)*	**10***		
Total Points	**100**		

Affective Behavior	***Directions:*** *Check behaviors observed during the role-play.*					
Tactfulness	**Negative, Unprofessional Behaviors**	**Attempt**		**Positive, Professional Behaviors**	**Attempt**	
		1	**2**		**1**	**2**
	Rude, unkind			Courteous, professional; assertive as required		
	Disrespectful, impolite			Polite, patient		
	Negative verbal communication (e.g., harsh words, disrespectful comments)			Professional verbal communication (e.g., respectful and understanding communication)		
	Brief, abrupt			Took time with person		
	Unconcerned with person's dignity			Maintained person's dignity		
	Negative nonverbal behaviors			Positive nonverbal behaviors		
	Other:			Other:		

Empathy	Distracted; not focused on the other person			Focused full attention on the other person		
	Judgmental attitude; not accepting attitude			Nonjudgmental, accepting attitude		
	Failed to clarify what the person verbally or nonverbally communicated			Used summarizing or paraphrasing to clarify what the person verbally or nonverbally communicated		
	Failed to acknowledge what the person communicated			Acknowledged what the person communicated		
	Rude, discourteous			Pleasant and courteous		
	Disregarded the person's dignity and rights			Maintained the person's dignity and rights		
	Other:			Other:		
Critical Thinking	Coached or told of an issue or problem			Independently identified the problem or issue		
	Failed to ask relevant questions related to the condition			Asked appropriate questions to obtain the information required		
	Failed to consider alternatives; failed to ask questions that demonstrated understanding of principles/concepts			Willing to consider other alternatives; asked appropriate questions that showed understanding of principles/concepts		
	Failed to make an educated, logical judgment/decision; actions or lack of actions demonstrated unsafe practices and/or did not follow the protocol			Made an educated, logical judgment/decision based on the protocol; actions reflected principles of safe practice		
	Other:			Other:		

Grading for Affective Behaviors		**Point Value**	**Attempt 1**	**Attempt 2**
Does not meet Expectation	• Response was insensitive and/or disrespectful. • Student demonstrated more than 2 negative, unprofessional behaviors during the interaction.	0		
Needs Improvement	• Response was insensitive and/or disrespectful. • Student demonstrated 1 or 2 negative, unprofessional behaviors during the interaction.	0		
Meets Expectation	• Response was sensitive and respectful; no negative, unprofessional behaviors observed. • More practice is needed for behavior to appear natural and for student to appear comfortable and at ease.	10		
Occasionally Exceeds Expectation	• Response was sensitive and respectful; no negative, unprofessional behaviors observed. • At times student appeared comfortable and at ease; but more practice is needed for behavior to become natural and consistent with a professional medical assistant.	10		
Always Exceeds Expectation	• Response was sensitive and respectful; no negative, unprofessional behaviors observed. • Student's behaviors appeared natural and comfortable. Behaviors are consistent with a professional medical assistant.	10		

Comments

CAAHEP Competencies	**Step(s)**
VII.P.3. Inform a patient of financial obligations for services rendered	5
A.1. Demonstrate critical thinking skills	Entire procedure
A.3. Demonstrate empathy for patients' concerns	7
A.7. Demonstrate tactfulness	9
ABHES Competencies	**Step(s)**
7. Administrative Procedures c. Perform billing and collection procedures	Entire procedure

Student Name________________________ Date______________

Patient Accounts and Practice Management

chapter **19**

CAAHEP Competencies	Assessment
VII.C.1.a. Define the following bookkeeping terms: charges	Skills and Concepts – A. 5
VII.C.1.b. Define the following bookkeeping terms: payments	Skills and Concepts – A. 6
VII.C.1.c. Define the following bookkeeping terms: accounts receivable	Skills and Concepts – A. 3
VII.C.1.d. Define the following bookkeeping terms: accounts payable	Skills and Concepts – A. 2
VII.C.1.e. Define the following bookkeeping terms: adjustments	Skills and Concepts – A. 4
VII.C.1.f. Define the following bookkeeping terms: end of day reconciliation	Procedure 19.4
VII.C.2.a. Identify precautions for accepting the following types of payments: cash	Skills and Concepts – B. 2
VII.C.2.b. Identify precautions for accepting the following types of payments: check	Skills and Concepts – B. 1
VII.C.2.c. Identify precautions for accepting the following types of payments: credit card	Skills and Concepts – B. 3
VII.C.2.d. Identify precautions for accepting the following types of payments: debit card	Skills and Concepts – B. 3
VII.C.3.a. Identify types of adjustments made to patient accounts including: non-sufficient funds (NSF) check	Skills and Concepts – A. 10
VII.C.3.b. Identify types of adjustments made to patient accounts including: collection agency transaction	Skills and Concepts – C. 4
VII.C.3.c. Identify types of adjustments made to patient accounts including: credit balance	Skills and Concepts – A. 9
VII.C.3.d. Identify types of adjustments made to patient accounts including: third party	Skills and Concepts – A. 8
VII.C.4. Identify patient financial obligations for services rendered	Workplace Applications – 1

CAAHEP Competencies	Assessment
VII.P.1.a. Perform accounts receivable procedures to patient accounts including posting: charges	Procedure 19.1
VII.P.1.b. Perform accounts receivable procedures to patient accounts including posting: payments	Procedures 19.1, 19.3
VII.P.1.c. Perform accounts receivable procedures to patient accounts including posting: adjustments	Procedure 19.3
VII.P.2. Input accurate patient billing information in Practice Management Systems (PMS)	Procedures 19.1, 19.3
VII.P.3. Inform a patient of financial obligations for services rendered	Procedure 19.2
A.3. Demonstrate empathy for patients' concerns	Procedure 19.2
A.7. Demonstrate tactfulness	Procedure 19.2
ABHES Competencies	**Assessment**
7. Administrative Procedures c. Perform billing and collection procedures	Procedures 19.1, 19.2, 19.3, 19.4

VOCABULARY REVIEW

Using the word pool on the right, find the correct word to match the definition. Write the word on the line after the definition.

Group A

1. The person legally responsible for the entire bill
   ____
2. A document sent by the insurance company to the provider and the patient explaining the allowed charge amount, the amount reimbursed for services, and the patient's financial responsibilities
   ____
3. The process of recording financial transactions
   ____
4. A manual bookkeeping system that uses a day sheet to record all financial transactions for the date of service and maintains patient account balances by using physical ledger cards
   ____
5. Poor, needy, impoverished ______________________
6. To come into or acquire ______________________
7. A list of fixed fees for services ______________________
8. A minor who has been granted emancipation by the court; the minor can assume the rights and responsibilities of adulthood
   ____
9. The amount of money the healthcare facility has in the bank that can be withdrawn as cash ______________________
10. A running balance of all financial transactions for a specific patient
   ____

Word Pool

- patient account
- bookkeeping
- cash on hand
- incurred
- pegboard system
- fee schedule
- explanation of benefits
- emancipated minor
- guarantor
- indigent

Group B

1. Something of value that cannot be touched physically ____________________
2. Hostile and aggressive ____________________
3. An imitation intended to be passed off fraudulently or deceptively as genuine; forgery ____________________
4. A chronologic file used as a reminder that something must be dealt with on a certain date ____________________
5. All property available for the payment of debts ____________________
6. An oath or swear word ____________________
7. Global technology that includes imbedded microchips that store and protect cardholder data; also called *chip and PIN* and *chip and signature* ____________________
8. Debt that is not guaranteed by something of value; credit card debt is the most common type ____________________
9. An individual assigned to make financial decisions about the estate of a deceased patient ____________________
10. The misuse of a healthcare facility's funds for personal gain ____________________embezzlement

Word Pool

- counterfeit
- EMV chip technology
- belligerent
- expletive
- embezzlement
- tickler file
- intangible
- executor
- assets
- unsecured debt

Group C

1. Money the bank pays the account holder on the amount in their account for using the money in the account ____________________
2. A special court established to handle small claims or debts, without the services of lawyers ____________________
3. Money in a bank account that is not assigned to pay for any office expenses ____________________
4. An individual or party who brings the suit to court ____________________
5. A fixed compensation periodically paid to a person for regular work ____________________
6. The central bank of the United States ____________________
7. The coordinator of financial resources assigned by the court during a bankruptcy case ____________________
8. An individual or business against whom a lawsuit is filed ____________________
9. To bring into agreement ____________________
10. A document guaranteeing payment of a specific amount of money to the payer named on the document ____________________

Word Pool

- trustee
- small claims court
- plaintiff
- defendant
- salaried
- reconciliation
- interest
- Federal Reserve Bank
- discretionary income
- negotiable instrument

ABBREVIATIONS

Write out what each of the following abbreviations stands for.

1. EOB ______________________________
2. A/R ______________________________
3. A/P ______________________________
4. NSF ______________________________
5. TILA ______________________________
6. FTC ______________________________
7. APR ______________________________
8. PIN ______________________________
9. POS ______________________________
10. EFT ______________________________
11. RTN ______________________________
12. ACH ______________________________

SKILLS AND CONCEPTS

Answer the following questions. Write your answer on the line or in the space provided.

A. Accounts Receivable

1. Examine the fee schedule and answer the following questions.

FEE SCHEDULE

BLACKBURN PRIMARY CARE ASSOCIATES, PC
1990 Turquiose Drive
Blackburn, WI 54937
608-459-8857

Federal Tax ID Number: **00-0000000**

BCBS Group Number: 14982
Medicare Group Number: 14982

OFFICE VISIT, NEW PATIENT

Focused, 99201	$45.00
Expanded, 99202	$55.00
Intermediate, 99203	$60.00
Extended, 99204	$95.00
Comprehensive, 99205	$195.00
Consultation, 99245	$250.00

OFFICE VISIT, ESTABLISHED PATIENT

Minimal, 99211	$40.00
Focused, 99212	$48.00
Intermediate, 99213	$55.00
Extended, 99214	$65.00
Comprehensive, 99215	$195.00

OFFICE PROCEDURES

ECG, 12 lead, 93000	$55.00
Stress ECG, Treadmill, 93015	$295.00
Sigmoidoscopy, Flex; 45330	$145.00
Spirometry, 94010	$50.00
Cerumen Removal, 69210	$40.00
Collection & Handling	
Lab Specimen, 99000	$9.00
Venipuncture, 35415	$9.00
Urinalysis, 81000	$20.00
Urinalysis, 81002 (Dip Only)	$12.00
Influenza Injection, 90724	$20.00
Pneumococcal Injection, 90732	$20.00
Oral Polio, 90712	$15.00
DTaP, 90700	$20.00
Tetanus Toxoid, 90703	$15.00
MMR, 90707	$25.00
HIB, 90737	$20.00
Hepatitis B, newborn to age 11 years, 90744	$60.00
Hepatitis B, 11-19 years, 90745	$60.00
Hepatitis B, 20 years and above 90746	$60.00
Intramuscular Injection, 90788	
Penicillin	$30.00
Cephtriaxone	$25.00
Solu-Medrol	$23.00
Vitamin B-12	$13.00
Subcutaneous Injection, 90782	
Epinephrine	$18.00
Susphrine	$25.00
Insulin, U-100	$15.00

COMMON DIAGNOSTIC CODES

Acute coronary thrombosis without myocardial infarction I24.0
Other forms of acute ischemic heart disease I24.8
Chronic ischemic heart disease I25.9
Essential hypertension (arterial)(benign) (essential)(malignant)(primary)(systemic) I10
Hypertensive heart disease with heart failure I11.0
Unspecified asthma, uncomplicated J45.909
Asthma with COPD J44.9
Other asthma J45.998
Unspecified asthma with status asthmaticus J45.902
Postural kyphosis M40.00
Osteoporosis M81.0
Acute otitis media H66.0
Chronic otittis media H66.3

a. What is the charge for a consultation? ____________________

b. What is the charge for CPT code 99203? ____________________

c. What is the most expensive procedure on the list? ______________________

d. Which injection is more expensive, insulin or vitamin B_{12}? ______________________

Match the following terms with the correct definition:

2. _____ Accounts payable
3. _____ Accounts receivable
4. _____ Adjustments
5. _____ Charges
6. _____ Payments

a. Money that is expected but has not yet been received
b. Fees applied to the patient account when services are rendered
c. The management of debt incurred and not yet paid
d. Money given to the provider in exchange for services
e. Credits posted to the patient account when the provider's fee exceeds the amount allowed stated on the EOB

7. What are the pitfalls of fee adjustments? ____

____

____

____

____

8. When a provider's fee exceeds the allowed amount stated on the explanation of benefits from the insurance company, a(n) ______________________ is posted to the patient account record for that difference.

9. When a patient has a credit balance on their account, what adjustment is posted to the account?

____

____

____

____

10. Describe the adjustments that are made to the patient's account when an NSF check is received by the healthcare facility.

____

____

____

____

11. What information should be included on the patient ledger? ______________________________

____

____

____

____

B. Patient Payment Management

1. Describe five precautions for accepting checks in the healthcare facility.

   a. ____________________

   b. ____________________

   c. ____________________

   d. ____________________

   e. ____________________

2. Describe four precautions to take if a patient is paying with cash.

   a. ____________________

   b. ____________________

   c. ____________________

   d. ____________________

3. Describe precautions to take when a patient pays with a debit card or a credit card. ____________________

   ____

   ____

   ____

   ____

   ____

C. Collection Procedures

1. Briefly explain how "skips" can be traced. ____________________

   ____

   ____

   ____

   ____

   ____

   ____

2. When a patient account is turned over to a collection agency, what adjustment is posted to the account?

   ____

   ____

D. Accounts Payable

1. Vendors supply which of the following?
   a. Parking lot maintenance
   b. Office supplies
   c. Cleaning services
   d. Utilities
   e. All of the above

2. If an employee is paid with a(n) ____________________, their ____________________ paycheck will always be the same dollar amount.

3. Each employee must complete a W-4 form. What information is indicated on that form? ____________

____

____

____

____

E. Banking Procedures in the Ambulatory Care Setting

1. Describe the banking procedures as related to the ambulatory care setting and include the medical assistant's role with each procedure.

   a. Making bank deposits: ____

   ____

   ____

   ____

   b. Preparing a bank deposit: ____

   ____

   ____

   ____

   c. Endorsing checks: ____

   ____

   ____

   ____

   d. Writing checks: ____

   ____

   ____

   ____

2. Describe three ways to do a mobile deposit of a check.

   a. ______________________________

   b. ______________________________

   c. ______________________________

3. Describe each type of endorsement.

   a. Blank endorsement: ______________________________

   ____

   ____

   ____

   b. Restrictive endorsement: ______________________________

   ____

   ____

   ____

   c. Special endorsement: ______________________________

   ____

   ____

   ____

4. List three reasons a stop-payment would be done.

   a. ______________________________

   b. ______________________________

   c. ______________________________

5. When preparing the bank deposit, you have the following in cash:

   (3) $50 bills
   (22) $20 bills
   (20) $10 bills
   (46) $5 bills
   (68) $1 bills

   What is the total for currency that you would record on the deposit slip? ______________

F. Banking in Today's Business World

1. In the ambulatory care setting, what is the checking account used for? ________________

____

____

2. In the ambulatory care setting, what is a savings account used for? ________________

____

____

3. You are a medical assistant in a small practice and have been told that you now have the responsibility for paying the bills by writing out and signing the checks. What is the first action you need to take before writing out the first check?

____

____

4. Name six activities that can be done with basic online banking services.

   a. ____

   b. ____

   c. ____

   d. ____

   e. ____

   f. ____

5. List the four requirements for a check to be negotiable.

   a. ____

   b. ____

   c. ____

   d. ____

CERTIFICATION PREPARATION

Circle the correct answer.

1. Which agreement for payment plans is *not* subject to Truth in Lending Act and does *not* require a signed Truth in Lending statement?
   a. Specific agreement for fewer than four installments and finance charge
   b. Specific agreement with more than four installments and finance charge
   c. Credit card or loan specifically for health-care treatment
   d. All of the above

2. What should be considered when using a collection agency?
   a. Net back
   b. Fee percentage
   c. Fee charged by the collection agency
   d. Both a and b

3. Accounts _____ are debts incurred but not yet paid.
   a. receivable
   b. delinquent
   c. payable
   d. bookkeeping

4. The recording of business and accounting transactions is called _____.
   a. receivables
   b. payables
   c. accounting
   d. bookkeeping

5. Which does *not* conform to the general rules for telephone collections?
   a. Call only between 8 AM and 9 PM.
   b. Assume a positive attitude.
   c. Leave a message at work revealing the nature of the call.
   d. Keep the conversation brief and to the point.

6. When should checks from patients and other sources be deposited?
   a. At the same time bills are paid
   b. The same day that they are received
   c. When the bank statement is reconciled each month
   d. At the end of the week

7. Which is *not* one of the four types of endorsements?
   a. Blank
   b. Quality
   c. Restrictive
   d. Special

8. A check drawn on the bank's own account and signed by an authorized bank official is called a _____.
   a. bank draft
   b. voucher check
   c. cashier's check
   d. certified check

9. The country is divided into how many Federal Reserve districts?
   a. 8
   b. 10
   c. 12
   d. 14

10. Which endorsement includes words specifying the person to whom the endorser makes the check payable?
    a. Blank endorsement
    b. Restrictive endorsement
    c. Qualified endorsement
    d. Special endorsement

WORKPLACE APPLICATIONS

1. Mr. Sanchez comes to the desk to check out after seeing the provider. When Laura tells him that his bill is $95, he complains that he only saw the provider for 10 minutes. The fee is in accordance with evaluation and management guidelines. Explain the fees to Mr. Sanchez.

____

____

____

____

2. In Laura's new role at Walden-Martin Family Medical Clinic, she will be writing checks to take care of the accounts payable for the clinic. A practicum student has just started at the clinic and will be working with Laura for the next several days. How should Laura describe this aspect of her job?

____

____

____

____

INTERNET ACTIVITIES

1. Using online resources, research the role of an accountant. Create a poster presentation, a PowerPoint presentation, or write a paper summarizing your research. Include the following points in your project:
   a. Why most healthcare providers employ one to handle financials for the office
   b. What an accountant does for the provider
   c. How a medical assistant helps the accountant do their job

2. Using online resources, research mobile deposit technology. Create a poster presentation, a PowerPoint presentation, or write a paper summarizing your research. Include the following points in your project:
   a. Describe three different mobile deposit technologies available for healthcare facilities.
   b. Describe which technology would work best for a small provider's office, large provider's office, and physical therapy rehabilitation facility.

Procedure 19.1 Post Charges and Payments to Patient Accounts

Name ______________________________ **Date** ____________ **Score** __________

Task: To enter charges into the patient account record manually and electronically.

Equipment and Supplies:
- Patient account ledger card (Work Product 19.1)
- SimChart for the Medical Office software
- Encounter form/superbill
- Provider's fee schedule

Scenario: Ken Thomas is a returning patient of Dr. Martin. He makes his $50 copayment at the time of the office visit.

Standard: Complete the procedure and all critical steps in _______ minutes with a minimum score of 85% within two attempts (*or as indicated by the instructor*).

Scoring: Divide the points earned by the total possible points. Failure to perform a critical step, indicated by an asterisk (*), results in grade no higher than an 84% (*or as indicated by the instructor*).

Time: Began_________ Ended_________ Total minutes: _________

Steps for Posting Charges Manually:	**Point Value**	**Attempt 1**	**Attempt 2**
1. For new patients, create the patient account by entering the following information on a patient account ledger card: • Patient's full name, address, and at least two contact phone numbers • Date of birth • Health insurance information, including the subscriber number, group number, and effective date • Subscriber's name and date of birth (if the subscriber is not the patient) For returning patients, review the account record to see whether a balance is due. If there is a balance, bring this to the patient's attention when they come for the appointment. Respectfully explain that the provider would appreciate a payment on the previous balance before they can care for the patient.	**50**		
2. After seeing the patient, the provider completes the encounter form, which includes all procedures and the associated fee schedule. Using the completed encounter form (see Figure 19.1 in textbook), enter the charges manually on the ledger card for the patient's account record. Total all the charges on the encounter form for the services rendered. Then subtract the copayment made from the total charges. The previous balance, if any, is added to this new total. Use the following worksheet to calculate the new balance. The new balance due amount should be presented to the patient before they leave the healthcare facility. TOTAL CHARGES: $__________ Amount paid (copayment): $__________ + Previous balance (if any): $__________ = New Balance Due: $__________	**50***		
Total Points	**100**		

Steps for Posting Charges in SimChart for the Medical Office			
1. After logging into SimChart, locate the established patient by clicking on Find Patient, enter the patient's name, verify DOB, and click on the radio button. This will bring you to the Clinical Care tab. If there is no encounter shown, create an encounter by clicking on Office Visit under Info Panel on the left, select a visit type, and click on Save. Once an encounter has been created, return to the Patient Dashboard and click on the Superbill link on the right (or click on the Coding and Billing tab).	**20**		
2. From the Superbill area, in the Encounters Not Coded section, click on the encounter (in blue). On page 1, enter the diagnosis in the Diagnosis field and document the services provided (additional services are found on pages 2-3 of the Superbill).	**20**		
3. Complete the information needed on page 4 of the Superbill and submit.	**20***		
4. Click on Ledger on the left and search for your patient. Once your patient has been located, click on the arrow across from the name in the ledger.	**20**		
5. Enter the payment received. The balance will be auto-calculated for you.	**20**		
Total Points	**100**		

Comments

CAAHEP Competencies	Step(s)
VII.P.1.a. Perform accounts receivable procedures to patient accounts including posting: charges	Manual: 2 SimChart: 2
VII.P.1.b. Perform accounts receivable procedures to patient accounts including posting: payments	Manual: 2 SimChart: 5
VII.P.2. Input accurate patient billing information in Practice Management Systems (PMS)	SimChart: 2-5
ABHES Competencies	**Step(s)**
7. Administrative Procedures c. Perform billing and collection procedures	Entire procedure

Work Product 19.1 Ledger

Ledger:

Blue Cross Blue Shield

ID # KT4496785

Group # 55124T

Subscriber: Ken Thomas Ken Thomas

398 Larkin Avenue

DOB: 10/25/1961 Anytown, Anystate 12345-1234

Date	Service Description	Charges	Payments	Adjustments	Balance

Procedure 19.2 Inform a Patient of Financial Obligations for Services Rendered

Name ______________________________ **Date** ____________ **Score** __________

Tasks: Inform a patient of his/her financial obligation and demonstrate professionalism and sensitivity when discussing the patient's billing record.

Equipment and Supplies:
- Copy of patient's insurance card (or see information in the scenario)
- Patient's account record (or see information in the scenario)

Scenario: Christi Brown is meeting with you regarding the bill she received in the mail. She called to make the appointment and she voiced her confusion about the bill. She stated that she thought her insurance covered everything. You check her record and see that she met her deductible and now needs to pay 20% of the billed amount. She owes $170.

Standard: Complete the procedure and all critical steps in _______ minutes with a minimum score of 85% within two attempts (*or as indicated by the instructor*).

Scoring: Divide the points earned by the total possible points. Failure to perform a critical step, indicated by an asterisk (*), results in grade no higher than an 84% (*or as indicated by the instructor*).

Time: Began_________ Ended_________ Total minutes: _________

Steps:	**Point Value**	**Attempt 1**	**Attempt 2**
1. Determine the patient's financial responsibility under the insurance plan by reviewing the copy of the patient's insurance card.	**20***		
2. Determine the amount the patient owes by reviewing the patient's account record.	**20***		
3. Discuss the situation with the patient. (Role-play the above scenario.)	**20**		
4. Demonstrate professionalism when discussing the situation with the patient. Verbal and nonverbal communication should demonstrate patience, understanding, and sensitivity. The medical assistant should refrain from inappropriate and unprofessional behavior, including eye rolling, harsh words, disrespectful comments, and similar behaviors.	**20***		
5. Demonstrate professionalism by respectfully providing the patient with payment options based on the clinic's policies and what the patient can pay on a monthly basis.	**20***		
Total Points	**100**		

Affective Behavior	***Directions:*** *Check behaviors observed during the role-play.*					
Tactfulness	**Negative, Unprofessional Behaviors**	**Attempt**		**Positive, Professional Behaviors**	**Attempt**	
		1	**2**		**1**	**2**
	Rude, unkind			Courteous, professional; assertive as required		
	Disrespectful, impolite			Polite, patient		
	Negative verbal communication (e.g., harsh words, disrespectful comments)			Professional verbal communication (e.g., respectful and understanding communication)		
	Brief, abrupt			Took time with person		
	Unconcerned with person's dignity			Maintained person's dignity		
	Negative nonverbal behaviors			Positive nonverbal behaviors		
	Other:			Other:		
Empathy	Distracted; not focused on the other person			Focused full attention on the other person		
	Judgmental attitude; not accepting attitude			Nonjudgmental, accepting attitude		
	Failed to clarify what the person verbally or nonverbally communicated			Used summarizing or paraphrasing to clarify what the person verbally or nonverbally communicated		
	Failed to acknowledge what the person communicated			Acknowledged what the person communicated		
	Rude, discourteous			Pleasant and courteous		
	Disregarded the person's dignity and rights			Maintained the person's dignity and rights		
	Other:			Other:		

Grading for Affective Behaviors		**Point Value**	**Attempt 1**	**Attempt 2**
Does not meet Expectation	• Response was insensitive and/or disrespectful. • Student demonstrated more than 2 negative, unprofessional behaviors during the interaction.	0		
Needs Improvement	• Response was insensitive and/or disrespectful. • Student demonstrated 1 or 2 negative, unprofessional behaviors during the interaction.	0		
Meets Expectation	• Response was sensitive and respectful; no negative, unprofessional behaviors observed. • More practice is needed for behavior to appear natural and for student to appear comfortable and at ease.	15		
Occasionally Exceeds Expectation	• Response was sensitive and respectful; no negative, unprofessional behaviors observed. • At times student appeared comfortable and at ease; but more practice is needed for behavior to become natural and consistent with a professional medical assistant.	15		
Always Exceeds Expectation	• Response was sensitive and respectful; no negative, unprofessional behaviors observed. • Student's behaviors appeared natural and comfortable. Behaviors are consistent with a professional medical assistant.	15		

Comments

CAAHEP Competencies	**Step(s)**
VII.P.3. Inform a patient of financial obligations for services rendered	3
A.7. Demonstrate tactfulness	5
A.3. Demonstrate empathy for patients' concerns	4
ABHES Competencies	**Step(s)**
7. Administrative Procedures c. Perform billing and collection procedures	Entire procedure

Procedure 19.3 Post Payments and Adjustments to Patient Account

Name ______________________________ **Date** __________ **Score** __________

Task: To post payments and adjustments to patient accounts accurately.

Equipment and Supplies:
- Patient account ledger card or SimChart for the Medical Office software

Scenario: Monique Jones (06/23/1985) was seen 6 months ago for a wellness visit and lab work. Her insurance had lapsed, and she is completely responsible for the bill. She did not make any payments and resisted all attempts at collection of the balance of $172.00. Her account was turned over to the collection agency and they were able to collect the balance in full. The collection agency retains 50% of what they collect as payment. Post the collection agency payment and adjustment to her account.

Standard: Complete the procedure and all critical steps in _______ minutes with a minimum score of 85% within two attempts (*or as indicated by the instructor*).

Scoring: Divide the points earned by the total possible points. Failure to perform a critical step, indicated by an asterisk (*), results in grade no higher than an 84% (*or as indicated by the instructor*).

Time: Began_________ Ended_________ Total minutes: _________

Steps:	**Point Value**	**Attempt 1**	**Attempt 2**
1. Look up the ledger card for the patient account (or the patient ledger in SimChart). Confirm that you have the correct patient account.	**30**		
2. Post an adjustment to reverse the adjustment done when the account was turned over to the collection agency.	**30**		
3. Post the payment and adjustment that reflects the actual dollar amount received from the collection agency and the amount that was retained as payment.	**40***		
Total Points	**100**		

Comments

CAAHEP Competencies	**Step(s)**
VII.P.1.b. Perform accounts receivable procedures to patient accounts including posting: payments	3
VII.P.1.c. Perform accounts receivable procedures to patient accounts including posting: adjustments	2, 3
VII.P.2. Input accurate patient billing information in Practice Management Systems (PMS)	2, 3
ABHES Competencies	**Step(s)**
7. Administrative Procedures c. Perform billing and collection procedures	Entire procedure

Procedure 19.4 End-of-Day Reconciliation

Name ______________________________ **Date** ____________ **Score** __________

Task: To complete the end-of-day reconciliation including preparing a bank deposit for currency and checks.

Equipment and Supplies:
- Daily transaction report (see scenario)
- Checks and currency for deposit (see scenario)
- Check for endorsement
- Calculator
- Paper method: bank deposit slip (Work Product 19.2)
- Electronic method: SimChart for the Medical Office (SCMO)

Scenario:
The following payments were received today at Walden-Martin Family Medical Clinic:

Cash:
Reuven Ahmad - $25.00
Amma Patel - $15.00
Ken Thomas - $40.00
Maude Crawford - $25.00
Al Neviaser - $30.00

At the start of the day, the cash drawer had 10 - $1 bills, 10 - $5 bills, 10 - $10 bills, 10 - $20 bills for a total of $360.00. At the end of the day, there is a total of $495.00.

Checks:
Julia Berkley - #3456 for $89.00
Jana Green - #6954 for $136.00
Kyle Reeves - #9854 for $1366.65
Truong Tran - #8546 for $653.36
Quinton Brown - #9865 for $890.22

The healthcare facility's name is Walden-Martin Family Medical Clinic, account number 123-456-78910, and the bank is Clear Water Bank, Anytown, Anystate.

Credit Cards:
Tai Yan - $150.00
Ella Rainwater - $300.00
Diego Miller - $75.00
Carl Bowden - $25.00
Noemi Rodriguez – $45.00

Daily Transaction Report:

Date	Patient	Account	Cash	Check	Debit/Credit
11/6/20XX	Reuven Ahmad	11872534	$25.00		
11/6/20XX	Amma Patel	12156063	$15.00		
11/6/20XX	Ken Thomas	11644627	$40.00		
11/6/20XX	Maude Crawford	12568850	$25.00		
11/6/20XX	Al Neviaser	11279412	$30.00		
11/6/20XX	Julia Berkley	12062515		$89.00	
11/6/20XX	Jana Green	10944532		$136.00	
11/6/20XX	Kyle Reeves	12073635		$1366.65	
11/6/20XX	Truong Tran	11726005		$650.36	
11/6/20XX	Quinton Brown	11272882		$890.22	
11/6/20XX	Tai Yan	12658901			$150.00
11/6/20XX	Ella Rainwater	11885104			$300.00
11/6/20XX	Diego Lupez	12530423			$75.00
11/6/20XX	Carl Bowden	11265329			$25.00
11/6/20XX	Noemi Rodriquez	11766543			$45.00
Total			$135.00	$3132.23	$595.00

Standard: Complete the procedure and all critical steps in _______ minutes with a minimum score of 85% within two attempts (*or as indicated by the instructor*).

Scoring: Divide the points earned by the total possible points. Failure to perform a critical step, indicated by an asterisk (*), results in grade no higher than an 84% (*or as indicated by the instructor*).

Time: Began_________ Ended_________ Total minutes: _________

Steps:	**Point Value**	**Attempt 1**	**Attempt 2**
1. Complete the starting cash portion of the cash reconciliation form (see Figure 19.12) using the information from the scenario.	**5**		
2. Complete the ending cash portion of the cash reconciliation form using the information from the scenario.	**5**		
3. Compare the cash taken in from the cash reconciliation form to the cash total from the daily transaction report. If the totals do not match, compare the individual transactions and determine where the error occurred.	**10***		
4. Compare the total from the credit card processing terminal and the debit/credit card total from the daily transaction report. if the totals do not match compare the individual transactions and determine where the error occurred.	**10***		
5. Gather the documents to be used to prepare the bank deposit. For the electronic method, enter the Simulation Playground in SCMO. Click on the Form Repository icon. On the INFO PANEL, click on Office Forms and then select Bank Deposit Slip.	**5**		

6. Enter the date on the deposit slip.	**5**		
7. Using the calculator, calculate the amount of currency to be deposited. Enter the amount in the CURRENCY line, completing the dollar and cent boxes.	**5**		
8. Enter the total amount in the TOTAL CASH line.	**5**		
9. For each check to be deposited, enter the check number, the dollars, and cents. List each check on a separate line.	**10***		
10. Calculate the total to be deposited and enter the number in the TOTAL FROM ATTACHED LIST box.	**10***		
11. Enter the number of items deposited in the TOTAL ITEMS box.	**5**		
12. Before completing the deposit slip, verify the check amounts listed and recalculate the totals. For the electronic method, click on SAVE.	**10***		
13. Place a restrictive endorsement on the check(s).	**5**		
14. Compare the total from the deposit slip to the total for checks from the daily transaction report. If the totals do not match, compare the individual transactions and determine where the error occurred.	**10***		
Total Points	**100**		

Comments

CAAHEP Competencies	**Step(s)**
VII.C.1.f. Define the following bookkeeping terms: end of day reconciliation	Entire procedure
ABHES Competencies	**Step(s)**
7. Administrative Procedures c. Perform billing and collection procedures	Entire procedure

Work Product 19.2 Bank Deposit Slip

DEPOSIT TICKET

WALDEN-MARTIN FAMLY MEDICAL CLINIC
1234 ANYSTREET
ANYTOWN, ANYSTATE 12345

DEPOSITS MAY NOT BE AVAILABLE FOR IMMEDIATE WITHDRAWAL

Clear Water Bank
Anytown, Anystate

ACCOUNT NUMBER: 123-456-78910

Endorse & List Checks Separately

DATE ________________				Dollars	Cents
CURRENCY					
COIN					
			TOTAL CASH		
1.					
2.					
3.					
4.					
5.					
6.					
7.					
8.					
9.					
10.					
11.					
12.					
			Less Cash Returned		
Total Items			Total Deposit		

Student Name________________________________ Date______________

Advanced Roles in Administration

chapter **20**

CAAHEP Competencies	Assessments
V.C.2 Identify communication barriers	Skills and Concepts – D. 4
X.C.7.i. Define: risk management	Skills and Concepts – B. 2
X.C.10a Identify: Health Information Technology for Economic and Clinical Health (HITECH) Act	Skills and Concepts – F. 1

VOCABULARY REVIEW

Using the word pool on the right, find the correct word to match the definition. Write the word on the line after the definition.

1. The environment where something is created or takes shape; a base on which to build ____________________
2. Obeying, obliging, or yielding ____________________
3. Sticking together tightly ____________________
4. Evidence of authority, status, rights, entitlement to privileges ____________________
5. Contains all documents related to an individual's employment ____________________
6. A relationship of harmony and accord between the patient and the healthcare professional ____________________
7. To appoint a person as a representative ____________________
8. A term referring to actions taken by management to keep good employees ____________________
9. General agreement ____________________
10. A steady employee whom a new staff member can approach with questions and concerns ____________________
11. Things that incite or spur to action; rewards or reasons for performing a task ____________________
12. Slighting; having a negative or degrading tone ____________________
13. Able to pay all debts ____________________

Word Pool

- consensus
- credential
- solvent
- matrix
- delegate
- incentive
- cohesive
- disparaging
- mentor
- retention
- human resources file
- compliant
- rapport

ABBREVIATIONS

Write out what each of the following abbreviations stands for.

1. HR ______
2. EHR ______
3. OCR ______
4. HITECH ______
5. PHI ______
6. ePHI ______
7. OSHA ______

SKILLS AND CONCEPTS

Answer the following questions. Write your answer on the line or in the space provided.

A. Medical Office Management

1. Describe the traits of a successful medical office manager. ______

2. Describe a good relationship between a manager and their employees. ______

B. Office Management Responsibilities

1. List five office management responsibilities.

   a. ______________________________

   b. ______________________________

   c. ______________________________

   d. ______________________________

   e. ______________________________

2. Risk management involves which of the following?
   a. Identifying, planning, and implementing strategies to minimize the risk of a lawsuit
   b. Creating policies and procedures
   c. Reviewing incident reports
   d. All of the above

C. Office Management Skills

There are 5 Cs of good communication. Match the C with the correct definition.

1. _____ Get to the point and do not wonder off topic.
2. _____ Be friendly, open, and honest.
3. _____ Use terms in the right way and use proper grammar.
4. _____ Use words that accurately convey your meaning.
5. _____ Provide the same message day to day.

a. clear
b. concise
c. consistent
d. correct
e. courteous

6. Characteristics of a good listener include all of the following *except*
   a. remain nonjudgmental and neutral.
   b. do not allow for silence.
   c. use appropriate eye contact.
   d. avoid distractions.
   e. all of the above.

7. When using the ABC method of time management, a(n) ______________________ is given to the most urgent or important task, a(n) ______________________ is given to less urgent or important tasks, and a(n) ______________________ is given those tasks that are the least important.

8. When staff members collaborate as a team in the healthcare workplace, communication ______________________.

9. When communication improves in the healthcare workplace, medical errors are ______________________ and patient satisfaction ______________________.

10. Employee morale can be improved when an office manager communicates openly and honestly through
    a. staff meetings.
    b. emails.
    c. memos.
    d. all of the above.

Match the following barriers with the way to overcome them.

11. _____ Physical separation barrier
12. _____ Language barriers
13. _____ Status barriers
14. _____ Gender difference barriers
15. _____ Cultural diversity barriers

a. Know that all employees, regardless of gender, feel empowered to communicate openly with others.
b. Encourage awareness and acceptance of everyone's language and culture differences will strengthen the team's communication
c. To help the team embrace the cultural differences among the members and educating the team on the differences can help promote understanding and cohesion.
d. Using technology (e.g., videoconferencing and webcams) can help employees interact and strengthen communication.
e. Promote awareness and acceptance that everyone counts and every position on the team is important

D. Finding the Right Employee for the Job

1. Effective methods for finding new employees include which of the following?
   a. Have medical assistants complete their practicum at the healthcare facility.
   b. Advertise on the local job boards.
   c. Post the job on the facility's website and link to other job boards.
   d. All of the above
   e. Only a and c

2. Which of the following is an illegal interview question?
   a. What motivates you to succeed?
   b. Why did you leave your last job?
   c. Do you have any children?
   d. Are you willing to work more than 40 hours a week?

3. Laws that affect employment include which of the following?
   a. Fair Labor Standards Act
   b. HIPAA
   c. Occupational Safety and Health Act
   d. Only a and c
   e. All of the above

4. State standards for minimum wage and overtime pay were established in the ________________________ Act.

5. Conditions affecting employees' safety and health in the workplace were established in the ________________________ Act.

6. ________________________ Act requires employers of 50 or more employees to offer up to 12 weeks of unpaid, job-protected leave to eligible employees for the birth of a child, an adoption, or a personal or family illness.

7. Follow-up activities after the interview include checking ________________________.

E: Working with New and Established Employees

1. Documentation for new employees would include which of the following?
   a. Form I-9
   b. W-4
   c. W-2
   d. a and b

2. A critical error with new employees is failing to provide them with a fair ____________________ and ____________________.

3. One type of benefit often offered to employees, where the employer pays a percentage of the employee's health insurance ____________________ premium is ____________________.

4. When providing remote/virtual training, the employer need to keep which of the following in mind?
   a. Equipment needs
   b. Internet access
   c. Learning styles
   d. All of the above

F. Policies and Procedures

1. List five items that should be included in a personnel policy manual.

   a. ____

   b. ____

   c. ____

   d. ____

   e. ____

2. ____________________ is defined by the U.S. Equal Employment Opportunity Commission as unwelcome sexual advances, requests for sexual favors, and other verbal and physical harassment of sexual nature.

3. The act that expanded on HIPAA is ____________________.

G. Generating and Using Reports

1. ____________________ is used to generate reports used to ensure that patients are getting all of the care that they need, and that the health care facility remains healthy financially.

2. Clinical reports that can be generated include
   a. symptoms of disease/illness.
   b. medications.
   c. laboratory tests.
   d. encounter summary.
   e. all of the above

3. ____________________ are used to make administrative decisions within a healthcare facility.

4. Part of ________________________ is when the practice management software uses claim scrubbers to evaluate the data entered for claim submission.

5. The process of extracting usable data from a larger set of raw data is referred to as ________________________.

CERTIFICATION PREPARATION

Circle the correct answer.

1. Which is a quality of an effective leader or office manager?
   a. Has a sense of fairness
   b. Has good communication skills
   c. Uses good judgment
   d. All of the above

2. Something that spurs an individual to action or rewards an individual for performing a task is called
   a. morale.
   b. incentive.
   c. appraisal.
   d. circumvention.

3. Which of the following protects the employee against unsafe workplaces?
   a. Fair Labor Standards Act
   b. Family and Medical Leave Act
   c. Occupational Safety and Health Act
   d. Age Discrimination Act

4. Some managers assign a person to assist new employees during the initial probationary period; this person is called a
   a. mentor.
   b. supervisor.
   c. coworker.
   d. subordinate.

5. A group of employees who stick together during difficult times could be called
   a. cohesive.
   b. adaptive.
   c. affable.
   d. meticulous.

6. Which subjects *cannot* be discussed in a job interview?
   a. Religion
   b. Work history
   c. Previous terminations of employment
   d. None of the above

7. The process of inciting a person to some action or behavior is called
   a. a reprimand.
   b. motivation.
   c. circumvention.
   d. an appraisal.

8. Which is a strong method of improving employee morale and encouraging outstanding performance?
   a. Incentives
   b. Recognition
   c. Fraternizing with subordinates outside work
   d. All of the above

9. Which is critical for good communication and smooth operation of a medical facility?
   a. Scheduling activities that involve the families of employees
   b. Holding regular staff meetings and sending regular emails and memos
   c. Shielding employees from negative information
   d. All of the above

10. Which employee behavior is grounds for immediate dismissal without warning?
    a. Embezzlement
    b. Insubordination
    c. Violation of patient confidentiality
    d. All of the above

WORKPLACE APPLICATIONS

1. Create a job description or job posting for a "dream" job of your choice. Make sure to include the duties, required education, and other details typically found in postings.

2. Create a plan of how to screen applications and résumés for a medical assistant job in a family practice department. Describe the process you would use to evidentially identify the few applicants who should be interviewed.

INTERNET ACTIVITIES

1. Using online resources, research team-building exercises designed to promote and build teamwork for a group of employees. Create a poster presentation, a PowerPoint presentation, or write a paper summarizing your research. Include the following points in your project:
   a. Describe three team-building activities.
   b. Why do you think each of these activities will promote and build teamwork?
   c. How would you make sure that these activities are relevant to working in healthcare?

2. Using online resources, research the I-9 form. Create a poster presentation, a PowerPoint presentation, or write a paper summarizing your research. Include the following points in your project:
   a. Describe the purpose of the form.
   b. Summarize the process for completing the I-9 form.
   c. Describe acceptable documentation used to complete the form.

Student Name____ Date____________________

Medical Emergencies

chapter 21

CAAHEP Competencies	Assessment
I.C.10.a. Identify the classification of medication, including: indication for use	Skills and Concepts – C. 9-18; Internet Activity – 3
I.C.10.b. Identify the classification of medication, including: desired effect	Skills and Concepts – C. 9-18; Internet Activity – 3
I.C.10.c. Identify the classification of medication, including: side effects	Internet Activity – 3
I.C.10.d. Identify the classification of medication, including: adverse reaction	Internet Activity – 3
I.C.12. Identify basic principles of first aid	Skills and Concepts – D. 2, 7, E. 7, 9-10, F. 8, G. 1-3, H. 6, 12, J. 2
XII.C.2.d. Identify safety techniques that can be used in responding to accidental exposure to: chemicals	Skills and Concepts – E. 10
I.P.13.a. Perform first aid procedures for: bleeding	Procedure 21.5
I.P.13.b. Perform first aid procedures for: diabetic coma or insulin shock	Procedure 21.1
I.P.13.c. Perform first aid procedures for: stroke	Procedure 21.3
I.P.13.d. Perform first aid procedures for: seizures	Procedure 21.3
I.P.13.e. Perform first aid procedures for: environmental emergency	Procedure 21.1
I.P.13.f. Perform first aid procedures for: syncope	Procedure 21.5
X.P.3. Document patient care accurately in the medical record	Procedures 21.1 to 21.6
A.1. Demonstrate critical thinking skills	Procedure 21.2

ABHES Competencies	Assessment
8. Clinical Procedures g. Recognize and respond to medical office emergencies	Procedures 21.1 through 21.7

VOCABULARY REVIEW

Using the word pool on the right, find the correct word to match the definition. Write the word on the line after the definition.

1. A self-refilling bag-valve-mask unit used for artificial respiration that is effective for ventilating and oxygenating intubated patients
____
2. Open _______________
3. A term used in healthcare settings to indicate an emergency situation and summon the trained team to the scene
____
4. Route for delivery of fluids and medications through a needle inserted into the marrow of certain bones
____
5. A patient without an appointment _______________
6. Tissue death _______________
7. Contraction of the muscles causing the narrowing of the inside tube of the vessel _______________
8. The application of manual chest compressions and ventilations to patients who are not breathing or do not have a pulse
____
9. Itching _______________
10. A position on the person's side that helps to keep the airway open and clear _______________

Word Pool

- Ambu bag
- cardiopulmonary resuscitation (CPR)
- code
- intraosseous
- necrosis
- patent
- pruritus
- recovery position
- vasoconstriction
- walk-in patient

ABBREVIATIONS

Write out what each of the following abbreviations stands for.

1. CPR _______________
2. ET _______________
3. LPN _______________
4. RN _______________
5. IV _______________
6. AED _______________
7. PPE _______________
8. %TBSA _______________
9. IM _______________
10. RICE _______________
11. CVA _______________
12. ED _______________

13. MI ______________________________

14. EAP ______________________________

15. POTS ______________________________

SKILLS AND CONCEPTS

Answer the following questions.

A. Emergencies In Healthcare Settings

Fill in the blank.

1. The medical assistant must follow the facility's ______________________ and they cannot assess the patient or give advice.

2. To sort out and classify the injured is called ______________________.

3. A written flow map to make triage decisions is called a(n) ______________________.

B. Roles and Documentation in Code Situations

Fill in the blank or select the correct answer.

1. A number of emergency procedures needed to ensure a person's immediate survival is called ______________________.

2. What procedures are included with basic life support?
   a. Cardiopulmonary resuscitation
   b. Controlling bleeding
   c. Treatment of shock and poisoning
   d. Stabilization of injuries and basic first aid
   e. All of the above

3. Which of the following activities can the medical assistant do in a code situation?
   a. Order treatments and procedures.
   b. Perform CPR and assist with treatments and procedures.
   c. Call 911 when the provider indicates it is needed.
   d. All of the above.
   e. Both b and c.

4. The documentation during a code will provide evidence that the ______________________ was met in the treatments given to the patient.

C. Emergency Equipment and Supplies

Fill in the blank or select the correct answer.

1. A(n) ______________________ is a rolling supply cart that contains emergency equipment.

2. The crash cart should be checked ______________________ by the supervisor or by two qualified employees.

3. Life-saving maneuver to resuscitate a person who has stopped breathing is called ______________________.

4. A device used to deliver a rescue breath is called a(n) ____________________________.

5. A soft flexible tube that is inserted in the nose and provides a patent airway is called a(n) ____________________________.

6. A catheter that is inserted into the trachea through the mouth and provides a patent airway is called a(n) ____________________________.

7. What equipment and supplies are needed when a provider performs an endotracheal tube intubation?
   a. Laryngoscope with either a curved (MacIntosh) or straight (Miller) blade
   b. ET tube in the appropriate size and stylet
   c. Ambu-bag
   d. Stethoscope
   e. All of the above

8. A(n) ____________________________ is a device that delivers an electrical shock to the heart muscle in an attempt to restore a normal heartbeat.

Match the desired effect and indication for use with the correct medication.

9. _____ Increases the stimulation of the heart muscle and is used to treat hypotension and heart failure.
10. _____ Blocks or reverses the opioid medication effects and is used for opioid overdose.
11. _____ An antihistamine that reduces the effects of histamine and is used to treat allergic reactions.
12. _____ Hormone that stimulates the liver to release glucose into the blood and is used to treat hypoglycemia.
13. _____ Increases the heart rate and is used to treat bradycardia.
14. _____ Increases the stimulation of the heart muscle and is also a vasoconstrictor and bronchial relaxant; used to treat anaphylaxis, cardiac arrest, severe asthma, and bronchospasms.
15. _____ A vasodilator that is used for congestive heart failure and angina.
16. _____ Slows the heart rate and allows blood to fill the ventricular chambers; treats ventricular tachycardia and ventricular fibrillation.
17. _____ Affects the chemicals in the brain and is used to treat seizures and agitation.
18. _____ Helps restore the regular heart rhythm and is used to treat ventricular arrhythmias.

a. amiodarone
b. atropine
c. diazepam
d. diphenhydramine
e. dopamine
f. epinephrine
g. glucagon
h. lidocaine
i. naloxone
j. nitroglycerin

D. Temperature-Related Emergencies

Fill in the blank or select the correct answer.

1. ____________________________ is caused by exposure to cold temperatures and the person may experience a pins-and-needles sensation followed by numbness in the affected area.

2. What is *not* a first aid procedure for frostbite?
   a. Move the person to a warmer location.
   b. Remove all wet clothing and cover with warm dry clothing.
   c. Observe for signs of hypothermia.
   d. Give the person alcohol to warm them quickly.

3. Which is *not* a sign or symptom of hypothermia?
   a. The core body temperature drops below 96° F
   b. Weak pulse, and slow, shallow breathing
   c. Clumsiness and slurred speech
   d. Drowsiness, confusion, and a loss of consciousness

4. Which of the following is *not* a risk factor for heat injuries?
   a. Dehydration, heart disease, and poor blood circulation
   b. Fever and sunburn
   c. Middle-aged and older adults
   d. Using alcohol and taking antidepressants, anticonvulsants, antipsychotics, and diuretics

5. ______________________________ is a mild heat-related illness that causes muscle pain and spasms in the abdomen, arms, and legs due to electrolyte imbalance.

6. Which is *not* a sign or symptom of heat exhaustion?
   a. Heavy sweating, muscle cramps, nausea, and vomiting
   b. Red, hot, dry skin
   c. Fast, weak pulse and fast, shallow respirations
   d. Tiredness, weakness, dizziness, headache, and fainting

7. Which is *not* a first aid procedure for heat stroke?
   a. Move the person to a shady or air-conditioned area.
   b. Spray or sponge down the person with cool water.
   c. Drink cool sports beverages.
   d. Seek medical attention immediately.

E. Other Environmental Emergencies

Match the description with the type of burn. Answers can be used more than once.

1. _____ Damage to the epidermis and part of the dermis; also called *partial-thickness burn*.
2. _____ Damage to the epidermis, dermis, and subcutaneous tissue; also called *full-thickness burn*.
3. _____ Damage to the epidermis; also called *superficial burn*.
4. _____ Burned area is red and tender; no scar development occurs.
5. _____ Burned area is not painful. Skin appears deep red, pale gray, brown, or black; scar formation is likely.
6. _____ Burned area is red and painful. Blisters may occur and a scar may develop.

a. first-degree burn
b. second-degree burn
c. third-degree burn

Fill in the blank or select the correct answer.

7. For minor burns, seek immediate medical attention and do not remove burned clothing stuck to the skin. For minor burns, soak area in ice water for at least 5 minutes.
   a. Both sentences are correct.
   b. Both sentences are incorrect.
   c. The first sentence is correct, and the second sentence is incorrect.
   d. The first sentence is incorrect, and the second sentence is correct.

8. Which is a sign or symptoms of poisonings?
   a. Bluish lips, cough, and difficulty breathing
   b. Heart palpitations and chest pain
   c. Nausea, vomiting, and abdominal pain
   d. Numbness, tingling, dizziness, weakness, double vision, drowsiness, irritability, and headache
   e. All of the above

9. First aid for poisonings includes checking and monitoring the person's airway, breathing, and pulse. First aid for poisoning also includes ensuring the person vomits the substance.
   a. Both sentences are correct.
   b. Both sentences are incorrect.
   c. The first sentence is correct, and the second sentence is incorrect.
   d. The first sentence is incorrect, and the second sentence is correct.

10. First aid for chemical exposure includes
    a. if the chemical is on the person's clothing, the clothing should be removed.
    b. if the chemical is airborne, bring the person to fresh air.
    c. for chemical exposures of the eye, flush the eye with cool water for 15 minutes while protecting the other eye from an accidental exposure.
    d. all of the above.

11. ______________________________ is a severe allergic reaction that can be life-threatening.

12. Epinephrine administered IM into the ______________________________ absorbs quicker than other sites.

13. A(n) ______________________________ vaccine booster maybe updated after a dirty or deep animal bite or a foreign body in the eye.

14. First aid for a foreign body in the eye is ______________________________.

F. Diabetic Emergencies

Fill in the blank or select the correct answer.

1. ______________________________ is severe hyperglycemia.

2. What causes hyperglycemia?
   a. Took too little insulin
   b. Ate too many carbohydrates
   c. Illness, trauma, or surgery
   d. Using an illegal drug
   e. All of the above

3. Signs and symptoms of hyperglycemia include
   a. very dry mouth, thirst, and frequent urination.
   b. nausea, vomiting, hunger, and stomach pain.
   c. fatigue, rapid pulse, and shortness of breath.
   d. all of the above.

4. IV fluids and insulin are used to treat ___________________________.

5. Severe hypoglycemia is called ___________________________.

6. What causes hypoglycemia?
   a. Took too little of insulin
   b. Ate too few carbohydrates
   c. Drank alcohol
   d. All of the above
   e. Both a and c

7. Signs and symptoms of hypoglycemia include
   a. double or blurry vision.
   b. fast pulse, palpitations.
   c. irritable, aggressive, nervous, headache, and unclear thinking.
   d. shaking, tired, hunger, sweaty, and cold skin.
   e. all of the above.

8. What is used to treat hypoglycemia?
   a. 6 ounces of fruit juice or regular soda
   b. 3 glucose tablets
   c. All of the above

G. Musculoskeletal Emergencies

Fill in the blank or select the correct answer.

1. Which is a first aid step for musculoskeletal emergencies?
   a. Elevate the legs of a person going into shock.
   b. Apply pressure to a bleeding wound with a clean cloth or sterile bandage.
   c. Immobilize the injured area.
   d. All of the above

2. To reduce or limit swelling, apply a(n) ___________________________ to the area.

3. Splint the body part in the position it is in and do not attempt to readjust the area or straighten it. Check the injured area for swelling, paleness, or numbness, which may indicate the ties are too tight.
   a. Both sentences are correct.
   b. Both sentences are incorrect.
   c. The first sentence is correct, and the second sentence is incorrect.
   d. The first sentence is incorrect, and the second sentence is correct.

H. Neurologic Emergencies

Fill in the blank or select the correct answer.

1. ___________________________ is a false sensation that you or your environment is spinning or moving.

2. A(n) ____________________________ is a traumatic brain injury caused by a blow to the head.

3. Signs and symptoms of a concussion include
   a. headache and temporary loss of consciousness right after the incident.
   b. confusion, amnesia, disorientation, irritability, and personality changes.
   c. nausea and vomiting.
   d. listlessness, tiredness, and concentration and memory problems.
   e. all of the above.

4. A(n) ____________________________ is a sudden increase of electrical activity in one or more parts of the brain and ____________________________ is a disorder that causes recurring seizures.

5. It is a medical emergency if the seizure lasts longer than _____ minutes or if a person has multiple seizures without becoming conscious between them.

6. What is the first aid for seizures?
   a. Place the person in the recovery position.
   b. Note the time the seizure began.
   c. Monitor the person's breathing and pulse.
   d. Protect the patient from harm.
   e. All of the above.

Match the description with the correct type of stroke.

7. _____ Occurs when an artery in the brain leaks or ruptures.
8. _____ A blood clot forms in an artery, blocking the blood flow to part of the brain.
9. _____ A blood clot or other debris forms elsewhere in the body and moves into the brain arteries, blocking the blood flow.
10. _____ Occurs when the arterial blood flow to part of the brain is blocked.

a. ischemic stroke
b. thrombotic stroke
c. embolic stroke
d. hemorrhagic stroke

Fill in the blank or select the correct answer.

11. Which are signs or symptoms of a stroke?
    a. Confusion, sudden severe headache, and speech problems
    b. Numbness of the face, arm, or leg
    c. Facial drooping or visual changes
    d. Trouble walking and lack of coordination or balance
    e. All of the above

12. First aid for stroke-type symptoms involves getting help (calling 911) immediately. There is a small window of time during which clot-dissolving medications can be given to help the body break down the clot that is blocking the artery.
    a. Both sentences are correct.
    b. Both sentences are incorrect.
    c. The first sentence is correct, and the second sentence is incorrect.
    d. The first sentence is incorrect, and the second sentence is correct.

I. Respiratory Emergencies

Fill in the blank or select the correct answer.

1. ____________________________, or over-breathing, is rapid and deep breathing.

2. Wheezing, breathlessness, chest tightness, and coughing are signs and symptoms of ____________________________.

3. ____________________________ inhalers, such as albuterol, will lessen an asthma attack within minutes.

4. Which is a sign of a total airway obstruction?
   a. Labored, noisy, or gasping breathing
   b. Stating they are choking
   c. Bluish skin color
   d. All of the above
   e. Both a and c

J. Cardiovascular Emergencies

Fill in the blank or select the correct answer.

1. ____________________________ means fainting, passing out, or having a temporary loss of consciousness.

2. Which is a first aid step for bleeding?
   a. Lower the bleeding extremity below the heart level.
   b. Hold direct pressure over the site and remove the initial gauze every 5 minutes to check the bleeding.
   c. All of the above.
   d. None of the above.

Match the description with the correct type of shock.

3. _____ Caused by a severe allergic reaction; blood pressure drops and the airway narrows.
4. _____ Due to a central nervous system injury and leads to vasodilation (not enough blood can return to the heart) and low blood pressure
5. _____ Due to heart muscle damage caused by a myocardial infarction
6. _____ Due to heavy bleeding or dehydration
7. _____ Caused by a severe infection that affects the functioning of vital organs.

a. cardiogenic shock
b. hypovolemic shock
c. anaphylactic shock
d. septic shock
e. neurogenic shock

Select the correct answer.

8. The most common symptom(s) of myocardial infarction include
   a. angina pectoris.
   b. cold sweats.
   c. heartburn.
   d. all of the above.

9. Which medication is used for myocardial infarction?
   a. Epinephrine
   b. Nitroglycerin
   c. Aspirin
   d. All of the above
   e. Both b and c

CERTIFICATION PREPARATION

Circle the correct answer.

1. What is considered a mild heat-related illness that causes muscle pains and spasms due to electrolyte imbalance?
   a. Heat stroke
   b. Heat exhaustion
   c. Heat cramps
   d. Hypothermia

2. What is considered a partial-thickness burn?
   a. First-degree burn
   b. Second-degree burn
   c. Third-degree burn
   d. Fourth-degree burn

3. Which type of burn causes erythema, tenderness, and physical sensitivity, but no scar development occurs?
   a. First-degree burn
   b. Second-degree burn
   c. Third-degree burn
   d. Fourth-degree burn

4. An adult has burns on his back, left arm and hand, and left foot and leg. Using the Rule of Nines, estimate the percentage of total burn surface area.
   a. 18%
   b. 27%
   c. 36%
   d. 45%

5. Which animal is *not* a common carrier of rabies?
   a. Guinea pig
   b. Raccoon
   c. Bat
   d. Fox

6. What is a symptom of a concussion?
   a. Confusion and amnesia
   b. Ringing in the ears
   c. Temporary loss of consciousness right after the incident
   d. All of the above

7. What is a symptom of a cerebrovascular accident?
   a. Confusion and speech difficulty
   b. Numbness of the face, arm, or leg
   c. Problem seeing in one or both eyes
   d. All of the above

8. What is *not* a sign of a partial airway obstruction?
   a. Forceful or weak coughing
   b. Bluish skin color
   c. Labored, noisy, or gasping breathing
   d. Panicked appearance, extreme anxiety, or agitation

9. What is a possible cause of syncope?
   a. Dehydration
   b. Standing up too quickly
   c. Drop in blood glucose
   d. All of the above

10. What is *not* a typical symptom of shock?
    a. Anxiety and agitation
    b. Chest pain
    c. Nausea
    d. Diaphoresis

WORKPLACE APPLICATIONS

1. A medical assistant suspects a patient is starting to have an allergic reaction. What should the medical assistant do? What will the provider order? How should the medication be administered?

____

____

____

2. Gabe was rooming Mr. Smith, who stated, "I think I am having a heart attack." What are the common symptoms of a myocardial infarction (MI)?

____

____

____

3. Dr. Walden ordered nitroglycerin for Mr. Smith. How does nitroglycerin work in the body? _______________

____

____

____

INTERNET ACTIVITIES

1. Using online resources, research one of the following conditions: seizures, cerebrovascular accident, asthmatic attack, and MI. Create a poster presentation, a PowerPoint presentation, or write a paper summarizing your research. Include the following points in your project:
   a. Description of the condition
   b. Etiology
   c. Signs and symptoms
   d. Diagnostic procedures
   e. Treatments
2. Using online resources, research a condition listed in #1. Create a patient education flyer based on your research. Include the following points in your flyer:
   a. Description of the condition
   b. Risks factors
   c. Warning signs and symptoms
   d. Actions the individual should take when experiencing the signs and symptoms
3. Research the following medications: diphenhydramine, epinephrine, glucagon, naloxone, and nitroglycerin. Using a reliable online drug resource, identify for each medication:
   a. Indication for use
   b. Desired effects
   c. Side effects
   d. Adverse reactions

   Write a short paper addressing each of these four areas for each medication.

Procedure 21.1 Provide First Aid for a Patient with an Environmental Emergency and Insulin Shock

Name ______________________ **Date** __________ **Score** __________

Task: Provide first aid to an individual who has a dog bite and hypoglycemia.

Background Information: For someone with hypoglycemic symptoms, test the blood glucose level. If the blood glucose is under 70 and the patient is conscious and able to swallow, give 4 ounces of fruit juice or regular soda or 3 glucose tablets. Test the blood glucose in 15 minutes. Continue with these steps until the glucose level is 70 or above.

Scenario: You are working with Dr. Martin, a family practice provider. Maude Crawford (date of birth [DOB} 12/22/19XX) is being seen for a dog bite on her left arm. The wound is still bleeding.

Directions: Role-play the scenario with a peer, who will be the patient, and you are the medical assistant.

Equipment and Supplies:
- Gloves and sterile gauze
- Sugary drink (4 oz. fruit juice or regular soda) or three glucose tablets
- Patient's health record

Standard: Complete the procedure and all critical steps in _______ minutes with a minimum score of 85% within two attempts (*or as indicated by the instructor*).

Scoring: Divide the points earned by the total possible points. Failure to perform a critical step, indicated by an asterisk (*), results in grade no higher than an 84% (*or as indicated by the instructor*).

Time: Began_________ Ended_________ Total minutes: _________

Steps:	Point Value	Attempt 1	Attempt 2
1. Wash hands or use hand sanitizer.	5		
2. Greet the patient. Identify yourself. Verify the patient's identity with full name and date of birth.	15		
3. Apply gloves. Place sterile gauze over the wound and apply direct pressure to control the bleeding.	20*		
4. Identify when the patient had her last tetanus booster.	10		
Scenario update: Mrs. Crawford has diabetes and states that she thinks she has low blood sugar. She has blurry vision, tremors, and a headache. She asks you for something to eat. According to the facility's policy, you check her blood glucose level, and it is 48 mg/dL. 5. Obtain a sugary drink or glucose tablets. Indicate how much to give to the patient.	20*		
Scenario update: After 15 minutes, her blood glucose level is 59 mg/dL. You notify the provider while a coworker stays with the patient. 6. Describe follow-up care for the patient. (See the background information.)	20		

Scenario update: After 15 minutes, her blood glucose level is 82 mg/dL. You notify the provider. 7. Document the situation in the patient's health record. Include the blood glucose levels, your actions, the provider who was notified, and the patient's response.	**10**		
Total Points	**100**		

Documentation

Comments

CAAHEP Competencies	Step(s)
I.P.13.b. Perform first aid procedures for: diabetic coma or insulin shock	5-6
I.P.13.e. Perform first aid procedures for: environmental emergency	3-4
X.P.3. Document patient care accurately in the medical record	7
ABHES Competencies	**Step(s)**
8. g. Recognize and respond to medical office emergencies	Entire procedure

Procedure 21.2 Incorporate Critical Thinking Skills When Performing Patient Assessment

Name ______________________________ **Date** ____________ **Score** __________

Task: Use critical thinking skills while performing a patient assessment regarding a neurologic emergency.

Scenario: You are working with Dr. Martin, a family practice provider. Maude Crawford's daughter calls concerned about her mother. The daughter stated that Maude Crawford (DOB 12/22/19XX) fell and hit her head.

Directions: Role-play the scenario with a peer. The peer will be the daughter, and you will be the medical assistant. The peer can make up information regarding the scenario. Your instructor will be the provider.

WMFM Clinic – Neurologic Emergency Phone Protocol:

Obtain the patient's name, date of birth, signs/symptoms, and the history of the situation. After call, document situation, symptoms, and action in the patient's health record.

If a patient reports the following neurologic concerns, send the patient to the emergency department via the ambulance immediately.

- Seizure or seizure like symptoms lasting 3 or more minutes
- Passing out or fainting; dizziness or weakness that does not go away
- Sudden or unusual headache that starts suddenly
- Unable to see or speak, sudden confusion
- Neck or spine injury
- Injuries that cause loss of feeling or inability to move
- Head injury with passing out, fainting, or confusion
- Facial drooping or sudden speech difficulties or visual problems

If a patient reports the following concerns, schedule a visit for the same day. If no appointments are available, consult the triage nurse or the provider regarding the situation.

- Headache/migraine
- Nonemergent neurologic concern such as muscle stiffness or rigidity that is progressively getting worse, insomnia, or a history of blurry or double vision.

Equipment and Supplies:

- Patient's health record
- Paper and pen
- Emergency Phone Protocol for clinic

Standard: Complete the procedure and all critical steps in _______ minutes with a minimum score of 85% within two attempts (*or as indicated by the instructor*).

Scoring: Divide the points earned by the total possible points. Failure to perform a critical step, indicated by an asterisk (*), results in grade no higher than an 84% (*or as indicated by the instructor*).

Time: Began________ Ended________ Total minutes: ________

Steps:	Point Value	Attempt 1	Attempt 2
1. Obtain the patient's name and date of birth.	20*		
2. Using critical thinking skills, ask appropriate questions to obtain information about the patient's condition. Write down the patient's issues or concerns or the situation. *(Refer to the Affective Behaviors Checklist – Critical Thinking and the Grading Rubric)*	20		
Scenario update: The daughter stated that Maude was "knocked out" for about a minute. She has been acting differently since the fall. You need to follow the Neurological Emergency Phone Protocol. 3. Complete the protocol and determine what actions to take using critical thinking skills. *(Refer to the Affective Behaviors Checklist – Critical Thinking and the Grading Rubric)*	20		
4. Instruct the caller on what should be done based on the protocol. Talk with the provider if needed.	20*		
5. Document the call in the patient's health record. Include the caller's name, the patient's condition (e.g., signs, symptoms, and concerns), name of the protocol used, information given to the caller, and the provider who was notified.	20*		
Total Points	100		

Affective Behavior	Affective Behaviors Checklist **Directions:** *Check behaviors observed during the role-play.*					
	Negative, Unprofessional Behaviors	**Attempt**		**Positive, Professional Behaviors**	**Attempt**	
		1	**2**		**1**	**2**
Critical Thinking	Coached or told of an issue or problem			Independently identified the problem or issue		
	Failed to ask relevant questions related to the condition			Asked appropriate questions to obtain the information required		
	Failed to consider alternatives; failed to ask questions that demonstrated understanding of principles/concepts			Willing to consider other alternatives; asked appropriate questions that showed understanding of principles/concepts		
	Failed to make an educated, logical judgment/decision; actions or lack of actions demonstrated unsafe practices and/or did not follow the protocol			Made an educated, logical judgment/decision based on the protocol; actions reflected principles of safe practice		
	Other:			Other:		

Grading Rubric for the Affective Behaviors Checklist **Directions:** *Based on checklist results, identify the points received for the procedure checklist. Indicate how the behaviors demonstrated met the expectations.*		**Points for Procedure Checklist**	**Attempt 1**	**Attempt 2**
Does not meet Expectation	• Response fails to show critical thinking. • Student demonstrated more than 2 negative, unprofessional behaviors during the interaction.	0		
Needs Improvement	• Response fails to show critical thinking. • Student demonstrated 1 or 2 negative, unprofessional behaviors during the interaction.	0		
Meets Expectation	• Response demonstrates critical thinking; no negative, unprofessional behaviors observed. • More practice is needed for behavior to appear natural and for student to appear comfortable and at ease.	20		
Occasionally Exceeds Expectation	• Response demonstrates critical thinking; no negative, unprofessional behaviors observed. • At times student appeared comfortable and at ease; but more practice is needed for behavior to become natural and consistent with a professional medical assistant.	20		
Always Exceeds Expectation	• Response demonstrates critical thinking; no negative, unprofessional behaviors observed. • Student's behaviors appeared natural and comfortable. Behaviors are consistent with a professional medical assistant.	20		

Documentation

Comments

CAAHEP Competencies	Step(s)
X.P.3. Document patient care accurately in the medical record	5
A.1. Demonstrate critical thinking skills	3
ABHES Competencies	**Step(s)**
8.g. Recognize and respond to medical office emergencies	Entire procedure

Procedure 21.3 Provide First Aid for a Patient With a Stroke and Seizure Activity

Name ______________________________ **Date** ____________ **Score** __________

Tasks: Provide first aid to an individual having a stroke and seizure activity. Document care in the health record.

Scenario: You are working with Dr. Martin, a family practice provider. Walter Biller (DOB 1/4/19XX) arrives for his appointment.

Directions: Role-play the scenario with a peer, who will be the patient, and you are the medical assistant.

Equipment and Supplies:
- Watch, stethoscope, and sphygmomanometer
- Folded towel, blanket, or coat
- Patient's health record
- Gloves and other personal protective equipment (as required)

Standard: Complete the procedure and all critical steps in _______ minutes with a minimum score of 85% within two attempts (*or as indicated by the instructor*).

Scoring: Divide the points earned by the total possible points. Failure to perform a critical step, indicated by an asterisk (*), results in grade no higher than an 84% (*or as indicated by the instructor*).

Time: Began_________ Ended_________ Total minutes: _________

Steps:	**Point Value**	**Attempt 1**	**Attempt 2**
1. Wash hands or use hand sanitizer.	**5**		
2. Greet the patient. Identify yourself. Verify the patient's identity with full name and date of birth.	**5**		
Scenario update: As you room Mr. Biller, you notice that he seems to be dragging his left leg when walking, the left side of his face is drooping, and he states his left arm is weak. You suspect that he might be having a stroke. He asks for a drink of water when you get to the exam room. 3. You call for help and assist the patient onto the examination table. Place the patient in the recovery position with his head slightly raised.	**10***		
4. Monitor the patient's airway. Obtain the patient vital signs.	**10**		
5. Speak calmly to the patient. Do not give the patient anything to drink.	**10**		
Scenario update: While you are waiting for the provider, Mr. Biller starts to jerk his arms and he becomes unresponsive. 6. Keep the patient in the recovery position. Note the time when the seizure started. Gently raise the chin to tilt the head back slightly to open the airway. Yell for help if help has not arrived.	**15***		
7. Continue to monitor his pulse rate and respiration rate. Put on gloves and other personal protective equipment as needed.	**10**		
8. Clear any hard or sharp items away from the patient. Place a soft, folded towel, blanket, or coat under the patient's head.	**10**		

9. Remove the patient's glasses (if on) and loosen any constrictive clothing around the neck. Stay with the person until they are fully awake and continue to monitor the respiration and pulse rates.	**10**		
10. Document the first aid measures you provided in the order that they occurred. In addition, document the seizure activity you witnessed, the length of the episode, and the provider notified.	**15**		
Total Points	**100**		

Documentation

Comments

CAAHEP Competencies	Step(s)
I.P.13.c. Perform first aid procedures for: stroke	Entire procedure
I.P.13.d. Perform first aid procedures for: seizures	6-9
X.P.3. Document patient care accurately in the medical record	10
ABHES Competencies	**Step(s)**
8.g. Recognize and respond to medical office emergencies	Entire procedure

Procedure 21.4 Provide First Aid for a Choking Patient

Name ______________________________ **Date** ____________ **Score** __________

Tasks: Provide first aid to a conscious adult who is choking. Document it in the health record.

Scenario: You are working with Dr. Martin, a family practice provider. As you return from lunch, you notice that an adult visitor is having an issue. It appears that she had been eating fast food and now she is holding her neck with both hands. She appears to be panicking.

Directions: Role-play the scenario with a peer. The peer will be the visitor, and you will be the medical assistant.

Equipment and Supplies:
- Patient's health record
- Gloves
- Mannequin

Standard: Complete the procedure and all critical steps in _______ minutes with a minimum score of 85% within two attempts (*or as indicated by the instructor*).

Scoring: Divide the points earned by the total possible points. Failure to perform a critical step, indicated by an asterisk (*), results in grade no higher than an 84% (*or as indicated by the instructor*).

Time: Began_________ Ended_________ Total minutes: _________

Steps:	Point Value	Attempt 1	Attempt 2
1. Approach the person and ask, "Are you choking?"	10		
Scenario update: She nods her head yes and cannot speak. She is standing. 2. Yell for help. Put on gloves if available. Stand behind the victim with your feet slightly apart. Reach your arms around the person's waist.	15*		
3. Make a fist and place it just above the person's navel. Make sure your thumb side is next to the person. Grasp the fist tightly with your other hand.	15*		
Scenario update: The next steps must be done on a mannequin. 4. With the correct hand position, make quick, upward and inward thrusts with your fist. Do 5 abdominal thrusts before doing back blows.	15*		
5. Stand behind the person and wrap one arm around the person's upper body. Position the person so they are bent forward with the chest parallel to the ground.	15		
6. Use the heel of your other hand to give a firm blow between the shoulder blades. Check to see if the object dislodges. If not, continue by giving another 4 back blows.	10		
7. Continue to give 5 abdominal thrusts followed by 5 back blows until the object is dislodged or the person loses consciousness. Note: If the person faints or loses consciousness, lower the person to the floor. Call 911 (or the local emergency number) or have someone else call. Begin CPR, starting with chest compressions. Check to see if the item is in the airway. Remove it only if it is loose.	10		

Scenario update: After two sets of abdominal thrusts and back blows, the woman coughs out a piece of food. She can now talk. 8. Arrange for the person to be seen by the provider. Document the first aid measures you provided in the order that they occurred.	**10**		
Total Points	**100**		

Documentation

Comments

CAAHEP Competencies	Step(s)
X.P.3. Document patient care accurately in the medical record	8
ABHES Competencies	**Step(s)**
8.g. Recognize and respond to medical office emergencies	Entire procedure

Procedure 21.5 Provide First Aid for a Patient With a Bleeding Wound, Fracture, or Syncope

Name ______________________________ **Date** __________ **Score** __________

Tasks: Provide first aid to an individual with a suspected fracture, a bleeding wound, and syncope. Document the first aid you provide.

Scenario: You are returning from lunch and see a person fall at the entrance of the healthcare facility. He is an older man and complains of pain in his right lower arm. His arm looks deformed and is bleeding. You call for help. A provider comes, and coworkers bring supplies. The provider tells you to care for the wound and splint the arm before moving the individual. You have a coworker helping you.

Directions: Role-play the situation with two peers. One peer will be the patient and the other peer will be a coworker. You will be the medical assistant.

Equipment and Supplies:
- Gloves
- Sterile gauze
- Bandage
- Splinting material (e.g., SAM splint)
- Coban wrap or gauze roll

Standard: Complete the procedure and all critical steps in _______ minutes with a minimum score of 85% within two attempts (*or as indicated by the instructor*).

Scoring: Divide the points earned by the total possible points. Failure to perform a critical step, indicated by an asterisk (*), results in grade no higher than an 84% (*or as indicated by the instructor*).

Time: Began_________ Ended_________ Total minutes: _________

Steps:	**Point Value**	**Attempt 1**	**Attempt 2**
1. Wash your hands or use hand sanitizer if possible. Identify yourself to the patient. Obtain the patient's name and date of birth as you put on gloves.	10		
2. Using sterile gauze, apply direct pressure over the wound to stop the bleeding. Make sure to immobilize the injured arm as you apply pressure. If possible, elevate the arm to help slow the bleeding. If the blood seeps through the gauze, apply another layer of gauze on the initial one. Continue with the direct pressure until the bleeding stops.	15*		
3. Once the bleeding has stopped, cover the dressing with a bandage. Remember to immobilize the injured arm as you work.	10		
Scenario update: As you apply the bandage to the injured arm, the patient states he does not feel good. He says he feels dizzy and thinks he is going to pass out. Your peer takes over by supporting his arm, and the man faints. He is still breathing and has a pulse. 4. Position the patient on his back. Continue to check his respirations and pulse rates.	15*		
5. Loosen any constrictive clothing around the neck and chest. Raise the legs above the heart level (about 12 inches).	15*		

Scenario update: After a few minutes, he starts to come around. He jokes that blood makes him faint. As he is lying on his back talking with you, you need to splint his injured arm. 6. Use the splint material and shape it to the injured arm. Do not straighten the arm. Apply the splint beyond the joint above and the joint below the injury.	**15***		
7. Use Coban or a gauze roll to secure the splint in place. Encourage the patient to hold the injured arm against his chest as he moves.	**10***		
8. Document the first aid measures you provided in the order they occurred. Note that the provider was at the scene.	**10**		
Total Points	**100**		

Documentation

Comments

CAAHEP Competencies	Step(s)
I.P.13.a. Perform first aid procedures for: bleeding	2, 3
I.P.13.f. Perform first aid procedures for: syncope	4, 5
X.P.3. Document patient care accurately in the medical record	8
ABHES Competencies	**Step(s)**
8.g. Recognize and respond to medical office emergencies	Entire procedure

Procedure 21.6 Provide First Aid for a Patient With Shock

Name ________________________________ **Date** ____________ **Score** __________

Tasks: Provide first aid to an individual who is in shock. Document the first aid you provide.

Scenarios: You are working with Dr. Julie Walden. The administrative medical assistant at the reception desk notifies you that Robert Caudill (DOB 10/31/19XX) is here and looks very ill. You bring the patient and his wife immediately back to the procedure room because it is the only available room. He asks to move to the exam table, and you assist him as he transfers to the table. You obtain his vital signs, which are P 92, irregular, 1+; R 26, regular, shallow; BP 72/48 RA, lying; and T 103.2° F.

Directions: Role-play the scenario with two peers. One peer will be the patient and the other will be the wife. You will be the medical assistant.

Equipment and Supplies:

- Stethoscope
- Watch
- Pen
- Sphygmomanometer (blood pressure cuff)
- Pillows, blankets, or small stool to help elevate the feet
- Exam table

Standard: Complete the procedure and all critical steps in ______ minutes with a minimum score of 85% within two attempts (*or as indicated by the instructor*).

Scoring: Divide the points earned by the total possible points. Failure to perform a critical step, indicated by an asterisk (*), results in grade no higher than an 84% (*or as indicated by the instructor*).

Time: Began________ Ended________ Total minutes: ________

Steps:	**Point Value**	**Attempt 1**	**Attempt 2**
1. Call for help. Monitor the patient's breathing and pulse until the provider arrives.	**10**		
Scenario update: The provider examines the patient and suspects septic shock. You administer 2 L of oxygen per nasal cannula as the provider ordered. The triage RN inserts an IV and administers IV fluids. The provider directs another medical assistant to call 911. 2. Raise the patient's legs 12 inches.	**15***		
3. Make sure the patient's head is flat on the bed.	**10***		
4. Loosen the person's clothing. Make sure the clothing does not restrict the neck and chest area.	**15***		
5. Obtain a pulse rate, respiration rate, and blood pressure. Continue to monitor the patient's airway, pulse rate, and respiration rate.	**15**		
6. While monitoring the patient, speak calmly with him. Use a gentle tone of voice. Demonstrate calming body language (e.g., do not appear scared, rushed, or out of control).	**15**		
7. Talk calmly with the patient's wife and explain what is occurring. Answer any questions the wife may have.	**10**		

8. Document the first aid measures you provided in the order they occurred. Indicate which provider examined the patient. In addition, document the administration of oxygen and the vital signs obtained.	**10**		
Total Points	**100**		

Documentation

Comments

CAAHEP Competencies	Step(s)
X.P.3. Document patient care accurately in the medical record	8
ABHES Competencies	**Step(s)**
8.g. Recognize and respond to medical office emergencies	Entire procedure

Procedure 21.7 Provide Rescue Breathing, Cardiopulmonary Resuscitation (CPR), and Automated External Defibrillator (AED)

Name ______________________________ **Date** __________ **Score** ________

Tasks: Perform rescue breathing and CPR. Use the AED machine.

Scenario: You are in the healthcare facility parking lot and find a person on the ground. No one is around.

Directions: Role-play the scenario with a peer. Your peer will be the person on the ground. You will be the medical assistant.

Equipment and Supplies:
- AED machine with adult pads
- Barrier ventilation device
- Mannequin
- Gloves (if available)

Standard: Complete the procedure and all critical steps in _______ minutes with a minimum score of 85% within two attempts (*or as indicated by the instructor*).

Scoring: Divide the points earned by the total possible points. Failure to perform a critical step, indicated by an asterisk (*), results in grade no higher than an 84% (*or as indicated by the instructor*).

Time: Began_________ Ended_________ Total minutes: _________

Steps:	**Point Value**	**Attempt 1**	**Attempt 2**
1. Check the scene for safety. Is it safe to approach and provide help to the victim?	**5**		
2. Check the person's response. Tap the individual on the shoulder and shout, "Are you all right?" Pause for a few moments for a response.	**5**		
Scenario update: There is no response from the individual. A bystander comes up and you direct that person to find an AED machine. 3. Call 911 and answer the questions from the dispatcher.	**10**		
4. Put on gloves if available. Roll the person over if the person is face down. Roll the person as an entire unit, supporting the head, neck, and back. Open the airway and assess the respirations and the pulse for 10 seconds. Note: Occasional gasping is not considered breathing. *a. Person is breathing and has a pulse*: Monitor the person until the emergency responders arrive. If needed and if no head, neck, or spinal injury is suspected, place the patient in the recovery position. *b. Person is not breathing and has a pulse*: Give 1 breath every 5-6 seconds. Check the pulse every 2 minutes. If pulse remains, continue with rescue breathing. If pulse is absent, start CPR. *c. Person is not breathing and has no pulse:* Give CPR, starting with compressions. Give 15 compressions and 2 breaths.	**20***		

Scenario update: The individual has a weak pulse and is not breathing. (Use a mannequin for the following steps.) 5. Use a barrier device if available. Pinch the person's nose and give each rescue breath over 1 second. Watch for the chest to rise. Give the appropriate amount of ventilations for the person's age. Continue to monitor the pulse as you give rescue breaths. *Note:* If the person had been choking, look in the mouth before giving a rescue breath. If you see the object, sweep it out with your finger. You can also provide nose ventilation if the mouth is injured. Stoma ventilation must be done if the person has a stoma (in the throat area).	**10***		
Scenario update: When you check the pulse again, there is no pulse. 6. Place your hands at the correct location on the chest. Bring your shoulders directly over the victim's sternum as you compress downward. Keep your elbows locked.	**10**		
7. Give 15 compressions at the appropriate depth. Give two ventilations and watch for the chest to rise. Continue with the cycle. Give approximately 100 compressions per minute to an adult.	**10***		
Scenario update: After two cycles, a bystander brings an AED but does not know how to use it. The bystander also does not know CPR. You need to stop the CPR and use the AED. 8. Turn on the AED and follow the directions. Attach the AED pads to the individual's bare dry chest. Attach the pads to the machine if required. *Note*: Make sure to remove any medication patches and medication residue from the chest before applying the pads.	**10***		
9. Have everyone stand back from the patient by announcing, "Stand clear." Push the analyze button and allow the machine to analyze the heartbeat.	**10***		
10. Follow the prompts on the AED machine. *a.* *Shock advised:* Announce, "Stand clear" and make sure no one is touching the individual. Press the shock button. After the shock, do CPR for 2 minutes, starting with compressions. Continue following the prompts until the emergency responders arrive. *b.* *Shock not advised:* Continue doing CPR for 2 minutes, starting with compressions. Continue following the prompts until the emergency responders arrive.	**10***		
Total Points	**100**		

Comments

ABHES Competencies	Step(s)
8.g. Recognize and respond to medical office emergencies	Entire procedure

Student Name____ Date____________________

Skills and Strategies

chapter **22**

CAAHEP Competencies	Assessment
X.C.9. Identify legal and illegal applicant interview questions	Skills and Concepts – K. 3-5; Certification Preparation – 7
ABHES Competencies	**Assessment**
10. Career Development a. Perform the essential requirements for employment, such as resume writing, effective interviewing, dressing professionally, time management, and following up appropriately	Procedures 22.1 through 22.6
b. Demonstrate professional behavior	Procedure 22.5
c. Explain what continuing education is and how it is acquired	Certification Preparation – 10; Internet Activities – 3

VOCABULARY REVIEW

Using the word pool on the right, find the correct word to match the definition. Write the word on the line after the definition.

1. Allowing the listener to recap and review what was said ______________________
2. Rewording a statement to check the meaning and interpretation; also shows you are listening and understanding the speaker ______________________
3. The ability to communicate and interact with others; sometimes referred to as *soft skills* ______________________
4. Websites where employers post jobs ______________________
5. Putting words to the patient's emotional reaction, which acknowledges the person's feelings ______________________
6. The act of working with another person or multiple individuals ______________________
7. Allows the listener to get additional information by explaining a specific statement or topic ______________________
8. Exchange of information among others in your field ______________________

Word Pool

- clarification
- collaboration
- compassion
- counteroffer
- dignity
- interpersonal skills
- job boards
- mock
- networking
- paraphrasing
- proofread
- reflecting
- reverse chronologic order
- skill set
- summarizing

9. The inherent worth or state of being worthy of respect
   ____
10. To have a deep awareness of another's suffering and the desire to lessen it ______________________
11. The most recent item is listed first, and the oldest item is last
   ____
12. To read and mark corrections ______________________
13. Simulated; intended for imitation or practice
   ____
14. A person's abilities, skills, or expertise in an area
   ____
15. Return offer made by one who has rejected an offer or a job
   ____

ABBREVIATIONS

Write out what each of the following abbreviations stands for.

1. CPR ______________________
2. CMA ______________________
3. BLS ______________________
4. AAMA ______________________
5. RMA ______________________
6. AMT ______________________
7. CCMA______________________
8. NHA ______________________
9. NCMA ______________________
10. NCCT ______________________
11. HIPAA ______________________
12. CMAC______________________
13. AMCA ______________________

SKILLS AND CONCEPTS

Answer the following questions. Write your answer on the line or in the space provided.

A. Understanding Personality Traits Important to Employers

Fill in the blank or select the correct answer.

1. Which traits help new employees blend with the existing staff?
   a. Collaboration and interpersonal skills
   b. Professionalism and compassion
   c. Genuine interest in the job
   d. All of the above

2. Which interpersonal skill(s) should a new employee have?
   a. Flexible and dependable
   b. Supportive of peers
   c. Remain calm under pressure
   d. All of the above

3. Effective ________________________ communication involves using clear, thoughtful, and easily understood language.

4. ________________________ communication relays more information to others than any words you could use and includes eye contact, posture, voice, and gestures.

5. Which is *not* a trait of effective nonverbal communication?
   a. Being focused, calm, and polite
   b. Being distracted and rushed
   c. Showing interest in the other person

6. For communication to be effective, ________________________ must occur and this can be shown by asking appropriate questions that can draw others into the conversation.

7. A person can demonstrate professionalism by
   a. being flexible, punctual, and honest.
   b. paying attention to details.
   c. using time-management skills.
   d. demonstrating the ability to follow directions and prioritize.
   e. all of the above.

B. Assessing Your Strengths and Skills

Fill in the blank, select the correct answer, or answer the question.

1. Describe four personality traits you have and list the "evidence" to support your claim. ________________

   ____

   ____

   ____

2. Which are *not* technical skills of a medical assistant?
   a. Phlebotomy and injections
   b. Electrocardiograms and obtaining vital signs
   c. Compassion and flexibility
   d. Software proficiency and reception duties

3. List at least four technical skills you possess and indicate where you developed each skill.____________

____

____

____

____

4. ____________________ job skills are developed in one job or experience that can be transferred to another job.

5. List at least two transferable skills that you have and indicate where you developed each skill.

____

____

C. Identifying Career Objectives and Personal Needs

Answer the question.

1. Identify career objectives for yourself.

   a. What area and skills did you enjoy in class and/or in practicum? ____________________

   ____

   b. Where do you want to be in 5 years? ____________________

   ____

   c. Where do you want to be in 10 years? ____________________

   ____

   d. What additional skills do you need to get where you want to go? ____________________

   ____

   e. Based on these answers, describe at least two goals you have for yourself. ____________________

   ____

   ____

2. Identify your personal needs by answering the following questions.

   a. Do you need a specific wage and/or benefits? If so, describe your needs. ____________________

   ____

   b. Do you need specific hours? If so, describe the hours. ____________________

   ____

   c. How far are you willing to travel? ____________________

   ____

d. Do you have a reliable mode of transportation?______________________________

____

____

D. Finding Job Openings

Match the credentialing examinations with the correct agency.

1. _____ National Certified Medical Assistant
2. _____ Certified Clinical Medical Assistant
3. _____ Certified Medical Assistant
4. _____ Clinical Medical Assistant Certification
5. _____ Registered Medical Assistant

a. American Association of Medical Assistants
b. American Medical Technologists
c. National Healthcareer Association
d. National Center for Competency Testing
e. American Medical Certification Association

Fill in the blank, select the correct answer, or answer the question.

6. ______________________ is the exchange of information among others in your field.
7. Larger healthcare facilities post job openings on their websites, and these are considered ______________________ job boards.
8. ______________________ job boards contain jobs from a variety of employers.
9. List four possible job search methods you can use in your area. These can include job boards, newspapers, and so on.

____

____

____

____

E. Developing a Resume

Fill in the blank or select the correct answer.

1. A(n) ______________________ summarizes your qualifications, education, and experience and its purpose is to "market" yourself.
2. A(n) ______________________ resume is the most popular format and focuses on the person's employment history.
3. A(n) ______________________ resume; also called a *hybrid resume,* lists a person's abilities and skill sets, along with listing the employment history.
4. A(n) ______________________ resume is customized to a unique job posting
5. What information is found in the education section on a resume?
   a. Schooling after high school
   b. Coursework completed
   c. Diplomas obtained and academic recognition
   d. Practicum information
   e. All of the above

6. What is *not* included in the work experience information on a resume?
   a. The reason you left
   b. The name of the facility and the city and state
   c. Dates in that position
   d. Title of the position held

7. For those in the workforce for a decade or more, employers want to see _____ years of employment information.

8. What information should be included for certifications?
   a. Title of the certification or license
   b. Awarding agency
   c. Expiration date
   d. All of the above

9. How should a person create a visually appealing resume?
   a. Bold only important information.
   b. Use simple bullets to help organize information.
   c. Change font size in certain areas to emphasize more important elements.
   d. Pay attention to the spacing and avoid too much "white space."
   e. All of the above.

F. Developing a Cover Letter

Fill in the blank or select the correct answer.

1. The goal of the ______________________ is to create enough interest that the reader wants to look at the resume.

2. Which strategy can be used to create a professional cover letter?
   a. Match the appearance of the cover letter and resume.
   b. Address the inside address and the salutation to a specific person.
   c. Be professional and sell yourself to the reader.
   d. Reaffirm that you are an excellent match for the job.
   e. All of the above

3. The cover letter should include the ______________________ and posting number.

G. Completing Online Profiles and Job Applications

Fill in the blank or select the correct answer.

1. What is the advantage of online profiles?
   a. An applicant completes the profile once and updates the information as needed.
   b. The employer can track the activities of applicants.
   c. The employer can easily read a person's information.
   d. The employer can advertise new postings to potential applicants whose profiles meet certain requirements.
   e. All of the above.

2. If you need to complete an application before an interview, come prepared with your information and arrive at least _____ minutes before the interview so you can complete the application.

3. What information is needed when completing an application or profile?
   a. Educational institution's name and address with dates and titles of coursework or diploma
   b. Past and present job information
   c. Certifications and credentials
   d. References
   e. All of the above

4. What information is *not* required for references?
   a. Person's name and title
   b. Email address
   c. Social media sites
   d. Contact information

5. Before using a person as a reference, they must be ______________________ and agree to be a reference.

H. Career Portfolios

Fill in the blank or select the correct answer.

1. The ______________________ is a tool that can show a potential employer that a person has the skills required for the job.

2. Which education-related documents could be included in a career portfolio?
   a. Copies of letters of recommendation
   b. Copies of transcripts, awards, and honors
   c. A list of the courses successfully completed with a short description of each course
   d. Copies of student clinical experience evaluation forms and skill document form
   e. All of the above

3. What information could be included in a career portfolio?
   a. Prior employment documents, such as letters of recommendation and employment evaluations
   b. References
   c. Certifications
   d. All of the above

I. Preparing for the Interview

Select the correct answer.

1. What should a job seeker do to prepare for an interview?
   a. Research the facility.
   b. Practice answering potential questions.
   c. Select interview attire.
   d. Prepare for the day of the interview.
   e. All of the above.

2. What should the job seeker research about the healthcare facility?
   a. Mission and value statements
   b. Size of the organization
   c. Size of the department with the open position
   d. Names and types of providers in the department
   e. All of the above

3. What should *not* be worn to an interview?
   a. A business suit
   b. Ripped jeans and flipflops
   c. Clean, wrinkle-free, and well-fitting dress pants and shirt/blouse

4. What should be brought to an interview?
   a. An interview portfolio
   b. A copy of your cover letter and resume for each interviewer
   c. A notepad and pen to take notes
   d. A list of references on resume paper and a list of questions for the interviewer
   e. All of the above

J. Types of Interviews

Fill in the blank or select the correct answer.

1. During a face-to-face interview, do not fidget and maintain good ______________________ contact.

2. Why might phone interviews be done?
   a. To screen applicants and narrow the candidate pool
   b. To provide additional information and verify that the applicant wants an interview
   c. To replace a face-to-face interview
   d. All of the above

3. When finishing a phone interview, the job seeker should ______________________ the interviewer at the end of the call.

4. The benefit of a virtual interview over a phone interview is that the interviewer can actually see the interviewee and allow the interviewer to assess the ______________________ and the ______________________ being presented.

5. When participating in a virtual interview, the camera is positioned to show your ______________________ and ______________________.

K. Professionalism During and After the Interview

Select the correct answer.

1. How should a job seeker answer a question such as "Tell me about yourself"?
   a. Inform if you are married or single
   b. Describe your hobbies and social activities
   c. Describe your career to date
   d. Detail your personal life
   e. All of the above

2. What should the job seeker do during the interview?
   a. Pause before simple, straightforward questions.
   b. Fill in silence with filler words such as "um."
   c. Be honest, and do not exaggerate experiences or length of employment.
   d. Share negative experiences about past employers.

3. Which question is considered legal during an interview?
   a. When did you move to this country?
   b. Who will look after your infant when you are at work?
   c. What medications are you taking?
   d. Can you work the weekend?
   e. All of the above.

4. Which question is considered illegal during an interview?
   a. Have you ever been arrested?
   b. Have you ever been convicted of a crime?
   c. Are you 18 or older?
   d. Are you eligible to work in this state?

5. Which question is considered legal during an interview?
   a. How old are you?
   b. Where do you attend church services?
   c. Can you perform the essential job functions with or without reasonable accommodation?
   d. Have you ever been convicted of a crime?
   e. Both c and d.

L. Improving Your Opportunities

Fill in the blank or select the correct answer.

1. When a person is not having success with the job search, what should be reevaluated?
   a. Am I being too selective?
   b. Am I looking for the correct job title?
   c. Can the geographic search area be enlarged?
   d. All of the above.

2. When a person is not getting calls for interviews, what should be reevaluated?
   a. Is the cover letter, resume, online profile, or application negatively affecting the job search?
   b. Are there spelling and grammar errors in the information?
   c. Do the cover letter and resume need to be reformatted or revised?
   d. Are the cover letter and resume customized to the job posting?
   e. All of the above

3. ______________________ interviews can help you refine your interview skills and behavior.

M. Starting and Keeping Your Job

Match the description to the correct form.

1. _____ Used to check the person's past for criminal activity and listing in sex offender database
2. _____ Required to be completed so funds can be transferred into the employee's bank account instead of the employee receiving a paper paycheck
3. _____ Completion of paperwork is required as part of the insurance enrollment activities
4. _____ Newly hired employee must sign forms related to the Health Insurance Portability and Accountability Act and computer security
5. _____ Used to verify a person's identity and employment authorization
6. _____ New hires must provide their tax status and how many withholding allowances they are claiming, which is used to withhold money from their paycheck

a. Form I-9
b. Form W-4
c. insurance benefit form
d. background check form
e. direct deposit form
f. agreement forms

Fill in the blank.

7. The purpose of the ______________________ period is to see if the new employee is the right fit for the job.
8. With _____-degree style performance appraisals, supervisors evaluate their employees based on their observations of job performance over a given time period.
9. With _____-degree style performance appraisals, supervisors gather input from your coworkers and others with whom you interact on a regular basis.
10. Always offer at least _____ weeks notice when resigning from a job, since you would want this length of notice from your employer if your job was terminated.

CERTIFICATION PREPARATION

Circle the correct answer.

1. ______ means to have a deep awareness of another's suffering and a desire to lessen it.
   a. Interpersonal skills
   b. Reflecting
   c. Compassion
   d. Dignity
2. "Communicates well" is a ______.
   a. technical skill
   b. personality trait
   c. transferable job skill
   d. both a and b
3. What is the best and most effective way to find employment?
   a. Checking job boards and newspaper ads
   b. Using the school career placement office
   c. Networking and checking job boards
   d. Using employment agencies
4. Which is the most popular type of resume that is used when people are seeking employment in the same field as their education or experience?
   a. Reverse chronologic
   b. Chronologic
   c. Combination
   d. Targeted

5. What is true regarding the header in the resume and cover letter?
   a. The information should appear on all pages of the cover letter and resume.
   b. Contains the person's name and mailing address.
   c. Contains a phone number and a professional email address.
   d. All of the above are true.

6. Which item is typically presented in a reverse chronologic order on a resume?
   a. Education information
   b. Work experience
   c. Skills
   d. Both a and b

7. What is an illegal interview question?
   a. "Are you eligible to work in this state?"
   b. "Who looks after your children when you work?"
   c. "Are you able to work 8 AM to 3 PM on the weekends?"
   d. "Have you ever been convicted of a federal offense?"

8. Form ______ is the Employee's Withholding Allowance Certificate.
   a. W-3
   b. W-2
   c. I-9
   d. W-4

9. Form ______ is the Employment Eligibility Verification Form.
   a. W-3
   b. W-2
   c. I-9
   d. W-4

10. What is the importance of continuing education for a medical assistant?
    a. Helps keep the person updated and current
    b. Needed to maintain a certification or registration
    c. Important for professional development
    d. All of the above

WORKPLACE APPLICATIONS

1. Select six interview questions from Figure 22.7 and write a response for each question. Your answer should be at least five sentences in length.

____

____

____

____

____

____

____

____

____

2. During an interview, Michelle was asked her age. Michelle knew this was not a legal interview question. If you were in this situation, how would you respond?

____

____

____

INTERNET ACTIVITIES

1. Using appropriate online resources, research one of the five national certification exams:
   - Certified Medical Assistant (CMA) through the American Association of Medical Assistants (AAMA)
   - Registered Medical Assistant (RMA) through the American Medical Technologists (AMT)
   - Medical Assistant Certification (CCMA) through the National Healthcareer Association
   - Medical Assistant (NCMA) through the National Center for Competency Testing (NCCT)
   - Clinical Medical Assistant Certification (CMAC) through the American Medical Certification Association (AMCA)

   In a PowerPoint presentation, poster, or paper, address the following points:
   a. List the credential and the sponsoring agency
   b. Describe the exam (e.g., number of questions, coverage of topics, time limit)
   c. Describe the registration process
   d. Describe the requirements for maintaining the credential (e.g., continuing education, fees, retaking the exam)

2. Using online resources, identify four potential job openings that interest you. Describe each position in a brief paper and provide the websites for the openings.

3. Using online resources, identify two resources for continuing education for medical assistants. Briefly describe the resources and list the websites.

4. Using online resources, identify 8-10 potential job postings that interest you.

Procedure 22.1 Prepare a Chronologic Resume

Name ______________________________ **Date** ____________ **Score** __________

Task: Write an effective resume for use as a tool in obtaining employment.

Equipment and Supplies:
- Computer with word processing software and a printer
- Current job posting
- Resume paper
- Paper and pen

Standard: Complete the procedure and all critical steps in _______ minutes with a minimum score of 85% within two attempts (*or as indicated by the instructor*).

Scoring: Divide the points earned by the total possible points. Failure to perform a critical step, indicated by an asterisk (*), results in grade no higher than an 84% (*or as indicated by the instructor*).

Time: Began_________ Ended_________ Total minutes: _________

Steps:	Point Value	Attempt 1	Attempt 2
1. Apply critical thinking skills as you create a list of the personality traits (wanted by employers), technical skills, and transfer job skills that you possess. Also write down your career goal(s).	5		
2. Using the current job posting, identify the required and recommended qualifications and credentials needed for the position.	10		
3. Using the computer with word processing software, create a professional-looking header for your document. Include your name, address, telephone number(s), and email address. Select an appropriate font style for your name and a smaller font size for your contact information.	10		
4. Create a section header for "Education." For the learning institution(s) you attended, list the school's name, city and state, degree obtained or coursework successfully completed, and the year. Include any additional educational information, such as awards and the student clinical experience information.	10		
5. Create a section header for "Healthcare Experience" and/or "Work Experience." Provide details about your work experience, including the facility's name, city and state, title of your position, start and end date (month and year), and job duties. The job duties must start with an active verb using the appropriate tense (e.g., a past job would have past tense verbs and a current job would include present tense verbs).	10		
6. Create a section header for "Special Skills," and list your special language skills, computer proficiencies, and other unique skills you possess that relate to the position.	10		
7. Create a section header for "Certifications and Credentials," and list the active credentials and certifications you have. Include the title of the certification, awarding agency, and the expiration date. *Note:* You may want to consider adding the date you are taking a credentialing examination. Employers like to know the status of your credentialing examination.	10		

8. All information on the resume needs to appear in reverse chronologic order (i.e., newest information is listed first). Work experiences should include both the start and end month and year.	**10**		
9. The resume needs to look professional and interesting. Use font styles (e.g., bold, underline, italic) to emphasize important words and phrases. Use professional-looking bullets to list job duties and other information. Use the key words from the posting throughout the resume.	**15***		
10. Proofread the resume. Correct any spelling, grammar, punctuation, or sentence structure errors you find. If time allows, have another person review your resume, and use the feedback to revise it.	**5**		
11. Print the resume on resume paper, and proofread it one final time. Any errors should be corrected and the document should be reprinted or emailed to the instructor.	**5**		
Total Points	**100**		

Comments

ABHES Competencies	Step(s)
10. Career Development a. Perform the essential requirements for employment, such as resume writing, effective interviewing, dressing professionally, time management, and following up appropriately	Entire procedure

Procedure 22.2 Create a Cover Letter

Name ______________________________ **Date** ____________ **Score** __________

Task: Write an effective cover letter that will accompany the resume.

Equipment and Supplies:
- Computer with word processing software and a printer
- Current job posting
- Resume paper
- Pen

Standard: Complete the procedure and all critical steps in _______ minutes with a minimum score of 85% within two attempts (*or as indicated by the instructor*).

Scoring: Divide the points earned by the total possible points. Failure to perform a critical step, indicated by an asterisk (*), results in grade no higher than an 84% (*or as indicated by the instructor*).

Time: Began_________ Ended_________ Total minutes: _________

Steps:	Point Value	Attempt 1	Attempt 2
1. Using the job posting, read through the job description. With a pen, circle the position requirements and the key phrases.	5		
2. Using the computer with word processing software, create a professional-looking header in the document's header that matches your resume header. Include your name, address, telephone number(s), and email address.	10		
3. Type the date in the correct location using the correct format. Have one blank line between the date line and the last line of the letterhead.	10		
4. Type the inside address using the correct spelling, punctuation, and location for the information. Leave 1 to 9 blank lines between the date and the inside address, depending on the location of the body of the letter.	10		
5. Starting on the second line below the inside address, type the salutation using the correct format. Use a colon after the person's name.	10		
6. Type the message in the body of the letter using the proper location and format. There should be a blank line after the salutation and between each paragraph. The message should be clear, concise, and professional. Use proper grammar, punctuation, capitalization, and sentence structure.	10		
7. The first paragraph should contain the title and number of the job posting. The middle paragraph(s) should summarize your strengths and include key phrases from the posting. The final paragraph should discuss your availability for an interview. The body should end with an expression of gratitude to the reader.	10		
8. Type a proper closing, leaving one blank line between the last line of the body and the closing. Use the correct format and location.	10		
9. Type the signature block using the correct format and location. There should be four blank lines between the closing and the signature block.	10*		
10. Spell-check and proofread the document. Check for proper tone, grammar, punctuation, capitalization, and sentence structure. Check for proper spacing between the parts of the letter.	10		

11. Make any final corrections. Print the document on resume paper and sign the letter or email the document to your instructor or potential employer.	**5**		
Total Points	**100**		

Comments

ABHES Competencies	Step(s)
10. Career Development a. Perform the essential requirements for employment, such as resume writing, effective interviewing, dressing professionally, time management, and following up appropriately	Entire procedure

Procedure 22.3 Complete a Job Application

Name ______________________________ **Date** __________ **Score** __________

Task: Complete an accurate, detailed job application legibly to secure a job offer.

Equipment and Supplies:
- Pen
- Application form
- Information regarding your past education, job experiences, and the skill sets you have developed (e.g., computer skills, keyboarding speed)
- Contact information for former supervisors and references
- Current resume

Standard: Complete the procedure and all critical steps in _______ minutes with a minimum score of 85% within two attempts (*or as indicated by the instructor*).

Scoring: Divide the points earned by the total possible points. Failure to perform a critical step, indicated by an asterisk (*), results in grade no higher than an 84% (*or as indicated by the instructor*).

Time: Began_________ Ended_________ Total minutes: _________

Steps:	**Point Value**	**Attempt 1**	**Attempt 2**
1. Read the entire job application before completing any part of the document.	**5**		
2. Refer to your information on past jobs, education experiences, and skill sets you have developed as you complete the application. Answers to the questions need to be accurate and honest.	**45**		
3. Use proper grammar, sentence structure, punctuation, spelling, and capitalization. Handwriting should be legible to the reader.	**15**		
4. Do not leave any space blank. Answer each question on the document. If the question does not apply, write "not applicable."	**10**		
5. Do not write "See resume" anywhere on the document.	**5**		
6. Include information on the application that exhibits dependability, punctuality, teamwork, attention to detail, a positive work ethic and initiative, the ability to adapt to change, a responsible attitude, and use of technology.	**10**		
7. Sign the document and date it.	**5**		
8. Proofread the document and make sure none of the information conflicts with the resume.	**5**		
Total Points	**100**		

Comments

ABHES Competencies	**Step(s)**
10. Career Development a. Perform the essential requirements for employment, such as resume writing, effective interviewing, dressing professionally, time management, and following up appropriately	Entire procedure

Work Product 22.1 Job Application

To be used with Procedure 22.3.

Name ______________________ **Date** __________ **Score** __________

WALDEN-MARTIN
FAMILY MEDICAL CLINIC
1234 ANYSTREET | ANYTOWN, ANYSTATE 12345
PHONE 123 123 1234 | FAX 123 123 5678

APPLICATION FOR EMPLOYMENT

Walden-Martin Family Medical Clinic is an equal opportunity employer and upholds the principles of equal opportunity employment. It is the policy of Walden-Martin Family Medical Clinic to provide employment, compensation and other benefits related to employment based on qualifications and performance, without regard to race, color, religion, national origin, age, sex, veteran status or disability, or any other basis prohibited by federal or state law. As an equal opportunity employer, Walden-Martin Family Medical Clinic intends to comply fully with all federal and state laws, and the information requested on this application will not be used for any purpose prohibited by law. Disabled applicants may request any needed accommodation. Please complete this application using ink, answer all questions completely, and sign the application.

Date: ______________________

Name: (First, Middle Initial, Last) ______________________

Social Security No.:______________ Phone: ______________

Address:______________________

City, State, Zip: ______________________

Have you been previously employed by Walden-Martin Family Medical Clinic?
☐ Yes ☐ No

If "Yes", when and job title?

How did you learn of the position for which you are applying?

☐ Newspaper/Print Advertisement ☐ Friend/Relative ☐ Employment Agency
☐ Job Service

☐ Radio/TV Advertisement ☐ Clinic Staff Person Name:

EMPLOYMENT DESIRED

Position(s) applied for: ____

☐ Full-time ☐ Part-time (If "Part time", number of shifts/hours desired _____)

Date available to start: ______________ Salary requested: ____________

PERSONAL HISTORY

Are you a United States citizen or do you have an entry permit which allows you to lawfully work in the U.S.? ☐ Yes ☐ No

If applicable, Visa Type: ______________ Immigration No.: ________________

Are you at least 18 years old? ☐ Yes ☐ No

Are you ineligible to be employed with an AnyState licensed health care entity as a result of being found guilty by a court of law for abusing, neglecting, or mistreating individuals in a health care related setting? ☐ Yes ☐ No

If "Yes," please explain: ____

Are you able to perform all of the duties required by the position for which you are applying, without endangering yourself or compromising the safety, health, or welfare of the patients or other staff member? ☐ Yes ☐ No

If "No," please explain:____

EDUCATION

	Name, City, State	Graduation Date	Course of Study/ Degree Obtained
High School:			
College:			
Other:			

LICENSURE/CERTIFICATION/REGISTRATION

Type of Certification, License or Registration	Agency/State	Registration Name

List any special skills or qualifications which you possess and feel are relevant to health care and the position for which you are applying.

____

____

____

____

____

MILITARY SERVICE

From: ____________ To: ________

Branch: ________________________

Duties: ________________________

Did you receive any specialized training? ☐ Yes ☐ No
If "Yes", describe: ____________________________________

EMPLOYMENT HISTORY

Please give accurate and complete information. Start with present or most recent employer.
May we contact and communicate with your present employer? ☐ Yes ☐ No

Employer:		**Phone:**	
Address:		**Supervisor:**	
Employed	Start: Month/Year: ____________ Ended: Month/Year: ____________	**Hourly Pay:**	Start: ______ Ended: ______
Position title and responsibilities:			
Reason for leaving:			

Employer:		**Phone:**	
Address:		**Supervisor:**	
Employed	Start: Month/Year: ____________ Ended: Month/Year: ____________	**Hourly Pay:**	Start: ______ Ended: ______
Position title and responsibilities:			
Reason for leaving:			

Employer:		**Phone:**	
Address:		**Supervisor:**	
Employed	Start: Month/Year: ______________ Ended: Month/Year: ______________	**Hourly Pay:**	Start: _______ Ended: ______
Position title and responsibilities:			
Reason for leaving:			

Employer:		**Phone:**	
Address:		**Supervisor:**	
Employed	Start: Month/Year: ______________ Ended: Month/Year: ______________	**Hourly Pay:**	Start: _______ Ended: ______
Position title and responsibilities:			
Reason for leaving:			

REFERENCES

Names of co-workers (no relatives) you have worked with and whom we may contact for a reference.

Name:	
Address:	
Phone:	
Job Title:	

Name:	
Address:	
Phone:	
Job Title:	

Name:	
Address:	
Phone:	
Job Title:	

Please read the following statements completely and carefully before you sign your name.

The Applicant HEREBY CERTIFIES that the answers given on this Application For Employment, including any statements or answers provided by the Applicant during interview, are true and correct. The Applicant fully authorizes Walden-Martin Family Medical Clinic to contact any references, past and present employers, persons, schools, law enforcement agencies and any other sources of information which may be relevant to the Applicant and this Application For Employment. It is understood and agreed that any misrepresentation, false statement, or omission by the Applicant will be sufficient reason for rejection of the Application For Employment or for dismissal from employment at any time, without recourse or liability to Walden-Martin Family Medical Clinic.

I have read, understand and agree to the above statement.

Sign: ______________________________

Date: ________________

Procedure 22.4 Create a Career Portfolio

Name ______________________________ **Date** ____________ **Score** __________

Task: Create a custom portfolio that provides potential employers evidence of your skills and knowledge as a medical assistant.

Equipment and Supplies:
- Three-ring binder or folder
- Plastic sleeves for the three-ring binder
- Dividers with tabs for the three-ring binder
- Current resume and cover letter
- Documents providing evidence of your skills and knowledge (e.g., transcripts, job evaluations, student clinical experience evaluation forms and skill checklist, projects completed in school, letters of recommendation, and copies of certifications [e.g., CPR card])

Standard: Complete the procedure and all critical steps in ______ minutes with a minimum score of 85% within two attempts (*or as indicated by the instructor*).

Scoring: Divide the points earned by the total possible points. Failure to perform a critical step, indicated by an asterisk (*), results in grade no higher than an 84% (*or as indicated by the instructor*).

Time: Began________ Ended________ Total minutes: ________

Steps:	**Point Value**	**Attempt 1**	**Attempt 2**
1. Group documents in a logical manner, putting similar documents together. Identify the arrangement for the portfolio. An arrangement could include cover letter and resume, education section (e.g., transcript, evaluation form and skills checklist, awards), prior job-related documents (e.g., evaluations), reference letters, and work products (e.g., projects you created in your medical assistant program).	25		
2. Insert one document per plastic pocket. Place all documents in plastic pockets.	15		
3. Neatly write the topic area on the tab of the dividers. Insert the tabbed dividers in the binder or folder.	15		
4. Place all documents in the binder or folder behind the correct divider. Place your cover letter and resume in the front of all the other documents.	15		
5. Create a table of contents to identify the tabbed areas.	15		
6. After the portfolio is assembled, review the entire portfolio to ensure it looks professional and the documents provide positive support of your skill set and knowledge.	15		
Total Points	**100**		

Comments

ABHES Competencies	Step(s)
10. Career Development a. Perform the essential requirements for employment, such as resume writing, effective interviewing, dressing professionally, time management, and following up appropriately	Entire procedure

Procedure 22.5 Practice Interview Skills During a Mock Interview

Name ______________________________ **Date** ____________ **Score** __________

Tasks: Project a professional appearance during a job interview and be able to express the reasons the medical assistant is the best candidate for the position.

Equipment and Supplies:
- Current job posting
- Resume
- Cover letter
- Interview portfolio (optional)
- Application (optional)
- Interviewer
- Mock interview questions

Standard: Complete the procedure and all critical steps in _______ minutes with a minimum score of 85% within two attempts (*or as indicated by the instructor*).

Scoring: Divide the points earned by the total possible points. Failure to perform a critical step, indicated by an asterisk (*), results in grade no higher than an 84% (*or as indicated by the instructor*).

Time: Began_________ Ended_________ Total minutes: _________

Steps:	**Point Value**	**Attempt 1**	**Attempt 2**
1. Wear interview-appropriate attire and be groomed professionally.	**15**		
2. Portray a professional image by shaking hands firmly prior to the start of the interview. Ensure that each interviewer has a copy of your resume and cover letter. Refrain from nervous behaviors (e.g., saying "um," tapping a pen or your foot) during the interview.	**10**		
3. Answer introductory questions by providing only professional information. This may include information about your education, experience, and career goals.	**10**		
4. Answer interview questions with open, honest, and positive responses. Completely answer questions, provide information or examples, and do not answer in single sentences or with limited responses.	**25**		
5. Use key words from the job posting when answering the interview questions.	**10**		
6. Ask the interviewer two to three appropriate questions about the facility or the position.	**20**		
7. Express interest in the job, and politely complete the interview by shaking hands and thanking the interviewer for the opportunity for the interview.	**10**		
Total Points	**100**		

Comments

ABHES Competencies	Step(s)
10. Career Development a. Perform the essential requirements for employment, such as resume writing, effective interviewing, dressing professionally, time management, and following up appropriately	Entire procedure
10. b. Demonstrate professional behavior	Entire procedure

Procedure 22.6 Create a Thank-You Note for an Interview

Name ______________________________ **Date** ____________ **Score** __________

Task: Create a meaningful, thank-you note to be sent after the interview process.

Equipment and Supplies:
- Computer with word processing software and a printer
- Job description
- Contact name from interview

Standard: Complete the procedure and all critical steps in ______ minutes with a minimum score of 85% within two attempts (*or as indicated by the instructor*).

Scoring: Divide the points earned by the total possible points. Failure to perform a critical step, indicated by an asterisk (*), results in grade no higher than an 84% (*or as indicated by the instructor*).

Time: Began________ Ended________ Total minutes: ________

Steps:	Point Value	Attempt 1	Attempt 2
1. Using word processing software, compose a professional letter using the business letter format. Include all of the required elements in the letter. Use correct spacing between the elements.	30		
2. Emphasize the particulars of the interview in the body of the letter.	20		
3. Include positive information you wish you had covered in the interview.	20		
4. Create a message that is concise and to the point.	20		
5. Proofread the letter and make any revisions as needed. Sign and send the thank-you note.	10		
Total Points	**100**		

Comments

ABHES Competencies	Step(s)
10. Career Development a. Perform the essential requirements for employment, such as resume writing, effective interviewing, dressing professionally, time management, and following up appropriately	Entire procedure

Notes

Notes